SHEEP NUTRITION

Sheep Nutrition

Edited by

M. Freer and H. Dove

CSIRO Plant Industry
Canberra
Australia

CABI *Publishing*
in association with
CSIRO PUBLISHING

CABI is a trading name of CAB International

CABI Head Office
Nosworthy Way
Wallingford
Oxfordshire OX10 8DE
UK

Tel: +44 (0)1491 832111
Fax: +44 (0)1491 833508
Email: cabi@cabi.org
Web site: www.cabi.org

CABI North American Office
38 Chauncey St
Suite 1002
Boston, MA 02111
USA

Tel: +1 617 395 4056
Fax: +1 617 354 6875
Email: cabi-nao@cabi.org

Published exclusively in Australia and New Zealand by:
CSIRO PUBLISHING
PO Box 1139 (150 Oxford Street)
Collingwood VIC 3066
Australia
Tel: (03) 9662 7666 Int: +(613) 9662 7666
Fax: (03) 9662 7555 Int: +(613) 9662 7555
E-mail: publishing.sales.csiro.au
Web site: www.publish.csiro.au

A catalogue record for this book is available from the British Library, London, UK.

Library of Congress Cataloging-in-Publication Data
Sheep nutrition / edited by Mike Freer and Hugh Dove.
p. cm.
Includes bibliographical references (p.).
ISBN 0-85199-595-0 (alk. paper)
1. Sheep-Feeding and feeds. 2. Sheep-Nutrition. I. Freer, Mike. II. Dove, Hugh.
SF376 .S555 2002

20020000680

ISBN-13: 978-0-85199-595-3

First printed 2002
Transferred to print on demand 2014

Printed and bound by CPI Group (UK) Ltd, Croydon, CR0 4YY

Contents

Contributors

N.R. Adams, *CSIRO Livestock Industries, Centre for Mediterranean Agricultural Research, Private Bag 5, Wembley, WA 6913, Australia*

E.F. Annison, *Faculty of Veterinary Science, University of Sydney, Camden, NSW 2570, Australia*

A.J. Ball, *Meat and Livestock Australia, c/o Animal Science, University of New England, Armidale, NSW 2351, Australia*

G. Caja, *Departamento de Ciencia Animal y de los Alimentos, Facultad de Veterinaria, Universidad Autonoma de Barcelona, 08193 Bellaterra, Cerdanyola, Spain*

S.W. Coleman, *USDA-ARS Subtropical Agricultural Research Station, 22271 Chinsegut Hill Road, Brooksville, FL 34601, USA*

R.L. Coop, *Moredun Research Institute, Pentlands Science Park, Bush Loan, Penicuik, Midlothian EH26 0PZ, UK*

J.L. Corbett, *Animal Science, University of New England, Armidale, NSW 2351, Australia*

H. Dove, *CSIRO Plant Industry, GPO Box 1600, Canberra, ACT 2601, Australia*

J.M. Forbes, *Centre for Animal Sciences, Leeds Institute of Biotechnology and Agriculture, University of Leeds, Leeds LS2 9JT, UK*

M. Freer, *CSIRO Plant Industry, GPO Box 1600, Canberra, ACT 2601, Australia*

D.A. Henry, *CSIRO Livestock Industries, Centre for Mediterranean Agricultural Research, Private Bag 5, Wembley, WA 6913, Australia*

P.I. Hynd, *Department of Animal Science, Adelaide University, Roseworthy Campus, Roseworthy, SA 5371, Australia*

G.J. Judson, *South Australian Research and Development Institute, 33 Flemington Street, Glenside, SA 5065, Australia*

A.V. Klieve, *Agency for Food and Fibre Sciences, Animal Research Institute, Locked Mail Bag No. 4, Moorooka, Qld 4105, Australia*

S.O. Knowles, *AgResearch Limited, Grasslands Research Centre, Private Bag 11008, Palmerston North, New Zealand*

J. Lee, *AgResearch Limited, Grasslands Research Centre, Private Bag 11008, Palmerston North, New Zealand*

D.B. Lindsay, *66 Lantree Crescent, Trumpington, Cambridge CB2 2NJ, UK*

R.I. Mackie, *Department of Animal Sciences, University of Illinois at Urbana-Champaign, 1207 W. Gregory Drive, Urbana, IL 61801, USA*

D.G. Masters, *CSIRO Livestock Industries, Centre for Mediterranean Agricultural Research, Private Bag 5, Wembley, WA 6913, Australia*

R.W. Mayes, *Macaulay Land Use Research Institute, Craigiebuckler, Aberdeen AB15 8QH, UK*

N.P. McMeniman, *School of Veterinary Science, University of Queensland, Brisbane, Qld 4072, Australia*

C.S. McSweeney, *CSIRO Livestock Industries, Long Pocket Laboratory, Meiers Rd, Indooroopilly, Qld 4068, Australia*

T.G. McEvoy, *Animal Biology Division, Scottish Agricultural College, Craibstone Estate, Bucksburn, Aberdeen AB21 9YA, UK*

J.V. Nolan, *School of Rural Science and Agriculture, University of New England, Armidale, NSW 2351, Australia*

V.H. Oddy, *Meat and Livestock Australia, Locked Bag 991, North Sydney, NSW 2059, Australia*

P.J. O'Reagain, *Queensland Beef Industry Institute, Department of Primary Industries, PO Box 976, Charters Towers, Qld 4820, Australia*

J.J. Robinson, *Animal Biology Division, Scottish Agricultural College, Craibstone Estate, Bucksburn, Aberdeen AB21 9YA, UK*

J.A. Rooke, *Animal Biology Division, Scottish Agricultural College, Craibstone Estate, Bucksburn, Aberdeen AB21 9YA, UK*

R.D. Sainz, *Department of Animal Science, University of California, Davis, CA 95616-8521, USA*

A.R. Sykes, *Animal and Food Sciences Division, PO Box 84, Lincoln University, Canterbury 8150, New Zealand*

T.T. Treacher, *51 Western Road, Oxford OX1 4LF, UK*

G.C. Waghorn, *AgResearch Limited, Grasslands Research Centre, Private Bag 11008, Palmerston North, New Zealand*

R.H. Weston, *45 Park Street, Glenbrook, NSW 2773, Australia*

D.R. Woodfield, *AgResearch Limited, Grasslands Research Centre, Private Bag 11008, Palmerston North, New Zealand*

Preface

There are over 1 billion sheep in the world, with almost one-third of these located in China, Australia, New Zealand and the UK. The global production of wool (2.3 million t) and sheep meat (7.6 million t) tends to be concentrated in these countries. However, the developing countries of the world also have substantial populations of sheep and it is these which contribute the bulk of the world's sheep milk production (8.2 million t). Regardless of country or production system, a feature common to most of the world's sheep is that they rely very substantially, at times exclusively, on pasture, sown or natural, as their source of nutrients.

Advances in nutrition science in the last half of the 20th century have helped us to define the processes of ruminant digestion and the nutrient requirements of the sheep. We know that short-chain (volatile) fatty acids, not glucose, are the product of ruminant carbohydrate digestion, and we can quantify the processes involved. With the current rapid advances in cellular genetics, we are increasingly able to define which rumen microorganisms are responsible for which processes. We have quantified much about the processes of protein breakdown in the rumen and the incorporation of the resultant ammonia into microbial protein. Together, these processes of fibre digestion and microbial protein production are the processes which allow ruminants to survive on low-quality roughages. Challenges remain in quantifying the importance of the synchrony of these processes under grazing conditions and in defining how we might breed pasture plants that achieve better synchrony.

Perhaps an even greater challenge is that the reliance of the world's sheep on pasture as their source of nutrients places a major constraint on our capacity to specify their daily intake of nutrients, especially in more extensive grazing systems. This, in turn, constrains our ability to predict absorption of nutrients, their interaction with body reserves of nutrients, and ultimately the way in which the grazing sheep partitions its nutrient supply between the processes of maintenance, production and reproduction. Reliance upon pasture also means that the grazing sheep is 'at the mercy' of any nutrient deficiency or toxicity present in the pasture and, as it consumes pasture, can also consume a raft of parasites that hinder health and production.

These are not just academic issues, but issues of major economic importance. Sheep producers in developed countries increasingly face declining 'terms of trade', that is, reduced returns in the face of increasing costs. A worldwide reaction to this has been to seek to produce higher-value wool, meat and dairy products, while also reducing the cost and the environmental risks of sheep production systems. At the same time, increasing per capita incomes in both developed and especially developing nations are already increasing the demand for more and better meat and fibre products. In developing nations, this is manifest as increased demand for meat and for better-quality meat, while, in developed nations, there is increasing demand for meat products better attuned to consumer demands for a healthy diet.

There is no doubt that issues such as these will be addressed by developing sheep genotypes better suited to new production systems, either by introducing new genotypes or by breeding within existing genotypes. Equally, there is no doubt that challenges remain for the science of nutrition. For example, in grazing systems, in which it is so difficult to define the nutrients actually consumed by sheep, how might we combine improved understanding of nutrient supply and of the mechanisms of growth at the cellular level to produce sheep meats with a nutrient composition, especially a lipid content and composition, more suited to human dietary goals? Similarly, how might we manipulate the diet of the grazing sheep to ensure the cheaper production of heavier fleeces with finer fibre diameters, to improve the incomes of wool producers?

In assembling this book, our target reader has been the senior undergraduate or postgraduate student in animal science, the very population which, as animal nutrition professionals, will have to face and give advice to producers about the nutritional challenges facing sheep production systems in the future. As editors, we in turn challenged our chapter authors to produce 16 chapters that placed their respective facets of sheep nutrition in the context of the nutritional challenges faced by the grazing sheep. We thank all our contributors for so admirably achieving this, and hope that the resultant text will prove interesting and stimulating to students and practitioners of sheep nutrition science worldwide.

M. Freer and H. Dove
CSIRO Plant Industry
Canberra
Australia

1 Nutritive Value of Herbage

S.W. COLEMAN[1] AND D.A. HENRY[2]

[1]*USDA-ARS, Subtropical Agricultural Research Station, Brooksville, Florida, USA;* [2]*CSIRO Livestock Industries, Wembley, Western Australia, Australia*

Introduction

Herbage, the primary food for sheep, belongs to the group of feeds described as roughages. Roughages, in contrast to concentrates, are derived from the leaves and stems of pasture and crop plants and their dry matter (DM) contains a significant amount of cellulose (> 180 g kg^{-1}). As herbage is grazed or cut from maturing and regrowing plants, the composition of the feed and, with it, the ability of the feed to supply nutrients to the animal are in a continual state of change. For example, a young growing pasture may support weight gains in excess of 300 g day^{-1} in young lambs, whereas a mature pasture may fail to maintain the weight of an adult sheep. This highlights the importance of establishing a robust system for defining the value of herbage for animal production, understanding how this value changes with the growth of the herbage and the needs of the animal and developing rapid methods for predicting changes that are occurring in the field.

What is Nutritive Value?

Nutritive value (NV) is a term used to quantify the presence and availability in a feed of nutrients that are required by the animal and to predict the productive output from the animal to which it is fed. It depends on the following:

1. The concentration of nutrients in the feed.
2. The availability of these nutrients to the animal.
3. The efficiency with which the absorbed nutrients are used by the animal.
4. The effect of feed composition on the voluntary intake of the feed.

Nutritive value must be expressed in standard units that can be applied also to the nutrient requirements of the animal. The most common feeding standard systems in use today specify the major nutrients in the feed DM in terms of protein (g kg^{-1}) and either metabolizable energy (ME/DM or M/D) (MJ kg^{-1}), as in the Australian and British systems (SCA, 1990; AFRC, 1993), or net energy (NE/DM) (Mcal kg^{-1}), as used in the USA (NRC, 1985).

Nutrient content of herbage

The lipid and protein concentrations in herbage DM are usually less than 30 and 250 g kg^{-1}, respectively, so the gross energy (GE) (heat of combustion) content of herbage DM mainly reflects the energy content of the carbohydrates: it varies little from 18.4 MJ kg^{-1}. The distribution of carbohydrates between the relatively soluble cell-content material (sugars, fructans and starch) and the cell-wall constituents (cellulose and hemicellulose), which are more slowly available through the action of cellulolytic organisms in the rumen, is information that can be gained only from chemical analysis. The same is also true of the protein.

The analysis of these chemical entities can be difficult and time-consuming, and various schemes have been developed which rapidly extract fractions that represent them. The 19th-century Weende system for the routine analysis of feeds measured crude protein (CP), crude fibre (CF), ether extract (fat), ash and, by difference, nitrogen-free extract. Determinations of CF have now been almost entirely replaced by extractions with neutral and acid detergents (Van Soest, 1967). These procedures separate the cell contents (neutral-detergent solubles (NDS)) from the total cell-wall material, comprising hemicellulose, cellulose and lignin, together defined as neutral-detergent fibre (NDF), or from the cellulose and lignin fraction, acid-detergent fibre (ADF). Assays for lignin, a polyphenol component of cell walls and an important indicator of their resistance to digestion, are not usually part of a routine analysis, mainly because of lack of agreement on a standard technique.

In routine analyses, the protein content of herbage is estimated as CP, which is the nitrogen (N) concentration multiplied by 6.25, because protein, on average, contains 16% N. Crude protein thus includes not only true protein but also simpler N compounds, such as urea and amides, which cannot be used directly by the animal but will augment the supply of N to the rumen microflora.

Availability of nutrients

In specifying the NV of a feed it is necessary to quantify the losses of energy and nutrients in excreta and to determine the amounts that remain available for productive purposes. The major and most variable losses are in the faeces (F), with the proportion of, for example, DM not excreted being termed digestibility (D). The losses can vary from less than 200 g kg^{-1} of the DM in young leafy herbage (D > 0.8) to more than 600 g kg^{-1} in dead stemmy pasture (D < 0.4). Since D, even within one forage, is so variable, tables of reference data, such as those compiled by the National Research Council (NRC, 1985), are of limited value and measurements or estimates are required for each forage. Depending on the measurements made, the digestible fraction may be calculated as digestible DM (DDM), digestible organic matter in the DM (DOMD) or digestible energy (DE) (see Fig. 1.1). It may also be useful to have information on the rate at which the DM, fibre or protein is digested in the rumen and procedures to obtain this information are discussed below.

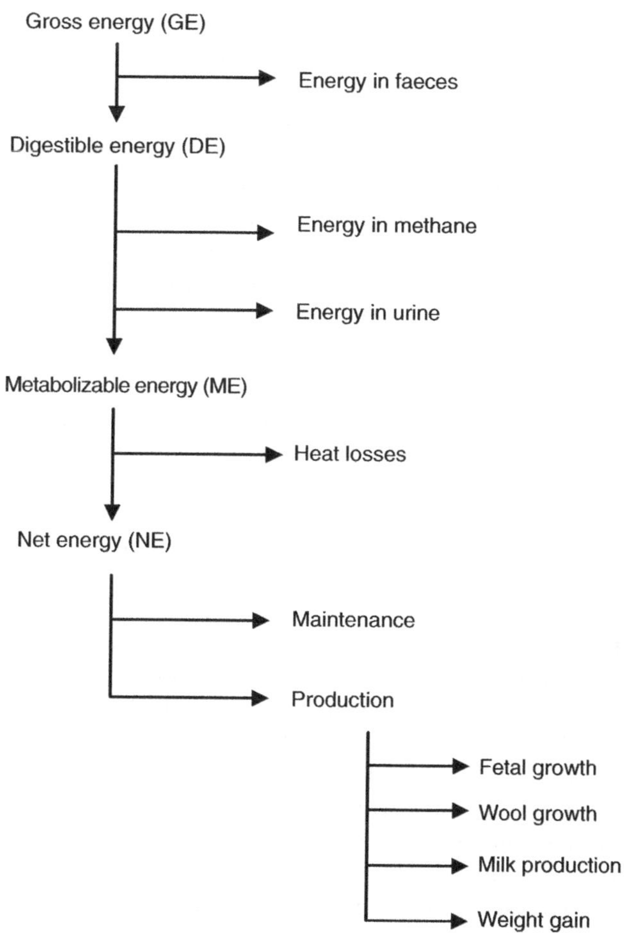

Fig. 1.1. Partition of feed energy.

Energy losses in urine (U) and methane (CH_4) produced during fermentation in the rumen are smaller and less variable than F, and together are generally about 19% of the DE. The remainder of the feed energy, GE minus (F + U + CH_4), is the metabolizable energy (ME). Based on the results of many animal-feeding trials, equations for predicting ME from DE, DDM or DOMD are given in NRC (1985) and by the Standing Committee on Agriculture (SCA, 1990). Values of M/D in herbage commonly range from > 12 MJ kg^{-1} in very young material to *c.* 5 MJ kg^{-1} in dead stemmy pasture residues.

The efficiency with which the sheep uses absorbed ME for its maintenance or for productive purposes is directly related to the M/D value of the herbage (see Annison *et al.*, Chapter 5, this volume). Metabolizable energy is used with different efficiencies for maintenance, milk production and weight gain and so the net energy (NE) value of herbage DM (Fig. 1.1) will be different for each purpose. These efficiency values, k_m, k_l and k_g, respectively, are predicted in the various feeding systems from M/D (e.g. SCA, 1990) and typical values are shown in Table 1.1.

Availability of CP in herbage is determined not only by its apparent digestibility in the whole alimentary tract but, more importantly, by the proportion that is degraded to simpler N compounds in the rumen. This proportion is high in young herbage, as most of the protein-rich cell contents are soluble and are released during initial chewing by the sheep. This fraction, rumen-degradable protein (RDP), is available to the rumen microbes for the synthesis of microbial CP (MCP) (see Annison *et al.*, Chapter 5, this volume); RDP not captured by the microbes is almost entirely lost to the animal as urea in the urine. True protein comprises part of the MCP and part of the relatively smaller amount of undegraded dietary protein (UDP) flowing from the abomasum. It is digested in and the amino acids are absorbed from the small intestine. The digestible portion of true protein (60–80% of the MCP and up to 85% of the UDP) makes up the protein available to the animal, usually referred to as metabolizable protein (MP). The primary protein limitation in mature herbage is usually an inadequate supply of RDP for efficient rumen function, whereas with young herbage it is occasionally the supply of UDP that may restrict animal performance.

The quality and efficiency with which the absorbed protein is used depends on the extent to which the proportions of individual amino acids in the MP meet the requirements of the sheep. As most of the MP derived from herbage is in the form of MCP, which has suboptimal proportions of methionine and lysine for wool growth and weight gain, respectively, changes to the plant's protein composition can have little effect on productivity unless the changes affect the UDP fraction. There is current interest in modifying herbage legumes, either through the inclusion of moderate levels of condensed tannins to reduce protein degradation (Waghorn *et al.*, 1999) or through genetic manipulation to increase the content of slowly degraded proteins rich in specific amino acids (Tabe *et al.*, 1993).

The voluntary intake of herbage

It is a common feature of most grazing systems that the intake of herbage by the sheep is restricted for much of the year, either by the supply of feed or by a grazing management policy aimed at the optimum use of the feed resource, e.g. in some wool production systems. However, when herbage is freely available, there are practical situations, e.g. weight gain in lambs, where the efficiency of animal production may be directly related to the amount of herbage consumed. The attributes that affect voluntary intake, such as the resistance of cell-wall material to breakdown during digestion, then become important components of NV (see Weston, Chapter 2, this volume). These attributes are closely related to those that determine the D and the efficiency of use of the nutrients in herbage. In other words, as the D of herbage increases, there is usually an increase in its voluntary intake by sheep, when offered *ad libitum*, so that, as well as a higher NV per mouthful, there are more mouthfuls. Conversely, the decrease in available energy and nutrients per unit of intake as D falls is compounded by decreasing intake. Although the relationship between intake and D shows a similar slope for many different herbage species, intercept values can vary widely (Freer and Jones, 1984).

What Influences Nutritive Value?

Different plant species differ inherently in their rate of reproductive development. This results not only in changes in chemical and anatomical characteristics, but also in the proportion of plant parts, e.g. leaf, stem, pseudostem, petiole, inflorescence, which in turn differ significantly in their quality attributes. Management and environment can then play a significant role in affecting NV, either by directly altering chemical and anatomical traits or by influencing the timing of changes in plant phenology.

Plant maturity

Advancing plant maturity is associated with a lowering of NV by virtue of a decrease in leafiness and an increase in the stem : leaf ratio, changes in the composition of the cell wall (Akin *et al.*, 1977) and a loss of cell contents with maturity (Ballard *et al.*, 1990). Typical values in maturing herbage are shown in Table 1.1.

The loss of cell contents during maturation is a major factor contributing to the decline in NV. This material, comprising water-soluble carbohydrates (WSC), proteins and lipids, is often assumed to be completely digestible by ruminants. However, the D of NDS, a measure of cell contents, can also decline. Ballard *et al.* (1990) reported a decline from 0.80–0.95 D of NDS in young *Lolium rigidum* (annual ryegrass) leaves to about 0.45 in senescent leaves. In contrast, the digestibility of NDS in the stem segment did not change from about 0.90–0.95.

Table 1.1. Typical values for the components of NV in the DM of mixed pasture herbage as it matures from young leafy material, stage 1, to mature stemmy flowering herbage, stage 4 (data from MAFF, 1990; equations from SCA, 1990).

	Stage			
	1	2	3	4
Crude protein (g kg^{-1})	190	150	120	84
Protein degradation[a] (h^{-1})	0.86	0.81	0.73	0.68
Neutral-detergent solubles (g kg^{-1})	465	418	373	291
Neutral-detergent fibre (g kg^{-1})	535	582	627	709
Acid-detergent fibre (g kg^{-1})	264	301	329	400
Ether extract (g kg^{-1})	25	21	19	14
DM digestibility[a]	0.79	0.72	0.65	0.52
ME/DM (MJ kg^{-1})	12.6	11.1	9.5	7.4
Efficiency of use of ME for:				
Maintenance, k_m	0.75	0.72	0.69	0.65
Milk production, k_l	0.65	0.62	0.59	0.55
Weight gain, k_g	0.51	0.43	0.35	0.23

[a]Measured at a feeding level adequate for maintenance only.

$k_m = 0.02M + 0.5$
$k_l = 0.02M + 0.4$
$k_g = (0.3L + 0.9)\ [0.043M + 0.01(15.4 - M)((\lambda/40)\sin(2\pi D/365) - 1.00)]$

where M is ME/DM; L is the proportion of legume in the herbage; D is the day of the year; λ is the latitude (+ in north; – in south). The estimates of k_g have been made for midsummer at 40°S, with a value of 0.3 for L.

Water-soluble carbohydrates can make up to 25% of some forages; high concentrations are positively related to efficient ruminant digestion (see Annison *et al.*, Chapter 5, this volume). They can also play a significant role in the preference and selection shown by ruminants (e.g. Ciavarella *et al.*, 2000). Although WSC concentrations vary markedly both within and between days, diurnal variation is not as large as between-species variation and plant breeders have found it a reliable trait for improvement through breeding (Humphreys, 1989).

Protein content of vegetative forage declines as the plant approaches maturity in a similar way to other cellular constituents. The CP content of *L. rigidum* leaves can decline from approximately 220 g kg^{-1} prior to anthesis to 130 g kg^{-1} 1 month after anthesis (Ballard *et al.*, 1990). The decline in protein in warm-season grasses, such as *Bothriochloa* spp. (old world bluestem), can be from 160 to 60 g kg^{-1} in leaves and from 11 to 3 g kg^{-1} in stems (Dabo *et al.*, 1988). The lower levels at plant maturity would be insufficient to supply the daily requirements for most classes of sheep.

Depending upon the stage of maturity, cell walls represent somewhere between 300 and 800 g kg^{-1} of plant DM, as reflected in measures of NDF. The structural links between cellulose, hemicellulose and lignin, which develop as the plant matures, reduce the D of cell walls. Levels of ADF, NDF and lignin all increase with maturity – examples in *Bothriochloa* spp.

include increases in ADF of stems from 400 to 500 g kg^{-1} and in NDF from 700 to 840 g kg^{-1} (Dabo *et al.*, 1988). Both cellulose and hemicellulose decrease in digestibility with plant maturation, and this decrease is closely linked to the degree of lignification. Cellulose, the predominant wall polysaccharide, has been shown to decrease from 0.83 digestibility at the youngest stage in sorghum to 0.37 at the milk-ripe stage of grain maturity (Goto *et al.*, 1991). Lignin is deposited in cell walls with the formation of the secondary wall and confers high resistance to digestion. Stems have a higher percentage of lignin than leaves and, as plants mature, the leaf : stem ratio decreases and hence the proportion of lignified tissue in the total biomass increases. For example, this is reflected in a decline in the D of whole *Bothriochloa* plants, with advancing maturity, from 0.65 to 0.45 (Dabo *et al.*, 1987).

The overall effect of these changes is a characteristic pattern of decline in D (Fig. 1.2) and CP content during the growing season.

Genetic variation

Plants have adapted to specific environments through evolution and those that have evolved under grazing have developed protective mechanisms against predatory attack (whether it be animal or insect). Some of these mechanisms include lignification, cutinization, silicification, secondary compounds, such as phenols and alkaloids, and prostrate growth architecture.

Fortunately, there is naturally occurring genetic variation that enables plant breeders to select and breed superior lines, whether they be superior in disease or pest resistance, agronomic traits or NV. However, care must be taken that selection for high yield, quality or disease or pest resistance does not inadvertently select against NV. This has led some plant breeders to include more intensive nutritive evaluation as part of their genetic engineering (Tabe *et al.*, 1993) and conventional breeding programmes (Ehlke *et al.*, 1986).

The photosynthetic mechanism typical of a plant species can also influence NV. C3 and C4 plant species are so called because their products of photosynthesis are, respectively, either three-carbon compounds (temperate grasses and dicotyledons) or four-carbon compounds (mostly tropical grasses). C4 plants are photosynthetically more efficient, and they tend to exhibit high DM accumulations that are often of lower NV (Minson, 1990) than C3 plants. C4 grasses have lower levels of non-structural carbohydrate, leading to decreased efficiency of microbial protein production in ruminants (Poppi *et al.*, 1999). In addition, the range of cell-wall content, measured as NDF, in C4 leaves is higher – 240 to 520 g kg^{-1} – than that found in C3 leaves – 230 to 400 g kg^{-1} (Ford *et al.*, 1979).

In general, legumes are higher in protein and lower in cell-wall content than grasses. However, the most significant difference is that, for a given D, the voluntary intake of legumes by ruminants can be 30% higher than that for grasses (Freer and Jones, 1984) and the digested material is used more

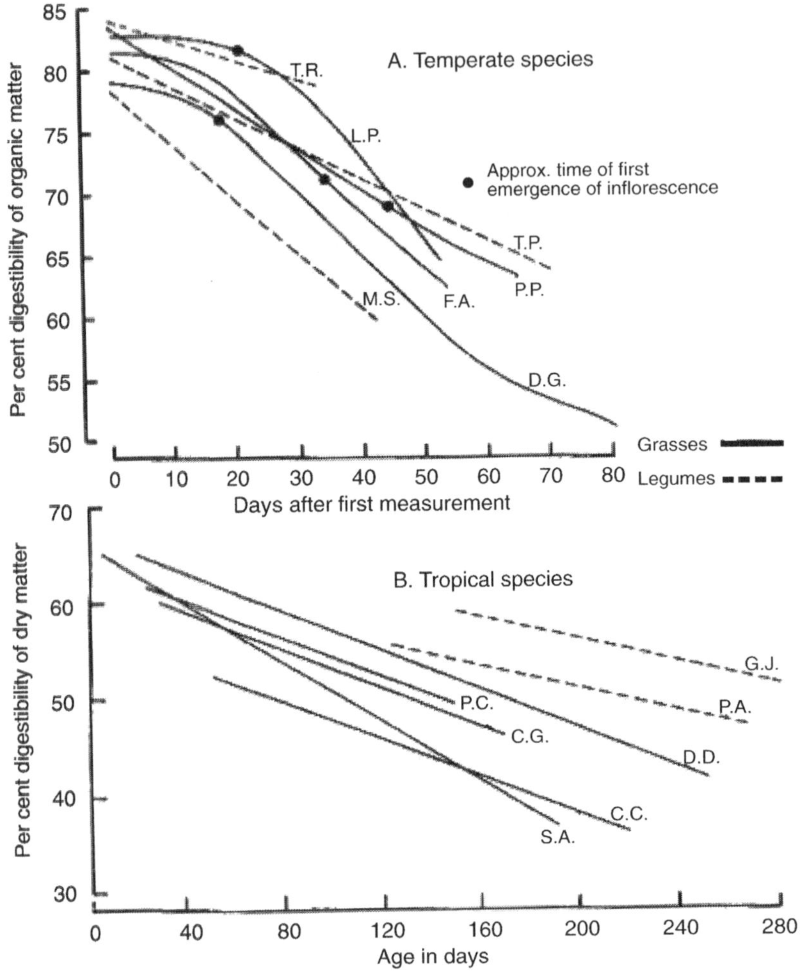

Temperate species. Spring growths; dates of first measurements varied between species and between localities.

L.P.	*Lolium perenne* var. S23 (ryegrass)
P.P.	*Phleum pratense* var. S48 (timothy)
F.A.	*Festuca arundinacea* var. S170 (tall fescue)
D.G.	*Dactylis glomerata* var. S37 (cocksfoot or orchard grass)
T.R.	*Trifolium repens* var. S100 (white clover)
T.P.	*Trifolium pratense* var. Ultuna (red clover)
M.S.	*Medicago sativa* var. Dupuits (lucerne or alfalfa)

Tropical species.

S.A.	*Sorghum almum*
C.C.	*Cenchrus ciliaris* var. Molopo (Buffel grass)
C.G.	*Chloris gayana* var. Callide (Rhodes grass)
P.C.	*Pennisetum clandestinum* (Kikuyu grass)
D.D.	*Digitaria decumbens* (Pangola grass)
P.A.	*Phaseolus atropurpureus* var. Siratro
G.J.	*Glycine javanica* var. Cooper

Fig. 1.2. Changes in digestibility of herbage from temperate and tropical species with increasing maturity (from Corbett, 1969).

efficiently by the sheep for weight gain. Table 1.2 shows typical differences in animal performance on grasses and legumes when compared relative to a base value of 100 for perennial ryegrass.

The difference in intake can be attributed in part to the shorter retention time in the rumen of the legume compared with the grass diet. The shorter retention time is due to more rapid breakdown of legume forage to particles of a size and effective density that allow them to be passed out of the rumen. This leads to a proportionately greater supply of undigested organic matter and protein for postruminal digestion from legume diets when compared with grass diets (Moseley, 1981). The ease of reduction of particle size is reflected in their biomechanical properties. Henry *et al.* (1997) reported that the intrinsic shear strength of grass leaves was 38–68 times that of legume leaves.

Environment

Temperature and light are probably the most important environmental factors that affect NV, both directly and indirectly. The temperature under which plants are grown has a direct effect on the concentration of chemical constituents, with genotype then determining exactly how different species change with increasing temperatures. Higher temperatures usually promote the accumulation of structural material (i.e. cell-wall material) and also more rapid metabolic activity, which decreases the pool size of cell contents. For example, Ford *et al.* (1979) reported that the cell-wall content of C3 grasses increased and that of C4 grasses decreased when the day/night temperature regime increased from 21/13°C to 32/24°C. More recently, Henry *et al.* (2000) showed that, when vegetative pasture species were grown in temperatures between 14 and 34°C, the lignin, cellulose and hemicellulose content of *Lolium multiflorum* (Italian ryegrass) increased

Table 1.2. Response of young sheep to pure pasture species grown in New Zealand (taken from Ulyatt, 1981).

Species	Relative liveweight gain
Perennial ryegrass	100
Short-rotation ryegrass	148
Italian ryegrass	160
Timothy	129
Browntop (*Agrostis tenuis*)	
Spring	100
Early summer	83
White clover	186
Lucerne	170
Lotus pedunculatus	143

markedly with increasing temperature and this was associated with a lower *in vitro* dry matter digestibility (DMD) (Fig. 1.3). However, in a C4 grass, *Thinopyrum ponticum* (tall couch grass), these constituents did not change with temperature. This genotype–environment interaction has been noted in numerous studies.

As a result of photosynthesis, there is diurnal variation in WSC levels, which rise to a peak during daylight hours (see Ciavarella *et al.*, 2000). This implies that makers of conserved fodder could capture the accumulation of WSC during the day by harvesting forage in the afternoon rather than in the morning. A further advantage is that ruminants prefer afternoon-cut hay compared with morning-cut hay (Fisher *et al.*, 1999), presumably because of the higher content of WSC (Ciavarella *et al.*, 2000).

Possibly the greatest effect of temperature and light on NV is their role in vernalization and photoperiodism, which changes the plant from vegetative to reproductive stages of development. The effect of changing maturity on NV is stronger than the effects of environment *per se*.

Once a plant has senesced and it is either standing dry feed or a conserved fodder, environment can still have a significant impact on NV. Rain can leach soluble matter from dry feed, while prolonged exposure to sunlight can bleach the material, causing a loss of carotenoids and vitamin A activity (see Lee *et al.*, Chapter 13, this volume). In hay, these risks are greatly increased before baling, due to the volume of material in a windrow exposed to weather; mechanical losses, which are mainly of leaf rather than stem, can also seriously reduce the NV of the final product.

When considering the environment in which forages are grown, it is also pertinent to consider the effects of soil type and moisture availability. Plants grown on different soils have different mineral nutrients available to them, which will influence both their growth and their composition. Different species vary in their genetic capacity to take up minerals and in their own requirements for growth, and the availability of soil minerals will be affected by fertilizer and other management decisions. It is important to note that mineral status adequate for plant growth is not necessarily adequate for animal growth or, alternatively, the uptake of minerals by the plant can be potentially toxic (see Lee *et al.*, Chapter 13, this volume).

Management

In grazed systems, the timing, frequency and intensity of grazing can all influence the botanical composition of the sward, the morphology and phenology of the plants present, the NV of the regrowth and the spatial heterogeneity of quality. Low stocking rates allow the grazing animal to be selective about what it consumes. This increases the variability across the paddock ('patchiness'), such that some patches tend to be grazed regularly; these maintain higher NV than ungrazed patches. High stocking rates force the animal to be less selective and to graze the sward to a lower residual height but result in the regrowth of material of more uniformly high

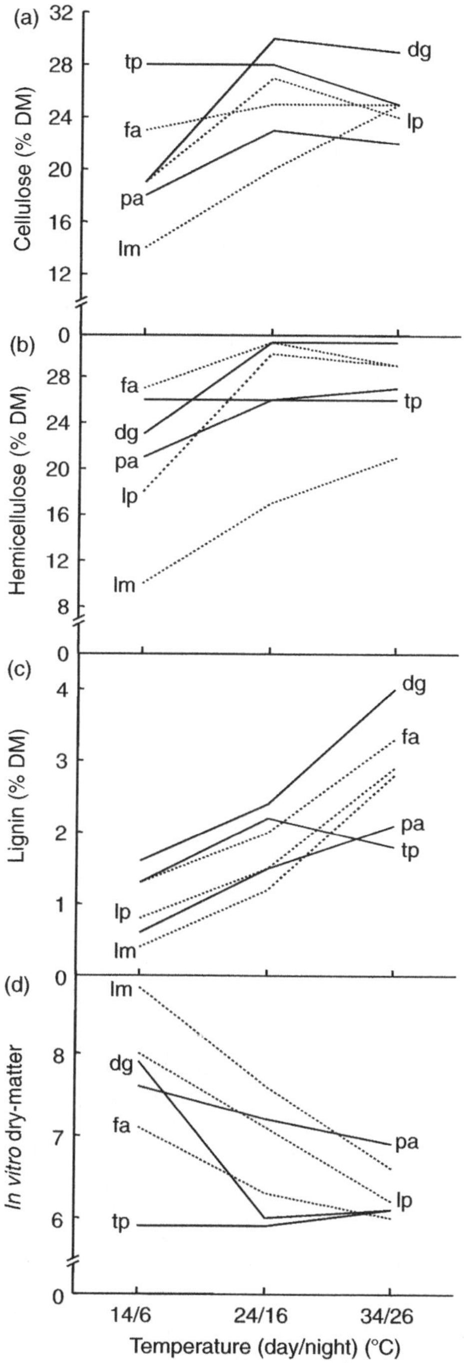

Fig. 1.3. Effect of temperature at which plants are grown on (a) percentage cellulose, (b) percentage hemicellulose, (c) percentage lignin and (d) *in vitro* dry-matter digestibility of leaf blades of six pasture grasses: *Dactylis glomerata* (dg), *Festuca arundinacea* (fa), *Lolium multiflorum* (lm), *Lolium perenne* (lp), *Phalaris aquatica* (pa), *Thinopyrum ponticum* (tp). *T. ponticum* is the only C4 grass.

NV. However, a caveat is that intake may be reduced at severe grazing pressure and plant regrowth rate is lower because of reduced leaf-area index.

Selective herbicides may be used to manipulate botanical composition and thus improve the NV of feed on offer; herbicides may also be used for 'spray topping' to conserve high-quality spring pasture as summer/autumn feed for livestock (Gatford *et al.*, 1999).

As has been appreciated for many years (see McIlroy, 1967), of the many factors in plant nutrition, the application of N has a major effect on NV, as distinct from forage yield. It influences botanical composition, particularly the legume : grass ratio, and increases the CP level in the forage, sometimes at the expense of WSC.

The Measurement of Nutritive Value

The direct estimation of NV involves at least the measurement of D. More detailed attributes of NV – the availability of digested nutrients and their efficiency of use by the animal – may either be measured directly or, more usually, predicted from D using standard equations derived from a large number of feeding trials, e.g. NRC (1985), SCA (1990) (Plate 1.1).

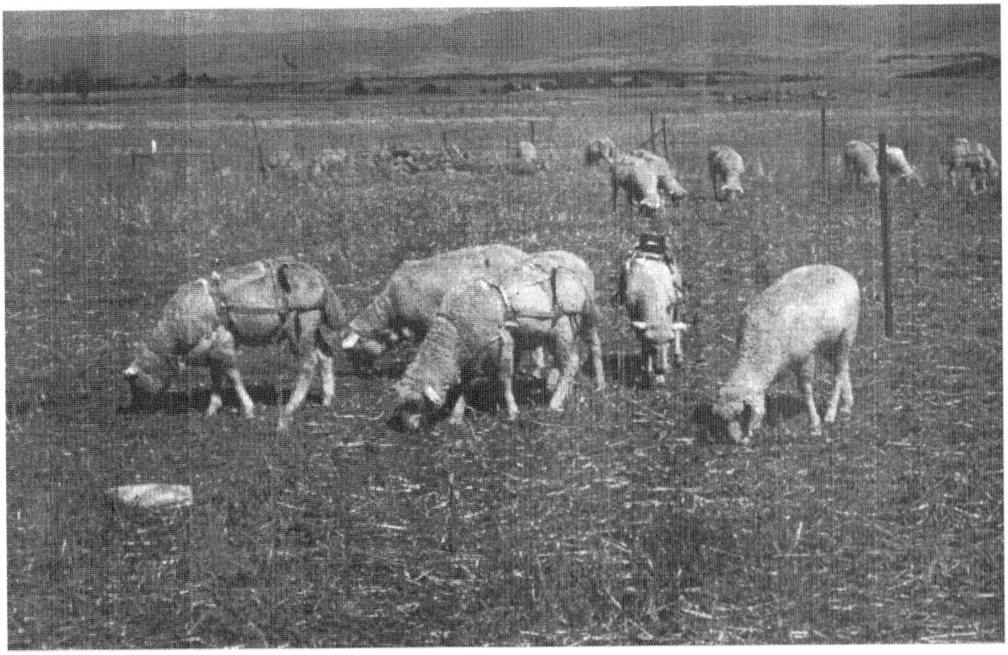

Plate 1.1. Sheep grazing cereal stubble in late summer near Canberra, Australia. Several of the animals are wearing equipment to permit total collection of faeces, as part of a study to assess the nutritive value of the cereal residues and summer-growing species. (Photo courtesy of J.B. Coombe, CSIRO Plant Industry, Canberra.)

Total collection

The usual method for direct measurement of D is a total-collection trial, in which animals are constrained and the entire amounts of feed eaten and faeces voided are weighed and analysed. The difference is assumed to be digested. Strictly speaking, the measurements are of apparent D since allowance is not made for faecal material not derived from the feed. Because of the variability that exists in D between animals given the same feed, three to six animals per feed are required to obtain a reliable estimate. As measurements must be made over 7–10 days, after a 10–14-day period of adaptation to the feed, tests with sheep are laborious and costly and require a large amount of herbage for the evaluation.

The D of a forage falls as the level of intake increases, because of the reduced time of retention of the feed in the gut. Therefore, when collecting data for calibrating *in vitro* or other indirect estimates of D, intake is usually standardized at a maintenance level of feeding. Minson (1990) showed that variability in the D of a forage was greater as its D decreased; a standard deviation of ±0.02 at a D above 0.650 increased to ±0.05 at a D of 0.50. This variability is important when trying to set acceptance criteria for methods to predict NV.

When feeds such as concentrates are given with forages, the D of the diet is not necessarily the weighted average of the diet components, because of associative effects (see Dove, Chapter 6, this volume). A forage should be fed as the sole dietary component to determine its NV, especially when collecting data from a group of forages for the calibration of indirect assay methods.

Marker techniques

When D estimates of diet consumed by grazing animals are desired, total-collection trials are difficult, so indirect methods, such as the use of markers, are suggested. This can be done either by the dosing of animals with markers to estimate both faecal output and intake (and thus D) or by employing markers that are part of the herbage. Marker-based techniques have a long history (see Dove and Mayes, 1991) and a recent development within this category has been the use of the hydrocarbons (*n*-alkanes) of plant wax, together with dosed synthetic alkanes, as markers to estimate diet selection, intake and digestibility (see Forbes and Mayes, Chapter 3, this volume).

How to Predict Nutritive Value

Due to the expense and time required to conduct animal trials, many procedures have been developed to estimate or predict NV, expressed in terms of D or the voluntary intake, or both. Coleman *et al.* (1999) reviewed methods for predicting NV, which included bioassays, chemical and structural characteristics and instrument-based methods, such as near-infrared reflectance spectroscopy (NIRS). Each method has advantages and disadvantages. For a method to find routine use among practitioners, producers and consulting nutritionists, it must be rapid, accurate and inexpensive. Accuracy is a description of how close to the actual value the predicted value is; precision is a measure of how repeatable a predicted value is. Robustness refers to whether a prediction equation accurately predicts samples not included in the calibration database. There are two steps involved in predicting NV: (i) selection of a reference forage sample database with known NV on which to base predictive relationships; and (ii) development and evaluation of prediction equations.

Database selection

Selection of an appropriate sample database with high-quality reference data is probably the most important part of the prediction process. The forage samples must have been fed in animal trials using standardized techniques to establish their known reference NV. The number of samples needed depends on the expected use of the equations, the importance of interfering matrix effects (i.e. environmental conditions) and the variability about the samples. For limited inference (i.e. research-plot samples), 100 samples may be sufficient to initiate calibration; 40 is a bare minimum. For predicting unknowns, such as producer samples, the database should probably have 500 or more samples produced under a diverse array of matrix effects. Variation in NV and in the forage characteristics used for regression are essential to develop a relationship, and the calibration-sample database should be selected to contain as much variability as possible in structural factors, such as plant species, time, climate and geographical location.

Development and evaluation of prediction equations

Common statistical methods for predicting NV from forage characteristics include simple or multiple regression, yielding empirical equations that are simple to construct, easy to use and easy to evaluate. Their greatest shortcoming is lack of robustness in their general applicability. Weiss (1993) proposed the use of theoretically based, rather than empirical, relationships or models to predict NV. Because empirical equations are based primarily on statistical relationships, cause and effect may or may not be present and use is typically limited to the population from which the calibration database was drawn. Theoretical models (e.g. Van Soest, 1967) seek to integrate biological mechanisms to predict NV more robustly, but their ability to predict NV accurately has thus far been limited.

Other, more elaborate statistical procedures, such as principal-component analysis (Stallcup *et al.*, 1983) or partial least-squares (PLS) regression

(Martens and Jensen, 1982), have been proposed to predict NV. These procedures share many of the shortcomings of multiple regression equations but appear to be more robust and tend to reduce the effects of autocorrelation between variables and overfitting, the phenomenon that occurs when too many independent variables are included in an equation, such that prediction accuracy is compromised rather than enhanced.

After an equation is developed, it must be validated, a procedure that requires using the equation to predict NV of samples that are unknown to the calibration data set. Proper validation was seldom practised prior to the use of NIRS. Since empirical equations (normally used for predicting NV) are valid only for the population of samples from which the calibration database was taken, that database must encompass the matrix of factors that influence either the dependent (NV) or independent (chemistry or near-infrared (NIR) spectra) variables. For herbage, these factors include season, maturity, species and location. When an equation is used to predict a group of unknown samples, it should be validated with a small number (10–20) of those samples to ensure that they are within the bounds of the calibration database, i.e. reference population. This is a difficult problem for predicting *in vivo* D and intake.

One method to validate an equation for NV using a structured database is to use the structure in a round-robin technique (or 'ring' test). Here, each of the factors that may influence NV (e.g. season) is validated in turn. In one example, four groups of grass silages (for a detailed description see Barber *et al.*, 1990) were fed to animals at three locations:

- Group 1 (pre-1980, n = 28) at the Agricultural Development and Advisory Service (ADAS), UK.
- Group 2 (post-1980, n = 72) at ADAS.
- Group 3 (n = 43) at the Rowett Research Institute, Scotland.
- Group 4 (n = 27) at the North of Scotland Agricultural College (NOSCA).

When *in vivo* measurements of organic-matter digestibility (OMD) were regressed on values predicted from NIR spectra, the r^2 and standard error (SE) were 0.79 and 30 g kg^{-1}, respectively (Fig. 1.4a). Only 4% of the samples were outside the acceptable (residual > 2 standard deviations (SD) or 10% of the mean OMD value) range. However, if the round-robin technique was used and the calibration repeated four times using three groups for calibration, with the fourth group reserved for validation (external), then the relationship between reference and predicted OMD was more diverse. The r^2 and SE were 0.50 and 42 g kg^{-1}, respectively. Furthermore, 25% of the samples were unacceptably predicted (> 2 SD). Part of the samples from ADAS post-1980 (below the unity line) and the Rowett Institute (above the unity line) were required in the calibration database for an acceptable calibration equation. However, both the ADAS pre-1980 and NOSCA samples could be well predicted using the other samples for calibration. Monitoring is required to test equations on any new population before it is used for predictions.

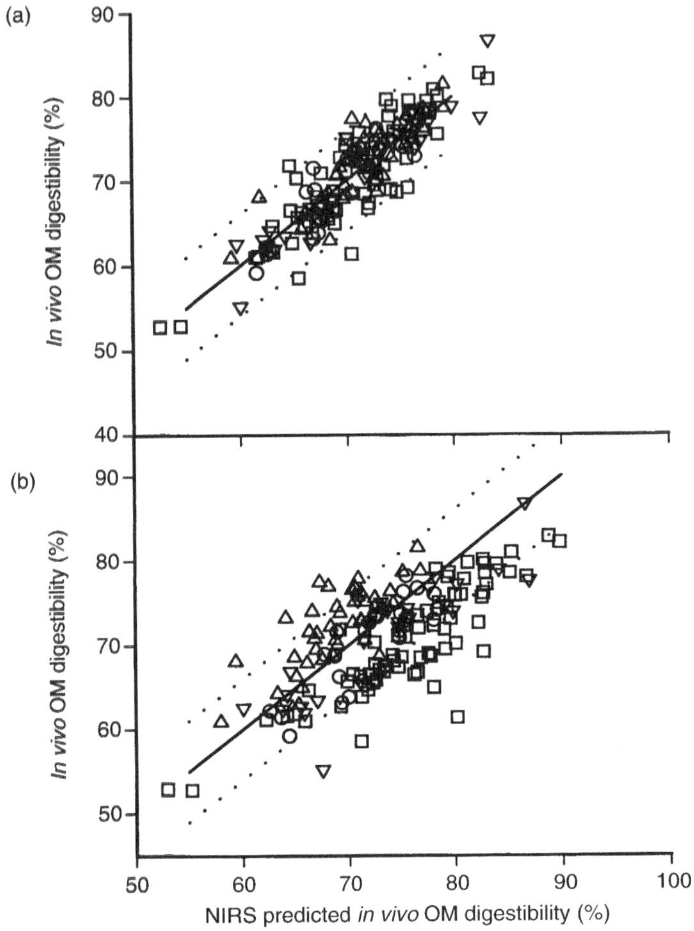

Fig. 1.4. The relationship between *in vivo* OMD of grass silages and that predicted using NIRS. Data points represent mean OMD from six sheep fed at: ADAS before 1980 (○); ADAS after 1980 (□); NOSCA (▽); and Rowett (△). Unity line (Y = X) (_______), or ± two SD of the mean (.......) (samples inside are acceptable, those outside are unacceptable). (a) Shows the values predicted from a single regression equation derived from all the samples; (b) shows the values predicted for each group of samples, from a regression equation based on the other three groups (external validation).

Chemical procedures

Van Soest (1994) and Minson (1990) have provided comprehensive reviews of the use of chemistry to predict NV. Three general conclusions can be drawn from their studies: (i) no single chemical constituent can be used to predict NV over a wide range of forage types; (ii) multiple regression equations including several chemical constituents improve but do not completely resolve this problem (Weiss, 1993); and (iii) empirical relationships in general are limited in their ability to predict across a wide range of forages (Mertens, 1973; Weiss, 1993).

Crude fibre in the Weende system of analysis has often been used as an index of NV, but the accuracy and precision of values predicted with this rough measure of cell walls are poor. As well as the uncertainties in the CF values obtained, the D of the cell-wall portion of forage plants varies between plant species and plant parts. For such reasons, a summative system based on digestible cell wall and cell contents was proposed (Van Soest, 1967). Cell contents are, under most circumstances, largely digestible (though see Ballard *et al.*, 1990) and the digestible cell-wall material may be estimated as part of the *in vitro* procedure of Tilley and Terry (1963), described below. Alternatively, the D of cell walls may be estimated from the lignin content, a less accurate procedure (Weiss, 1993; Van Soest, 1994).

In one of many examples of the use of chemical analyses, Moore *et al.* (1996) developed equations based on multiple forage constituents (CP, ADF, NDF and all possible interactions and quadratics) to predict intake and D. These equations satisfactorily fitted hay samples in their extensive database but, when applied to another database of D by sheep (Mertens, 1973), the same equations did not predict D well. Removing the effects of 'laboratory' by covariance improved the fit. Also, recalculating the equations using the same independent variables but based on the Mertens (1973) database indicated a reasonable relationship between chemistry and NV. This demonstrates two problems with developing equations from published data. The equations are largely limited to the sample population on which they were built, and differences in methods among laboratories for measuring NV contribute significant variation.

Biological procedures

Three bioassay techniques have been developed, with several variations of each, depending on the specific aim of the prediction: (i) *in vitro* D using rumen microorganisms; (ii) *in vitro* D using an enzyme preparation; and (iii) the *in situ* or nylon-bag technique.

In vitro *procedures using rumen microorganisms*

A major development since the early 1960s has been the two-stage *in vitro* system, consisting of 48 h incubation with rumen fluid followed by 24 h incubation of the residue in acid–pepsin solution (Tilley and Terry, 1963). The procedure has been generally accepted but suffers from a number of limitations (for a discussion of sources of errors, see Mertens, 1973). For instance, the constant 48 h incubation time does not account for variation in residence time caused by differences in level of intake, nor does the procedure account for differences between forages in the role that mastication plays in their digestion. Recent innovations include using freshly macerated herbage rather than dried, ground plant material (Barrell *et al.*, 2000) to mimic grazed herbage more closely.

Differences between *in vivo* and *in vitro* estimates of D are usually in the range of error for *in vivo* determinations (Van Soest, 1994), but it is important to include forages with known *in vivo* D as standards in each run. Weiss (1994) compiled reports of *in vitro* : *in vivo* relationships and found that, with D expressed as g kg^{-1}, the standard error of prediction ranged from 14.6 (C3 grasses) to 37.8 (C4 grasses) g kg^{-1}. The expected slope of such relationships is 1.0, but Weiss (1994) found that they ranged from 0.71 to 1.27; he emphasized that separate equations need to be developed for each laboratory and perhaps for species within each laboratory. In general, *in vitro* procedures based on rumen fluid are the most robust for predicting D, but run-to-run variability, the cost of maintaining a rumen-fistulated animal and slow turnaround severely limit their routine use for samples submitted by farmers.

Enzyme-based in vitro *procedures*

In an attempt to remove the need to maintain rumen-fistulated animals and the variability in rumen fluid, procedures have been developed using cellulolytic enzymes rather than rumen microbes. Early attempts with crude cellulase preparations gave poor results, but Jones and Hayward (1975) obtained good correlations with *in vivo* measurements by preceding cellulase digestion with a 24 h incubation in acid–pepsin. McLeod and Minson (1978) established and validated the routine procedure that is now widely used.

In situ *procedures*

The so-called *in situ* or *in sacco* procedures for measuring the rate of disappearance of DM or other feed components in the rumen involve suspending a number of samples (2–5 g DM) of the forage in the rumen, using bags made of nylon or other synthetic material with a mean pore width usually within the range 35–50 μm. Bags are removed, successively, after specified times, washed in a standard manner and then dried and weighed to estimate the loss of DM or its components for each time of incubation.

A typical disappearance curve for DM is shown in Fig. 1.5. The equations usually fitted to such curves (see the legend to Fig. 1.5) have coefficients that can provide information about both the potential extent and the rate of disappearance of the constituent in the rumen (Ørskov and McDonald, 1979). Apart from the limitation that the *in situ* technique measures disappearance only in the rumen, problems with the technique include the need to maintain rumen-fistulated animals, variability due to particle or microbial movement in or out of the bags and variation due to incomplete or excessive washing. However, this technique remains the standard procedure for estimating the rumen degradability of dietary CP.

Another approach to the measurement of the rate of disappearance of DM is the measurement of the rate of gas production during *in vitro* fermentation (Menke *et al.*, 1979). Although this is simple in principle, it is only recently that procedures have been developed that allow it to be done rou-

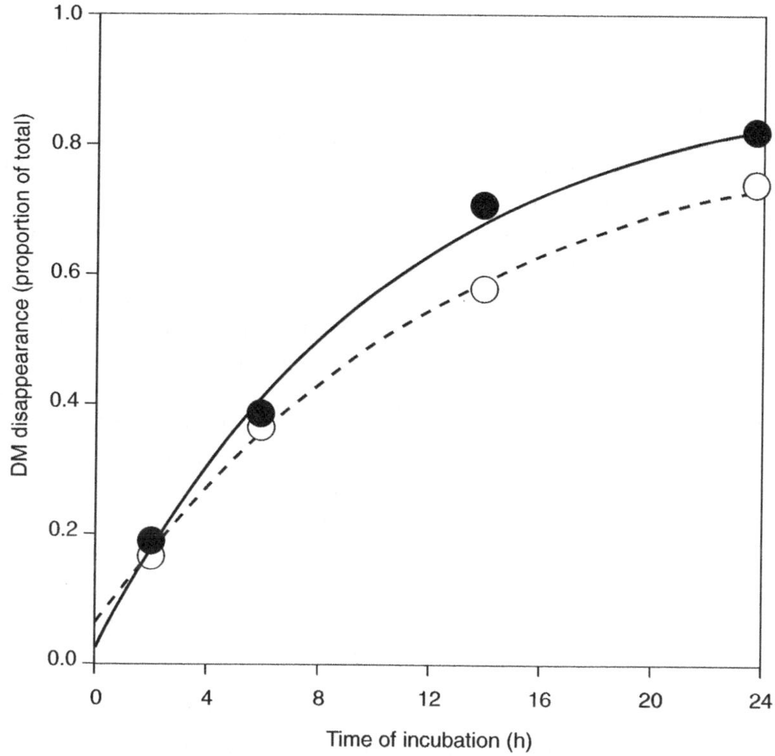

Fig. 1.5. Typical curves fitted to data for the proportional disappearance of herbage dry matter incubated in the rumen of sheep. Data points represent chopped samples of either forage-rape leaf (●) or stem (○) material, and are the means of six separate determinations (Dove and McCormack, 1986). The curves fitted to the data are of the form:

$$p = a - b(1 - \exp(-ct))$$

where p is the proportion of the constituent that disappears in time t; a is the proportion that disappears immediately; $(a - b)$ is the potential disappearance of the constituent; and c is the rate of disappearance per unit time. Values for the coefficients a, b and c are given in the original reference.

tinely. Cone *et al.* (1999) compared several variations of the *in vitro* with *in situ* procedures and found differences in absolute values for rate parameters but observed reasonable relationships among the techniques. Simple correlation coefficients ranged from 0.55 to 0.97 among rate parameters for *Lolium perenne* (perennial ryegrass) measured as either regrowth or silage samples.

Physical procedures

Near-infrared reflectance spectroscopy

Norris *et al.* (1976) were the first to report the use of NIRS to estimate chemical composition and NV of forages. The NIR spectral region (a part of the electromagnetic region) exists between the visible red and the mid-infrared (~1000–2500 nm). As monochromatic light interacts with the molecular structure of herbage the vibrational energy of groups of atoms (for example C–H, N–H) absorbs energy at wavelengths that harmonize with its vibrational frequency. The fingerprint of these absorptions is complex and consists of harmonic overtones and combination bands from the primary absorptions in the far and mid-infrared. The signal information is therefore ambiguous and must be teased out with statistical procedures. The combination of chemistry, physics and statistics has developed into the field known as chemometrics. Multiple regression was the earliest statistical method used, but more recently principal-components and PLS regression (Martens and Jensen, 1982) have gained wide acceptance.

Due to the simple sample preparation (dry and grind), non-destructive analysis, speed and ability to estimate many attributes, NIRS has found rapid acceptance. However, as it predicts NV only indirectly, the need to maintain a sample database with accurate reference values for NV has been a deterrent to uptake of the NIRS approach; the same requirement exists for other predictive methods, such as forage chemistry.

NIRS is most routinely used to predict chemical composition. Frequently, the chemical composition predicted by NIRS is later used in separate equations to predict NV and intake. However, it has been demonstrated that NIRS can also be used to predict intake directly (Coleman *et al.*, 1995) and NV (Barber *et al.*, 1990) without the use of two different steps. This avoids the problem that, when two prediction equations are used to predict a single value (NV), the errors about each equation are compounded. The results of some studies that have reported prediction of *in vivo* D from NIRS, *in vitro* D (rumen fluid or pepsin–cellulase) estimates or a number of chemical fractions – modified ADF or acetyl bromide lignin – are compiled in Table 1.3. In most cases, NIRS was as accurate (small bias) and precise (high r^2 and small SE of prediction) as *in vitro* or chemical procedures.

Coleman *et al.* (1995) advocated the use of faecal indices based on NIRS to estimate NV. When used together with markers such as alkanes, these faecal indices have the capability to greatly extend the number of animals and pastures that may be studied in an experiment.

Tensile or shear strength

Low voluntary intake by ruminants can be attributed in part to the resistance of the forage to breakdown during chewing and consequent long retention times in the rumen (Balch and Campling, 1962). This resistance to breakdown has been attributed to the physical strength of the material (i.e. the force or energy required to fracture the material) (Mackinnon *et al.*, 1988). The strength of plant material has been measured either as the energy or force required to fracture (e.g. grind or shear) a mass of plant material or to fracture individual plant parts. Fracture can be measured in shear (using cutting or punch-and-die apparatus), tension (breaking specimens by longitudinal pull) or compression, or by grinding (which is likely to be a mixture of fracture processes).

Table 1.3. Relative precision and accuracy for prediction of *in vivo* digestibility from NIRS and various conventional laboratory methods: *in vitro* estimates of dry-matter or organic-matter digestibility using rumen fluid (IVDMD and IVOMD, respectively), or using pepsin–cellulase (PC); or measurements of acetyl bromide lignin (ABLIG), modified acid-detergent fibre (MADF) or neutral-detergent cellulase digestibility (NDC).

Forage type and measure	Method	Calibration			Validation					Reference
		n	r^2	SEC	n	r^2	SEP	Slope	Bias	
Mixed DE (MJ kg^{-1})	NIRS	30	0.67	0.71	30	0.67	0.71	–	–	Eckman *et al.* (1983)
	IVDMD	30	0.59	0.84	30	0.76	0.50	–	–	
Grass silage OMD (g kg^{-1})	NIRS	122	0.85	25	48	0.76	26	0.93	−7.9	Barber *et al.* (1990)
	IVOMD	122	0.74	32	48	0.64	36	0.89	−18.5	
	PC	122	0.55	42	48	0.40	47	0.71	23.3	
	ABLIG	122	0.52	44	48	0.14	53	0.48	11.8	
	MADF	122	0.34	51	48	0.20	51	0.52	−5.9	
Straw OMD (g kg^{-1})	NIRS	81	0.74	33	42	0.65	37	0.99	−12.4	Givens *et al.* (1991)
	IVOMD	81	0.61	39	42	0.60	39	0.99	−9.0	
	NDC	81	0.61	39	42	0.48	49	1.12	−12.4	
	PC	81	0.60	39	42	0.51	44	0.95	−7.8	

SEC, standard error of calibration; SEP, standard error of prediction.

Foot and Reed (1981) reviewed attempts to directly correlate voluntary intake of forages with the energy required to grind a fixed weight of dried material through a laboratory mill. They concluded that, in addition to some technical constraints, the correlations were generally unsatisfactory for the prediction of intake (some correlation coefficients were as low as 0.41).

A punch-and-die apparatus has been described in which a known mass of material was compressed to a standard pressure and then sheared (Baker *et al.*, 1993). One advantage of this method over grinding energy is that it could be adapted to both dry and hydrated plant material (Henry *et al.*, 1996a). Also, it better defines the biomechanical character of shear, rather than grinding energy, which is an ill-defined mixture of fracture forces. This measure of shear energy accounted for a higher proportion of the variance of voluntary intake (r = 0.94) by sheep of dry, mature subterranean clover compared with other measures of grinding energy (r = 0.87–0.93) (Baker *et al.*, 1992).

There has been a proliferation of other instrumentation and methodology for measuring the strength of plant material, including the Warner–Bratzler shear apparatus, originally designed for measuring meat tenderness (e.g. Mackinnon *et al.*, 1988), instrumented scissors (e.g. Lucas and Pereira, 1990) and apparatus to measure tensile strength (e.g. Vincent, 1990). Many of the advantages and disadvantages of these methods are discussed by Henry *et al.* (1996b), who described a guillotine-type instrument to measure shear strength.

In leaves of grasses, shear strength is only weakly correlated with tensile strength ($r = -0.47$) (Henry *et al.*, 1996b), making the choice of which character to measure (and perhaps breed for) critical. The biological basis of this weak, negative relationship is unclear, but it is pertinent to remember that tensile fracture will occur at the weakest point, whereas shear fracture is usually orientated directly across the structural components.

The choice of which biomechanical character to measure will be influenced by both the ease and rapidity of measurement (here, the shear methods are superior) and the relationship to animal performance. It has been suggested that tensile strength may be important during prehension of leaves (Vincent, 1990), whereas shear strength may be important in chewing (Mackinnon *et al.*, 1988), although strong evidence for these contentions is lacking. The only published data on a relation between tensile strength and animal performance appear to be those of Voigt *et al.* (1970), who reported no relationship between the leaf tensile strength of weeping lovegrass (*Eragrostis curvula*) and 'palatability' (defined as a plant characteristic that determined whether and to what degree feed was attractive to animals). In contrast, shear strength has been shown to be negatively correlated with rate of DM consumption (Mackinnon *et al.*, 1988) and total voluntary intake (Baker *et al.*, 1992) by sheep.

Conclusion

Nutritive value of herbage is variable because of variation in plant genetics, the rate and degree of plant development, environmental conditions under which it is grown and management practices. In general, NV declines with maturity, is lower in tropical and subtropical forages than in temperate forages and is lower in plants grown under high temperatures. It is best assessed using animal trials, but these are laborious, expensive and time-consuming. Moreover, NV of grazed herbage cannot be assessed directly and can only be crudely estimated, using indirect techniques. Consequently, there is a need for accurate, rapid and inexpensive techniques to estimate or predict NV. Chemical composition, mechanical resistance, bioassays and instrument-based methods have all been proposed, each with advantages and limitations. The method based on NIRS shows great promise and offers the speed necessary for routine analytical laboratories. The limitations of predictive methods are the requirement of a large database of samples with known NV, along with information for prediction (herbage chemistry, physical constraints or spectra).

References

AFRC (1993) *Energy and Protein Requirements for Ruminants*. An advisory manual prepared by the AFRC Technical Committee on Responses to Nutrients, CAB International, Wallingford, UK, 159 pp.

Akin, D.E., Robinson, E.L., Barton, F.E. and Himmelsbach, D.S. (1977) Changes with maturity in anatomy, histochemistry, chemistry and tissue digestibility of bermudagrass plant parts. *Journal of Agricultural and Food Chemistry* 25, 179–186.

Baker, S.K., Klein, L., Minson, D.J. and Purser, D.B. (1992) Voluntary intake and the energy required to shear or comminute dry, mature subterranean clovers. *Proceedings of the Nutrition Society of Australia* 17, 74.

Baker, S.K., Klein, L., de Boer, E.S. and Purser, D.B. (1993) Genotypes of dry, mature subterranean clover differ in shear energy. In: *Proceedings of the XVII International Grasslands Congress, New Zealand*. New Zealand Grassland Association, Palmerston North, pp. 592–593.

Balch, C.C. and Campling, R.C. (1962) Regulation of voluntary food intake in ruminants. *Nutrition Abstracts and Reviews* 32, 669–686.

Ballard, R.A., Simpson, R.J. and Pearce, G.R. (1990) Losses of the digestible components of annual ryegrass (*Lolium rigidum* Gaudin) during senescence. *Australian Journal of Agricultural Research* 41, 719–731.

Barber, G.D., Givens, D.I., Kridis, M.S., Offer, N.W. and Murray, I. (1990) Prediction of the organic matter digestibility of grass silage. *Animal Feed Science and Technology* 28, 115–128.

Barrell, L.G., Burke, J.L., Waghorn, G.C., Attwood, G.T. and Brookes, I.M. (2000) Preparation of fresh forages for incubation and prediction of nutritive value. *Proceedings of the New Zealand Society of Animal Production* 60, 9–14.

Ciavarella, T.A., Dove, H., Leury, B.J. and Simpson, R.J. (2000) Diet selection by sheep grazing *Phalaris aquatica* L. pastures of differing water-soluble carbohydrate content. *Australian Journal of Agricultural Research*, 51, 757–764.

Coleman, S.W., Stuth, J.W. and Holloway, J.W. (1995) Prediction of intake by near-infrared spectroscopic analysis of fecal samples. In: Owens, F.N., Gill, D., Lusby, K. and McCollum, T. (eds) *Symposium: Intake by Feedlot Cattle*. Oklahoma Agricultural Experiment Station P-942, Stillwater, Oklahoma, pp. 145–155.

Coleman, S.W., Lippke, H. and Gill, M. (1999) Estimating the nutritive potential of forages. In: Jung, H.G. and Fahey, G.C. (eds) *Nutritional Ecology of Herbivores: Proceedings of the V International Symposium on the Nutrition of Herbivores*. American Society of Animal Science, Savoy, Illinois, pp. 647–695.

Cone, J.W., van Gelder, A.H., Soliman, I.A, de Visser, H. and van Vuuren, A.M. (1999) Different techniques to study rumen fermentation characteristics of maturing grass and grass silage. *Journal of Dairy Science* 82, 957–966.

Corbett, J.L. (1969) The nutritional value of grassland herbage. In: Cuthbertson, D.P. (ed.) *International Encyclopaedia of Food and Nutrition*, Vol. 17(2). Pergamon Press, Oxford, pp. 593–644.

Dabo, S.M., Taliaferro, C.M., Coleman, S.W., Horn, F.P. and Claypool, P.L. (1987) Yield and digestibility of old world bluestem grasses as affected by cultivar, plant part and maturity. *Journal of Range Management* 40, 10–15.

Dabo, S.M., Taliaferro, C.M., Coleman, S.W., Horn, F.P. and Claypool, P.L. (1988) Chemical composition of old world bluestem grasses as affected by cultivar and maturity. *Journal of Range Management* 41, 40–48.

Dove, H. and McCormack, H.A. (1986) Estimation of the ruminal degradation of forage rape after incubation in nylon bags in the rumen of sheep. *Grass and Forage Science* 41, 129–136.

Dove, H. and Mayes, R.W. (1991) The use of plant wax alkanes as marker substances in studies of the nutrition of herbivores: a review. *Australian Journal of Agricultural Research* 42, 913–952.

Eckman, D.D., Shenk, J.S., Wangsness, P.J. and Westerhaus, M.O. (1983) Prediction of sheep responses by near infrared reflectance spectroscopy. *Journal of Dairy Science* 66, 1983–1987.

Ehlke, N.J., Casler, M.D., Drolsom, P.N. and Shenk, J.S. (1986) Divergent selection for *in vitro* dry matter digestibility in smooth bromegrass. *Crop Science* 26, 1123–1126.

Fisher, D.S., Mayland, H.F. and Burns, J.C. (1999) Variation in ruminants' preference for tall fescue hays cut either at sundown or at sunup. *Journal of Animal Science* 77, 762–768.

Foot, J.Z. and Reed, K.F.M. (1981) The energy consumed in the grinding of herbage and its relationship to voluntary intake of herbage by ruminants. In: Wheeler, J.L. and Mochrie, R.D. (eds) *Forage Evaluation: Concepts and Techniques*. CSIRO, East Melbourne, pp. 121–129.

Ford, C.W., Morrison, I.M. and Wilson, J.R. (1979) Temperature effects on lignin, hemicellulose and cellulose in tropical and temperate grasses. *Australian Journal of Agricultural Research* 30, 621–633.

Freer, M. and Jones, D.B. (1984) Feeding value of subterranean clover, lucerne, phalaris and wimmera ryegrass for lambs. *Australian Journal of Experimental Agriculture and Animal Husbandry* 24, 156–164.

Gatford, K.L., Simpson, R.J., Siever-Kelly, C., Leury, B.J., Dove, H. and Ciavarella, T.A. (1999) Spray-topping annual grass pasture with glyphosate to delay loss of feeding value during summer. I. Effects on pasture yield and nutritive value. *Australian Journal of Agricultural Research* 50, 453–464.

Givens, D.I, Baker, C.W. and Adamson, A.H. (1991) A comparison of near-infrared reflectance spectroscopy with three *in vitro* techniques to predict the digestibility *in vivo* of untreated and ammonia-treated cereal straws. *Animal Feed Science and Techology* 35, 83–94.

Goto, M., Gordon, A.H. and Chesson, A. (1991) Changes in cell-wall composition and degradability of sorghum during growth and maturation. *Journal of the Science of Food and Agriculture* 54, 47–60.

Henry, D.A., Baker, S.K. and Purser, D.B. (1996a) Measuring the compression and shear energies of green plant material. *Proceedings of the Australian Society of Animal Production* 21, 497.

Henry, D.A., Macmillan, R.H. and Simpson, R.J. (1996b) Shear and tensile fracture properties of leaves of pasture grasses. *Australian Journal of Agricultural Research* 47, 587–603.

Henry, D.A., Macmillan, R.H. and Simpson, R.J. (1997) Intrinsic shear strength of leaves of pasture grasses and legumes. *Australian Journal of Agricultural Research* 48, 667–674.

Henry, D.A., Simpson, R.J. and Macmillan, R.H. (2000) Seasonal changes and the effect of temperature and leaf moisture content on intrinsic shear strength of leaves of pasture grasses. *Australian Journal of Agricultural Research* 51, 823–831.

Humphreys, M.O. (1989) Water-soluble carbohydrates in perennial ryegrass breeding. II. Cultivar and hybrid progeny performance in cut plots. *Grass and Forage Science* 44, 237–244.

Jones, D.I.H. and Hayward, M.V. (1975) The effect of pepsin pretreatment on the prediction of dry matter digestibility from solubility in fungal cellulase solutions. *Journal of the Science of Food and Agriculture* 26, 711–718.

Lucas, P.W. and Pereira, B. (1990) Estimation of the fracture toughness of leaves. *Functional Ecology* 4, 819–822.

Mackinnon, B.W., Easton, H.S., Barry, T.N. and Sedcole, J.R. (1988) The effect of reduced leaf shear strength on the nutritive value of perennial ryegrass. *Journal of Agricultural Science, Cambridge* 111, 469–474.

MAFF (1990) *UK Tables of Nutritive Value and Chemical Composition of Feedingstuffs*. Ministry of Fisheries, Agriculture and Food, Aberdeen, UK, 420 pp.

Martens, H.A. and Jensen, S.A. (1982) Partial least squares regression: a new two-stage NIR calibration method. In: Holas, J. and Kratchovil, J. (eds) *Proceedings of 7th World Cereal Congress, Amsterdam*. Elsevier, Amsterdam, pp. 607–647.

McIlroy, R.J. (1967) Carbohydrates of grassland herbage. *Herbage Abstracts and Reviews* 37, 79–87.

McLeod, M.N. and Minson, D.J. (1978) The accuracy of the pepsin–cellulase technique for estimating the dry matter digestibility *in vivo* of grasses and legumes. *Animal Feed Science and Technology* 3, 277–287.

Menke, K.H., Raab, L., Salewski, A., Steingass, H., Fritz, D. and Schneider, W. (1979) The estimation of the digestibility and metabolizable energy content of ruminant feedingstuffs from the gas production when they are incubated with rumen liquor *in vitro*. *Journal of Agricultural Science, Cambridge* 93, 217–222.

Mertens, D.R. (1973) Application of theoretical mathematical models to cell wall digestion and forage intake in ruminants. PhD dissertation, Cornell University, Ithaca, New York (*Dissertation Abstracts* 74–10).

Minson, D.J. (1990) *Forage in Ruminant Nutrition*. Academic Press, Sydney, 483 pp.

Moore, J.E., Burns, J.C. and Fisher, D.S. (1996) Multiple regression equations for predicting relative feed value of grass hays. In: Williams, M.J. (ed.) *Proceedings 1996 American Forage and Grassland Council, Georgetown, USA*. AFGC, Georgetown, Texas, pp. 135–139.

Moseley, G. (1981) The role of physical breakdown in controlling the nutritive quality of forages. In: *Annual Report of the Welsh Plant Breeding Station*. Welsh Plant Breeding Station, Aberystwyth, pp. 167–182.

Norris, K.H., Barnes, R.F., Moore, J.E. and Shenk, J.S. (1976) Predicting forage quality by infrared reflectance spectroscopy. *Journal of Animal Science* 43, 889–897.

NRC (National Research Council) (1985) *Nutrient Requirements of Sheep*, 6th edn. National Academy Press, Washington, DC, 97 pp.

Ørskov, E.R. and McDonald, I. (1979) The estimation of protein degradability in the rumen from incubation measurements weighted according to rate of passage. *Journal of Agricultural Science, Cambridge* 92, 499–503.

Poppi, D.P., McLennan, S.R., Bediye, S., de Vega, A. and Zorrilla-Rios, J. (1999) Forage quality: strategies for increasing nutritive value of forages. In: *Proceedings of XVIII International Grassland Congress, Calgary, Canada*. Association Management Center, Calgary, pp. 307–322.

SCA (1990) *Feeding Standards for Australian Livestock. Ruminants*. Standing Committee on Agriculture and CSIRO, Melbourne, 266 pp.

Stallcup, O.T., Brown, C.J., Johnson, Z.B., Kreider, D.L. and York, J.O. (1983) Use of principal-component analysis in summarizing nutritive and analytical characteristics of forages. In: *Proceedings of the XIV International Grassland Congress, Boulder, USA*. Westview Press, Boulder, Colorado, pp. 494–497.

Tabe, L.M., Higgins, C.M., McNabb, W.C. and Higgins, T.J.V. (1993) Genetic engineering of grain and pasture legumes for improved nutritive value. *Genetica* 90, 181–200.

Tilley, J.M.A. and Terry, R.A. (1963) A two-stage technique for the *in vitro* digestion of forage crops. *Journal of the British Grassland Society* 18, 104–111.

Ulyatt, M.J. (1981) The feeding value of temperate pastures. In: Morley, F.H.W. (ed.) *Grazing Animals*. World Animal Science, Vol. B1, Elsevier, Amsterdam, pp. 125–141.

Van Soest, P.J. (1967) Development of a comprehensive system of feed analyses and its application to forages. *Journal of Animal Science* 26, 119–127.

Van Soest, P.J. (1994) *Nutritional Ecology of the Ruminant*, 2nd edn. Cornell University Press, Ithaca, New York.

Vincent, J.F.V. (1990) Fracture properties of plants. *Advances in Botanical Research* 17, 235–287.

Voigt, P.W., Kneebone, W.R., McIlvain, E.H., Shoop, M.C. and Webster, J.E. (1970) Palatability, chemical composition and animal gains from selections of weeping lovegrass, *Eragrostis curvula* (Schrad.) Nees. *Agronomy Journal* 62, 673–676.

Waghorn, G.C., Reed, J. and Ndlovu, L.R. (1999) Condensed tannins and herbivore nutrition. In: *Proceedings of the XVIII International Grassland Congress, Calgary, Canada*, Vol. 3. Association Management Center, Calgary, pp.153–166.

Weiss, W.P. (1993) Symposium: prevailing concepts in energy utilization by ruminants: predicting energy values of feeds. *Journal of Dairy Science* 76, 1802–1811.

Weiss, W.P. (1994) Estimation of digestibility of forages by laboratory methods. In: Fahey, G.C., Moser, L.E., Mertens, D.R. and Collins, M. (eds) *Forage Quality, Evaluation, and Utilization*. American Society of Agronomy, Madison, Wisconsin, pp. 644–681.

2 Constraints on Feed Intake by Grazing Sheep

R.H. Weston

45 Park Street, Glenbrook, New South Wales, Australia

Introduction

Herbage obtained by grazing provides the major source of nutrients for most of the world's sheep. However, the intake of herbage generally falls well short of the amount they need to express their genetic potential for production.

Major constraints to pasture consumption can be related to: (i) the amounts and spatial distribution of the components of the pasture biomass; (ii) the chemical and physical properties of the herbage; and (iii) environmental attributes associated with climate, disease and sheep behaviour. Intakes commensurate with the achievement of high levels of production may be reached for only short periods of the year on the highest-quality temperate pastures. Such pastures generally contain appreciable quantities of legume leaf and provide herbage that is low in fibre, high in protein and readily broken down by chewing (comminution). These conditions rarely occur on tropical pastures.

Grazing ruminants, relative to omnivores, need very high feed intakes to achieve maximum production. These high intakes are necessary because the gross energy value of herbage is relatively low. In addition, 15–60% of this energy is lost via the faeces, up to 18% of the energy released during ruminal fermentation is lost as heat and combustible gases and the nutrient energy absorbed is inefficiently used in body-tissue synthesis, with more than half being lost as heat (see also Coleman and Henry, Chapter 1, this volume). Moreover, significant energy costs are incurred in grazing and ruminating and this energy also appears as heat.

It follows that the capacity of the sheep's gastrointestinal tract to cope with the ingestion of pasture and the resulting digesta could be expected to be involved in the constraint on intake. Furthermore, it might be expected that, with high-quality pasture, limitations on the ability to dissipate heat could act as an intake constraint at times of high production, such as during rapid lamb growth and at peak lactation.

Recent publications have comprehensively covered some areas relating to pasture intake constraints (Kennedy and Doyle, 1993; Ungar, 1996; Wilson and Kennedy, 1996; Pittroff and Kothmann, 1999; Hinch *et al.*, 2003). In this chapter, the emphasis will be on developing a conceptual scheme for forage intake constraint. However, it would be fair to say that a general consensus remains to be achieved about many aspects of intake regulation.

In the discussion that follows it will be assumed that the animals are healthy and that no deficiencies of minerals or vitamins exist. The terms intake constraint or intake regulation, as used here, refer to a longer-term situation (> 2–3 days), as distinct from individual meals or grazing periods. Optimal diet, as used here, refers to a palatable diet adequate with respect to essential nutrients and sufficiently digestible for its physical characteristics not to act to constrain intake; typically such a diet would be a ground and pelleted mixture containing lucerne hay (*Medicago sativa*) and concentrates (1 : 1) providing appropriate amounts of essential nutrients. The term rumen refers here to the reticulo-rumen, and metabolic body weight (MW) is equal to body weight (BW) expressed in $kg^{0.75}$. In estimating the quantity of protein apparently digested in the intestines, it has been assumed that 80% of crude protein (CP) (non-ammonia nitrogen × 6.25) entering the intestines is in the form of protein with an apparent digestibility of 0.74. Unless stated otherwise, the adult sheep referred to here has a BW of 50 kg (MW 18.8) and the weaner lamb a BW of 25 kg (MW 11.2).

The Regulation of Forage Intake

The framework of a conceptual model of forage-intake regulation, linking energy transactions and rumen function, is shown in Fig. 2.1 (see also Weston, 1996). As energy intake by the sheep eating forage generally fails to meet the potential need for energy, the regulation model contains an energy-deficit component (the animal's capacity to use energy minus useful dietary energy intake). The energy deficit is thought to generate hunger signal(s), the intensity of which is directly related to the size of the deficit. Constraints on the clearance of the digesta from the rumen, due to the level and properties of the herbage fibre, result in digesta accumulation in that organ. Hence, the regulation model contains a digesta-'load' component, which reflects sensory input to the central nervous system from the rumen mechanoreceptors. It is postulated that the load generates satiety signals, the intensity of which is directly related to the size of the load beyond a threshold value. With the energy-deficit and the digesta-'load' components operating, the overall feeding drive is overcome when the inhibitory signals from the 'load' and other constraints (see Fig. 2.1) more than balance the hunger signal(s) derived from the energy deficit.

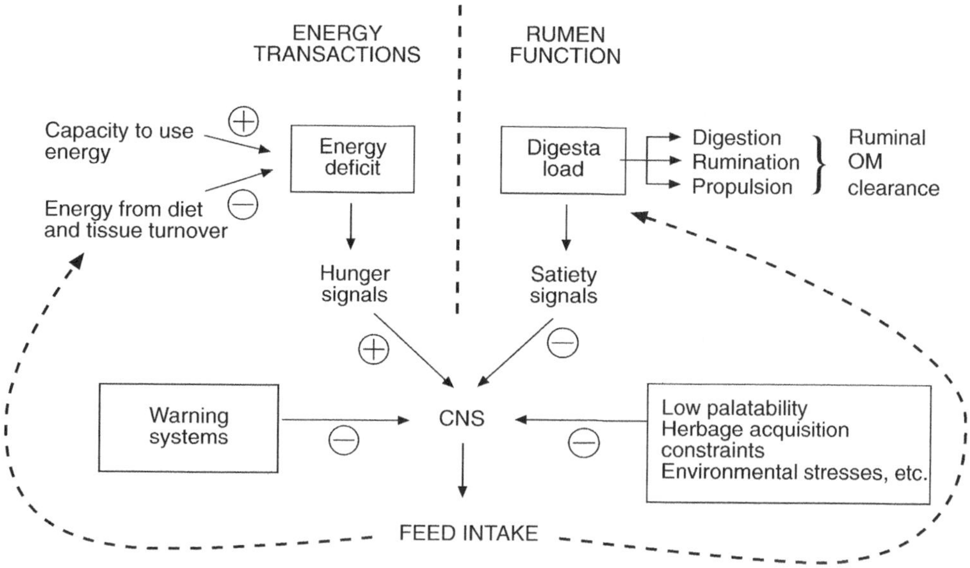

Fig. 2.1. Conceptual scheme for pasture-intake regulation. CNS, central nervous system.

This model implies that on abundant high-quality pasture, where net energy intake is high and accordingly energy deficit low, the rumen digesta 'load' needed to provide an overriding satiety signal will be relatively low. In contrast, with abundant lower-quality pasture the load could be expected to be higher, associated with a lower energy intake and an accompanying higher energy deficit. Inverse relationships have, in fact, been shown between the amount of digesta in the rumen and energy intake for weaner lambs fed *ad libitum* indoors on a narrow range of forages containing adequate essential nutrients (Fig. 2.2).

A feature of this model is that over a wide range of forage qualities both the sheep's capacity to use energy and the rate of digesta clearance from the rumen play a role in the intake regulation. However, within this range neither factor would be solely responsible for limiting intake. Accordingly, the hunger drive can be overcome at an intake level providing less energy than the animal is capable of using.

The conceptual model can be expanded to encompass a further range of dietary situations, as discussed by Weston (1996). For example, at very high levels of energy deficit, a physiological upper limit to digesta 'load' could possibly be reached; in these situations energy transactions would not influence the regulation, with intake being directly proportional to digesta clearance rate. Again, with very high-quality pasture, an intake adequate to satisfy the capacity to use energy may provide a digesta 'load' sufficiently low for the sensory input from the mechanoreceptors to be irrelevant. Further, a deficiency of essential nutrients or the presence of deleterious substances in the pasture herbage can modulate the intake via effects on rumen function, energy metabolism or pasture ingestion.

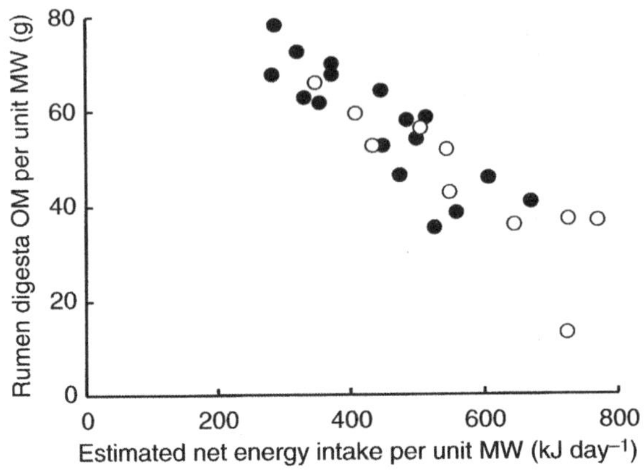

Fig. 2.2. The relationship between the quantity of digesta organic matter (OM) in the rumen per unit metabolic weight (MW) and the estimated intake of net energy per unit MW. The data are from studies with weaner lambs: (i) fed various forage diets (●) (Weston, 1996); or (ii) fed a basal forage diet and given varying quantities of a nutrient solution *per abomasum* (○) (Gherardi and Black, 1989).

Studies of meal eating indicate that a network of warning systems (Fig. 2.1) exists to protect the internal milieu from disturbance and the gastrointestinal tract from overload. This network comprises mechano-, osmo-, thermo- and chemoreceptors, together with a range of peptides that are produced in response to eating, and it acts mainly in influencing the termination of meal eating. Its operation in the longer-term regulation, as distinct from meal-eating regulation, would apply only in limited situations, such as where high electrolyte load or heat dissipation were relevant limitations.

Constraints

Capacity to use energy

Under optimal conditions the sheep appears to limit feed intake in relation to its capacity to dispose of energy via the pathways of oxidation and synthesis (Weston, 1996). We can think of this capacity as being equal to the sum of the energy needs for: (i) maintenance; (ii) sustaining growth or energy accretion at a rate consistent with a particular genetic programme; and (iii) reproduction activities. In the forage-fed sheep, a change in its capacity to dispose of energy, due for example to an alteration in its physiological state, will change the energy deficit and hence the magnitude of the hunger signal(s) (see Fig. 2.1) and the constraint on forage intake.

Differences in the sheep's potential to use energy are to be expected at different stages of growth and development. In crossbred sheep kept under optimal conditions the demand for energy per unit BW declined progressively with age and daily metabolizable energy (ME) intake per unit of MW decreased from about 1300 kJ in the early weeks of life to about 600 kJ at about 90 weeks of age (Weston and Poppi, 1987). Prolonged undernutrition, where the animal falls behind in its genetic programme relating to body size, results in an enhanced capacity to use energy. This is often reflected in compensatory growth and its attendant increase in feed intake (see Oddy and Sainz, Chapter 11, this volume). Again, this situation may be seen in comparisons of intakes per unit MW by sheep differing in body-fat content, these generally being lower with the fatter animals.

The ewe's capacity to use energy varies in the reproduction cycle. Daily milk production accounts for up to *c.* 500 kJ net energy per unit MW. In the first two trimesters of pregnancy, energy demand for the uterofetal complex is low; hence the capacity to use energy should show little change. However, observed decreases in the intake of optimal diets in late pregnancy suggest a reduced capacity to use energy at this time in ewes with adequate levels of body-tissue stores.

Although forage intake changes with the sheep's capacity to use energy, the size of the change is less with forage diets than with optimal diets and varies directly with forage quality. For example, at pasture, young sheep (*c.* 20 kg BW) consumed *c.* 150 kJ more ME per unit MW daily than their adult counterparts (Arnold, 1966). In contrast, the corresponding difference with an optimal diet was greater, at *c.* 310 kJ (see Weston and Poppi, 1987).

Few adequate data are available to indicate clearly how the sheep changes the components of its grazing behaviour to obtain more feed when its capacity to use energy is elevated. Increases in grazing time reported in three studies with lactating ewes have been 0–7%, 7–12% and 25–62% (e.g. Dulphy *et al.*, 1980). Ewes suckling twins graze longer than those with singles, in line with a higher energy demand. Changes in the rate of pasture consumption (i.e. g h^{-1}) have also been reported, with values ranging from 14 to 62%. Higher pasture intake in the thin sheep relative to its fatter counterpart has been found to be associated with a large increase in intake rate and only a small elevation in the time spent grazing.

Genotype and day length are likely to affect the capacity of the sheep to use energy and accordingly the degree of constraint on forage intake. Blaxter *et al.* (1966) in studies under optimal conditions found that feed intake per unit MW differed between six breeds of sheep (coefficient of variation 4.8%) and was proportional to their maintenance energy requirement. However, there appear to be no unequivocal data showing long-term differences in intake at pasture between commercial breeds of sheep. Problems exist experimentally in obtaining animals truly representative of breeds, in ensuring that all breeds have a comparable dietary history and in selecting an appropriate index of body size for making intake comparisons.

Indoor studies indicate that feed-intake constraint with some sheep genotypes occurs in winter in association with the short day length. For example, Scottish Blackface wethers were found to consume 20% less in winter than at peak times in spring/summer. Young (1987) has discussed possible explanations for such photoperiod effects, including the possibility that a reduced energy demand could be involved.

Physical Properties of Herbage

Physical properties of forages can constrain intake, as illustrated by the marked difference between forage diets and optimal diets in the relationship between intake and the useful (i.e. net) energy content of the diet. With optimal diets, generally based on ground ingredients, intake increases with decrease in net energy content; this compensatory change results in the maintenance of a high intake of net energy. In contrast, with forage diets, as fed in long or chopped form, such a decrease in net energy content is usually due to more fibre and is associated with a lower forage intake and, accordingly, a diminished net energy intake. The increases in forage intake that accompany grinding and pelleting, found to average 23 (standard deviation (SD) ± 10) g dry matter (DM) day^{-1} per unit MW in the data set examined by Minson (1990), illustrate the significance of physical considerations as intake constraints.

Resistance of digesta organic matter (OM) to removal from the rumen

The rumen has been identified as the compartment in the alimentary tract associated with constraint on forage intake. This constraint relates to the rate of clearance of particulate OM, as effected by digestion and by transfer to the omasum. Since the digestion rate of fibre is usually less than 0.08 h^{-1} (i.e. 8% of the fibre pool digested per hour), feed particles need to be retained in the rumen for a significant time period to permit adequate fibre digestion.

Direct relationships between forage intake and the clearance rate of OM from the rumen (Fig. 2.3) indicate that the clearance rate can act as an

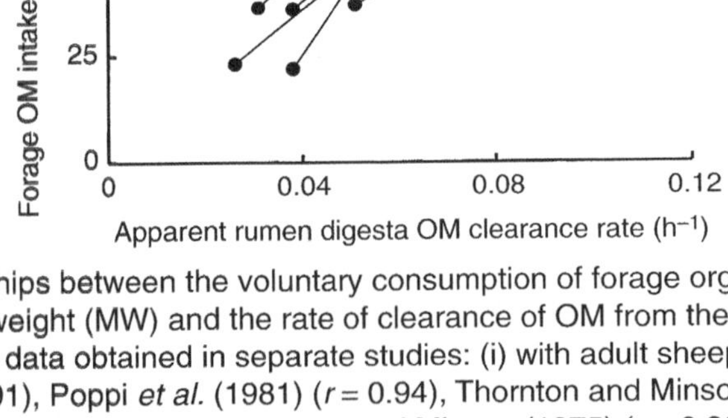

Fig. 2.3. Relationships between the voluntary consumption of forage organic matter (OM) per unit metabolic weight (MW) and the rate of clearance of OM from the rumen. The values are calculated from data obtained in separate studies: (i) with adult sheep (●) by Rees and Little (1980) ($r = 0.91$), Poppi *et al.* (1981) ($r = 0.94$), Thornton and Minson (1972) ($r = 0.95$), Laredo and Minson (1973) ($r = 0.90$), Laredo and Minson (1975) ($r = 0.90$) and Thornton and Minson (1973) ($r = 0.67$); and (ii) with weaner lambs (○) by Weston (1996) ($r = 0.94$).

intake constraint. However, although the correlations are high (usually ≥ 0.90), the absence of a single closely defined relationship between intake and clearance indicates the influence of other factors. These could include capacity to use energy, essential nutrient inadequacy and low palatability. The data obtained in these studies also indicate that there is no simple relationship between the voluntary intake of forage and rumen digesta load (Fig. 2.4), even though the amount and characteristics of the digesta could provide mechanoreceptor feedback signals in the intake regulation scheme.

Determinants of the clearance rate of digesta OM from the rumen

The rate of removal of OM from the rumen is determined by both the characteristics of the forage consumed and the physiological processes controlling digesta transactions in the rumen. Slow removal of OM from the rumen prevails with forages having a high resistance to degradation by chewing and a high content of components – generally fibre constituents – that are relatively slowly digested by the rumen microbiota. When digestibility is low, a high proportion of the OM has to be removed by onward passage, which is much slower than removal via the alternative routes of absorption and eructation. Particle-size constraints apply to the rate of clearance of OM by onward passage, as well as to the rate of microbial digestion. Accordingly, the resistance of the forage to fragmentation by chewing during eating and ruminating can be considered as a determinant of the rate of OM removal from the rumen.

The clearance rate of digesta to the omasum is essentially the ratio of outflow rate ($l\ h^{-1}$) to pool size (l). Accordingly, it can vary when physiological

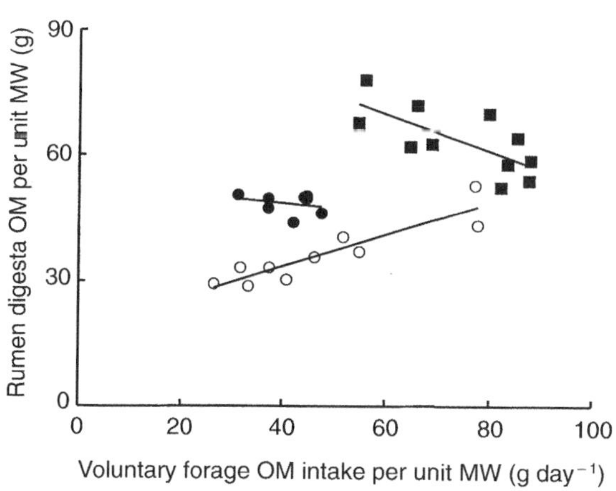

Fig. 2.4. Relationships between the quantity of digesta organic matter (OM) in the rumen per unit of metabolic weight (MW) and the voluntary consumption of forage OM per unit MW. The values were calculated from the data of Laredo and Minson (1973) (○), Poppi *et al.* (1981) (●) and Weston (1996) (■).

changes in the sheep result in changes in rumen digesta volume setting or digesta outflow per unit time. For example, rumen digesta volume decreases in late pregnancy in association with upward displacement of the rumen by the gravid uterus. However, the digesta outflow rate remains relatively constant; hence the clearance rate is increased. In contrast, increased clearance rates due to increased outflow but with relatively constant load setting have been reported in sheep during lactation and with high dietary electrolyte load.

The following factors have a role in determining digesta clearance rate.

Digesta-particle characteristics

The onward passage of digesta particles from the rumen depends on their physical characteristics, including size, shape and buoyancy. Before passage is possible, large particles have to be reduced appropriately in size and small particles need to be able to sediment, an attribute that depends on their shape and on the buoyancy associated with fermentation gases. Because the particles have irregular shapes, size is commonly defined in digestion studies in relation to passage or otherwise through sieves of defined apertures during agitation in water. Large particles, those retained by a 1200 μm sieve, have negligible clearance from the rumen to the omasum in sheep. Particles passing through a 1200 μm sieve are cleared from the rumen at rates inversely related to size; for example, those passing the 150 μm sieve have been found to be cleared from the rumen eight to 14 times faster than those isolated in the 1200 μm–600 μm sieve size fraction.

Feed-particle degradation by chewing

Chewing during forage ingestion and rumination is the major process involved in forage particle-size reduction. At pasture, grazing times of 13.7 h day^{-1} have been recorded, with the number of ingestion bites exceeding 56,000. Ingestive chewing is directed towards cropping the herbage and reducing the feed particles to dimensions permitting, under compression, the formation of a bolus suitable for swallowing. Accordingly, appreciable reduction in particle size is usually unnecessary and the extent of the fragmentation is variable. For example, ingestive chewing has been found to reduce the proportion of large particles by 50% or more with high-quality temperate forage but by only 19–34% with stem and leaf fractions of tropical grasses. Again, mastication is less when sheep graze rapidly due to time constraints and high energy deficits.

The feed-particle composition of the bolus regurgitated for rumination is considered to be similar to that in the reticulum, with the large-particle content being lower than that in the rumen. The bolus would have up to 20% of the OM as large particles and, during rumination, this would be reduced by 40–65%. Most particles are subjected to chewing in more than one rumination cycle, especially with high-fibre forages, where rumination time can be equivalent to 2.0 or more min g^{-1} forage fibre. With legumes, an average value of the breakdown rate of large particles reported by Kennedy and Doyle (1993) was 0.14 (SD ± 0.04) h^{-1}; with grasses the corresponding values ranged from 0.05 h^{-1} to 0.29 h^{-1}.

Variation between forages in resistance to degradation by chewing is related to forage physical properties, as illustrated in Fig. 2.5. Thus the time spent chewing can be directly related to the shear energy of the forage (see Coleman and Henry, Chapter 1, this volume). Again, the time spent chewing each rumination bolus increases with increase in forage comminution energy, resulting in fewer rumination boluses being processed per unit rumination time. Although the time spent chewing can also be related to forage fibre content, comminution energy at a given fibre level may vary between forage-plant genotypes and is higher for stem fractions than for leaf fractions of similar fibre content.

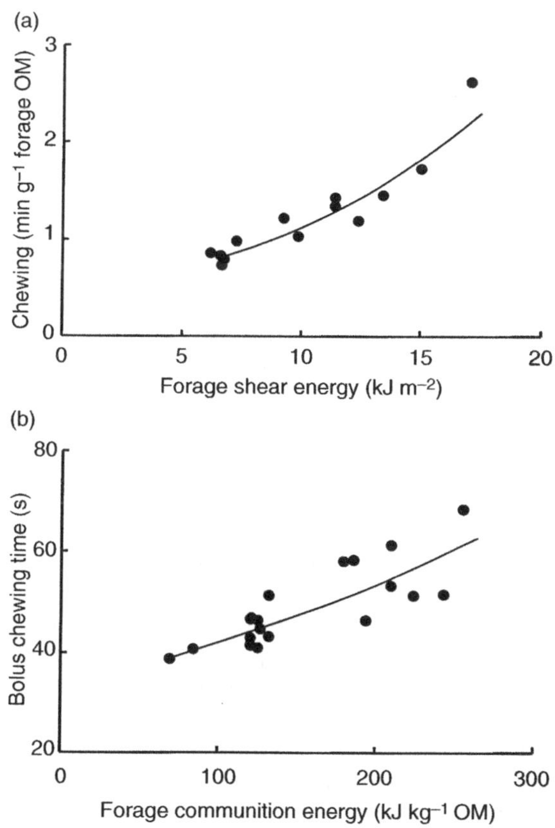

Fig. 2.5. The relationships between (a) time spent chewing and forage shear energy for adult sheep, and (b) time spent chewing rumination boluses and forage comminution energy for weaner lambs. The values are from unpublished data of D.A. Henry or from studies referred to in Weston (1996).

Anatomical differences between forage-plant genotypes partly explain corresponding variations between the forages in resistance to degradation by chewing (Wilson and Kennedy, 1996). Leaves of pasture legumes and grasses provide contrasting situations. Legume leaves have a reticulate venation, comprising a large central vascular bundle and a subsidiary network of fine bundles, with the latter being easy to degrade. Ingestive mastication of such leaves results in a predominance of irregularly shaped small blocky particles, which require little further degradation by rumination chewing. Grass leaves, on the other hand, have parallel venation, with each leaf containing several significant vascular bundles. During ingestive chewing, the grass leaf is mainly broken down longitudinally into long narrow particles, comprising one or more vascular bundles and adherent epidermis and mesophyll tissue; these need significant rumination chewing to effect transverse fracture and the release of the non-vascular tissue. Other anatomical features affecting rate of particle degradation include: (i) secondary cell-wall thickness, which increases with plant maturity; (ii) the proportion of vascular tissue, which is higher in tropical than in temperate pasture plants; (iii) type of epidermal tissue structure as it relates to ease of the removal of cuticle; (iv) the presence of those sclerenchyma bundles that effectively link vascular tissues with the epidermis, thus slowing leaf splitting during chewing; and (v) the degree of roughness of the fibre surface, which can constrain particle movement through the digesta.

Feed-particle degradation by digestion and attrition

Feed particles comprising tissues having cells with thin walls, e.g. the parenchyma in immature forages, are readily degraded in the rumen by microbial digestion and attrition due to mechanical abrasion of particles. However, with the more robust particles, attrition is of minor significance and microbial digestion contributes to degradation mainly in an indirect way – the reduction of particle resistance to breakdown by chewing.

Large particles subjected to microbial digestive processes by incubation with rumen digesta have been shown to have a reduced tensile strength and less resistance to breakdown by wet milling. Again, when microbial growth and, accordingly, ruminal fibre digestion are impaired, such as may occur with inadequate dietary essential nutrients, more time is spent chewing. For example, sheep were found to spend 29% more time ruminating and to perform 39% more bites per rumination bolus with a sulphur-deficient forage than with the same diet supplemented with inorganic sulphur (Weston *et al.*, 1988).

We now know that with high-fibre forages anaerobic fungi have an important role in reducing particle resistance to breakdown by chewing. The fungi produce a range of enzymes that degrade cell-wall polysaccharides and have the capacity to disrupt the covalent linkages that connect lignin and hemicellulose (see also Mackie *et al.*, Chapter 4, this volume).

Provided an optimal molecular environment exists in respect of essential nutrients, pH, etc., the main constraint to the microbial digestion rate of forage fibre is the accessibility of the fibre polysaccharides to the microbiota and their enzymes. Decrease in particle size enhances the accessibility of substrate per unit particle weight. Again, the highly branched nature of some of the cell-wall polymers limits access of the enzymes to susceptible bonds. Further, lignin forms a barrier to the accessibility of the cell-wall polysaccharides due to its linkage with hemicellulose.

Essential Nutrient Concentrations in Pasture Herbage

Constraints on pasture intake by sheep can occur with diets containing inadequate concentrations of minerals, vitamins and various sources of carbon and nitrogen. Thus feed-intake responses with appropriately deficient diets have been found to supplements providing essential amino acids, non-protein nitrogen, branched-chain fatty acids and many minerals.

Deficiencies of essential nutrients can be seen to constrain pasture intake mainly via effects on processes relating, either directly or indirectly, to: (i) the rate of degradation of feed particles in the rumen; (ii) the rates of synthesis of nutritionally useful compounds by the rumen microbiota; (iii) the capacity to dispose of nutrients via the various metabolic pathways of oxidation, synthesis and excretion; and (iv) the maintenance of the internal milieu.

Nitrogenous substances

Amounts of essential amino acids and ammonium ions inadequate for the sheep's body-tissue requirements or a deficiency of ammonium ions for the rumen microbiota result in constraint on herbage intake. The general form of the relationship between amino acid availability at the tissue level (represented by protein digested in the intestine) and the intake of an optimal diet is indicated in Fig. 2.6. Decrease in protein availability below a threshold level results in feed-intake decrease and accordingly decrease in digestible OM intake. The level of protein needed with a forage diet is less than that required with the optimal diet (Fig. 2.6). With the forage diet, physical factors constrain energy intake to a lower level and hence the level of production is lower; accordingly, less protein or essential amino acid is required per unit net energy for maximum forage intake to be achieved.

The intake of mature and senescent pasture herbage and other low-quality herbages can be limited by a deficiency of available nitrogenous substances. Data from a range of studies indicate that constraint on intake often prevails when the herbage contains less than 100–120 g CP kg^{-1} digestible OM. However, threshold values for adequacy could be expected to vary with the presence of various plant secondary metabolites. For example, tannins may, on the one hand, reduce the release of ammonia for the microbiota and, on the other hand, reduce plant protein degradation in the rumen and hence increase essential amino acid absorption.

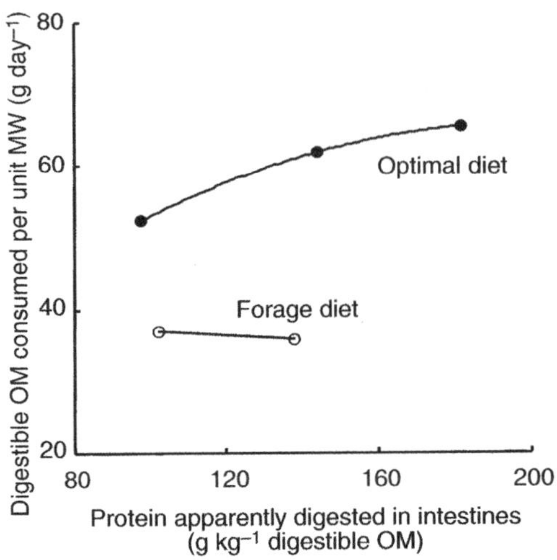

Fig. 2.6. The relationship between the consumption of digestible organic matter (OM) per unit metabolic weight (MW) and the quantity of protein apparently digested in the intestines, calculated as described in the text, for weaner sheep fed an optimal diet (BW *c.* 25 kg) or fed a forage diet (BW *c.* 37 kg). The data are from Weston (1971, 1973).

Few studies have been conducted to determine whether the intake of medium- or high-quality herbages could be limited by essential amino acid deficiency at the tissue level. Barry (1981) showed clearly that this deficiency did not apply with weaner lambs fed a high-quality fresh herbage diet (*c.* 260 g CP kg^{-1} digestible OM). However, the intake of digestible OM at *c.* 56 g day^{-1} per unit MW in this study was lower than that sometimes observed with high-quality herbages. Cruickshank *et al.* (1992) summarized data on the protein provided by high-quality herbage diets fed fresh or obtained by grazing. With 13 of the 14 diets considered, the mean quantity of CP entering the intestines was 273 (SD ± 28) g kg^{-1} digestible OM, with the mean for grasses (n = 6) being the same as for legumes (n = 7). It may be estimated that these amounts of CP would provide *c.* 162 ± 15 g protein apparently digested in the intestines kg^{-1} digestible OM, values similar to those found with high-quality grasses and clovers dried without heat (180 ± 17 g) (Weston and Hogan, 1971). On the basis of the data in Fig. 2.6, significant intake constraint with weaner lambs would not be expected with these 13 high-quality diets.

Although the herbage diet in the study of Barry (1981) and the 13 diets referred to above would appear to provide adequate protein for weaner lambs, we cannot assume that this situation will always prevail. Various studies have shown that, on occasion, rumen microbial protein synthesis can be significantly reduced with herbages that would otherwise have been assessed as high-quality on the basis of CP content and OM digestibility (e.g. SCA, 1990; Dove and Milne, 1994). For example, the ryegrass diet in the data set examined by Cruickshank *et al.* (1992) can be calculated to provide only *c.* 120 g apparently digested protein per kg digestible OM. Similarly, Dove and Milne (1994) found that with autumn vs. summer herbage of high N content and the same digestibility (0.88), microbial protein production per kg digestible OM was much higher in summer. Their data imply that this was a response to higher water-soluble carbohydrate (WSC) content in the summer herbage. However, further research is needed to define the optimum conditions of WSC content and protein availability per unit useful energy needed for the expression of maximum intake.

Most medium- and high-quality herbages probably meet the protein requirements for the expression of maximum feed intake in late pregnancy and lactation. Herbage diets provide more digested protein per unit digestible OM in late pregnancy and possibly in lactation than in the non-pregnant, non-lactating state, due to more rapid digesta clearance from the rumen.

In addition to ammonia, the rumen microbial population appears to need sources of the branched-chain fatty acids 2-methyl-butyrate, isobutyrate and isovalerate to digest fibre at the maximum rate. These compounds are derived mainly from dietary proteins; hence a deficiency is possible with herbages of low protein content or having proteins resistant to proteolysis in the rumen.

Minor nutrients

Some 18 chemical elements are required by sheep in addition to C, H, O and N. Deficiencies constraining feed intake by the grazing sheep are considered possible with only nine of these, namely, Na, Mg, Cu, Zn, Co, Se, P, I and S. With sheep at pasture, the sources of these elements are the herbage consumed, the drinking-water and soil and dust, either attached to the herbage eaten or directly ingested during grazing at ground level.

The relationship between the concentration of available elements in herbage and herbage intake is in most cases asymptotic up to levels where excess of the element is toxic. The threshold value for maximum intake obviously varies with the sheep's physiological state, being higher for producing animals. It will also be modulated by the degree of intake constraint and accordingly the energy availability that applies after deficiency of the element is remedied.

Accurate prediction of the intake constraint due to mineral inadequacy is generally not possible, because of the limitations of data on the sheep's requirements and the concentrations and availabilities of the elements in the ingesta. Again, the levels of available body reserves may affect the time needed for an intake response. Also, the requirement for the expression of maximum intake is often less than that needed for all body functions. Published estimates of the sheep's requirements (e.g. Underwood and Suttle, 1999) provide an initial reference source in assessing element adequacies, but note that published values are usually expressed on a feed DM basis rather than on more appropriate bases, such as net energy or ME.

The maximum constraints to feed intake due to deficiencies of essential elements could be expected to occur with Co and I. These elements are not required by plants; hence the concentrations therein will reflect soil status and may theoretically be zero in herbage that is otherwise of good quality. Very approximate estimates of the extent of intake constraints in the production situation can be made from the increases in growth rate that occur when the deficiencies are remedied. Data for penned sheep were summarized by Minson (1990) and show that remedying the deficiency in forages increased daily growth rate by 23–67 g with Na, 10–110 g with Co, 4–74 g with Se and 21–142 g with P. The herbage-intake enhancement corresponding to some of these increases could be relatively large. For example, with a medium-quality herbage (OM digestibility 0.65), some 250 g more feed OM would be needed daily for the 25 kg weaner lamb to increase the daily rate of body gain by 100 g. However, in the case of P, responses in grazing sheep have not been reported.

Impaired microbial digestion in the rumen due to herbage deficiencies of the chemical elements being discussed here has been shown only with respect to Mg and S. The microbiota require S in the synthesis of the S-amino acids and of biotin and thiamine. Remedying S deficiency in forages has been shown to increase OM intake (0–18 g day^{-1} $unit^{-1}$ MW), OM digestibility (4–7 units), digestible OM intake (4–12 g day^{-1} $unit^{-1}$ MW) and the quantity of CP entering the intestines per unit feed intake (13%) and its S-amino acid content (17%) (Weston *et al.*, 1988). It seems likely that the constraint on forage intake with S deficiency results initially from an impairment of the metabolism of the rumen microbiota rather than from body metabolic needs. It is pertinent that the presence of cyanogenic glycosides in forages reduces the availability of S to the microbiota, due to the formation of thiocyanate.

Climate

Grazing sheep can experience a wide range of climate conditions that could influence their herbage intakes. The thermal environment is of major significance in this respect, with either hot or cold conditions prevailing seasonally in many locations. The sheep, like other mammals, has to maintain its body temperature within narrow limits and this maintenance of thermal balance is affected by the many factors that contribute to heat input and heat dissipation, as discussed by Corbett and Ball (Chapter 7, this volume).

Heat input under most conditions is mainly affected by metabolic heat production and solar radiation. Metabolic heat input increases markedly with increase in forage quality and is higher at pasture than with indoor feeding, as eating time is longer and more locomotion heat is generated; solar heat input is dependent on solar elevation (Table 2.1) and accordingly varies with latitude and time of day. The ability to dissipate this heat load and thus reduce the potential constraint on grazing behaviour depends on the ambient temperature, humidity, air movement, etc.

Table 2.1. Indicative values of heat inputs for an adult sheep.

Source	Conditions	Heat input (W)
Mean metabolic heat input for a housed sheep offered feed *ad libitum*	Low-quality forage (OMD 0.5; OMI 0.8 kg day^{-1})	70
	High-quality forage (OMD 0.8; OMI 1.5 kg day^{-1})	140
Mean daily additional heat input due to grazing activity[a]	(i) Ample herbage – level land	20
	(ii) Poorer herbage – hilly land	30
Solar radiation from a clear sky to a fleeced sheep at right angles to the beam[b]	Solar elevation 10°	60
	40°	210
	90°	240

[a]Based on the energy costs of eating and walking (SCA, 1990) and using an efficiency of energy use of 0.73 in (i) and 0.65 in (ii). It is assumed that the additional times spent eating in (i) and (ii) were 7 h and 6 h, respectively, and that the corresponding additional walking activities were 3.0 km horizontal and 5.0 km horizontal + 0.2 km vertical, respectively.
[b]Based on solar heat inputs (Blaxter, 1989), assuming body-surface area to be 1.32 m^2 and that the solar beam is incident on one-half of the surface area.
OMD, organic matter digestibility; OMI, organic matter intake.

Behavioural adaptations to thermal stress by grazing sheep are well documented (e.g. Hinch *et al.*, 2003). In hot conditions, sheep reduce grazing activities in the middle of the day. To compensate, the initial grazing period begins earlier in the day, the onset of the afternoon grazing is delayed and night-time grazing is increased. The newly shorn sheep is particularly susceptible to thermal change. Relative to its unshorn counterpart, in hot weather the shorn animal seeks shade earlier in the day and in the cold spends less time grazing at night. Under cold conditions, it also spends more time grazing on the leeward side of the wind-breaks and seeks shelter earlier with the onset of windy conditions.

Although the effects of climate on sheep behaviour are well known, there are few data on the extent to which these responses change pasture intake. Increases in intake at pasture by newly shorn sheep have been recorded. Again, decreases with these animals have been found with severe cold, the responses being less with fat sheep, presumably due to their better tissue insulation (Young, 1987). Feed-intake data are available from indoor studies of ambient temperature effects, but these cannot be readily extrapolated to the pasture situation, due to the differences in solar heat input, air movement and heat production during feed acquisition. However, despite their limitations, indoor studies have illustrated the nature of the dietary intake response to different thermal conditions. For example, data from the indoor studies with weaner lambs fed an optimal diet at various ambient temperatures (Ames and Brink, 1977) show three response zones to thermal change (Fig. 2.7). A zone of thermal neutrality existed between about 5°C and 30°C. At lower temperatures, energy intake increased as temperature was reduced, presumably as the energy need for body-temperature maintenance increased and, accordingly, the animal's capacity to use energy was enhanced. Above 30°C, intake declined sharply, presumably due to the onset of heat-dissipation limitations.

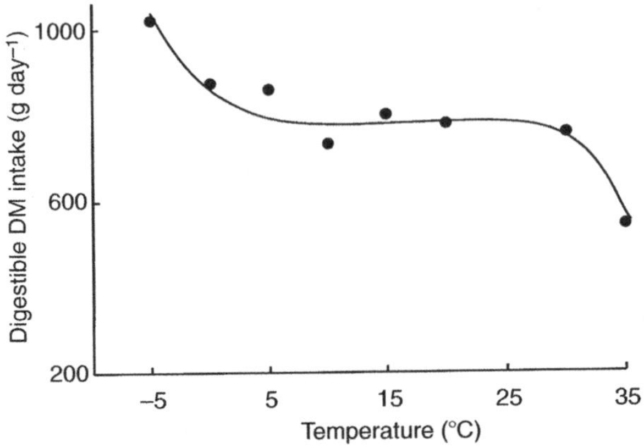

Fig. 2.7. The relationship between digestible dry matter (DM) intake and environmental temperature in weaner lambs fed an optimal diet. The data are from Ames and Brink (1977).

The lack of adequate heat-transaction data for grazing sheep precludes accurate prediction of heat-load effects on pasture intake. However, it can be deduced from the estimates of metabolic heat input given above that intake constraint will be greatest with high-quality pastures, which is important in respect of rates of milk production and lamb growth.

Palatability

Palatability in the present context is defined as the capacity of herbage to provide stimuli to the senses of sight, smell, taste and touch; it does not include the capacity to provide post-ingestive stimuli that could influence herbage acceptance. Both the chemical and physical properties of the herbage are relevant.

Various indoor studies indicate that pasture constraint due to low palatability might be expected given appropriate pasture conditions, as discussed by Weston (1996). For example, low palatability as an intake constraint was suggested in studies with mature *Trifolium subterraneum* forage and with a straw forage having a high resistance to structural degradation. Observed increases in the amount of digesta in the rumen, due to the enhanced intakes of some coarse forages following grinding and pelleting, may indicate constraint due to high resistance of the herbage to breakdown by ingestive mastication. Limited data suggest that constraint due to these physical properties may be greater in weaner lambs than in adults.

Data from short-term preference tests can indicate palatability differences between herbages, but this information is usually of little value as a guide to intake constraint over a significant time period. Sheep become accustomed to particular tastes and odours and hunger lowers sensory thresholds. However, palatability can be so low that herbage is rejected even when no other feed is available.

Although preference tests are generally of little relevance in the context of intake constraint, the consistent finding of selection against herbage with a lower proportion of WSC in the cell-content fraction may be significant (e.g. Ciavarella *et al.*, 2000). In studies of several days' duration, lower intakes (Hight *et al.*, 1964; Leury *et al.*, 1999) and lower preference (Leury *et al.*, 1999) have been observed for herbages with a lower WSC content. The intake effects observed may be more than would be expected by the accompanying differences in forage fibre content and OM digestibility, and a component of palatability may be involved.

Light Intensity and Herbage Water

Herbage grown under conditions of reduced light intensity has lower levels of WSC and higher levels of compounds including non-protein nitrogenous substances, organic acids and electrolytes. It also has higher levels of water and may have adherent water due to rain, dew and guttation through leaf pores.

Under appropriate conditions, the herbage DM content may fall below 100 g kg^{-1} and the intake of such material is often depressed. Limits must exist to the volume of fresh pasture and water that sheep can consume and handle. Wilson (1978) found that the critical herbage DM content in respect of intake constraint was between 125 and 145 g kg^{-1} but other studies have found constraint at up to 190 g kg^{-1}. Wilson (1978) also showed in two studies that, per unit MW, adult sheep could consume *c.* 680 g day^{-1} fresh forage, which included *c.* 100 g day^{-1} external water. In contrast, in other experiments where herbage DM content and DM intake were positively related, fresh forage intakes per unit MW were found to be much lower at *c.* 400, *c.* 350 and even *c.* 170 g day^{-1} (Lloyd Davies, 1962; John and Ulyatt, 1987). These differing values suggest that factors in addition to water and forage bulk could be involved in the constraint on intake with forages of low DM content.

At pasture, Orr *et al.* (1997) found bite mass and the rate of herbage intake (DM or fresh) to be low in the morning, when herbage DM content was depressed due to dew and guttation. The basis for these effects and whether or not they persist throughout the day in wet weather have yet to be established.

We need to know more about why low light intensity and high water content depress herbage intake. Although water is known to be released rapidly during ingestion of low-DM herbage, information on rumen water pools and rumen water transactions appears to be lacking.

Herbage Acquisition

The sheep at pasture, like its counterpart fed indoors, has a certain capacity to use energy, which in turn generates hunger signals. Accordingly, it is to be expected that the sheep will graze so that the extent and duration of hunger are minimized. Further, it could be expected that the animal will attempt to graze for the shortest time possible because the energy expenditure in eating is related to time rather than to ingested mass, and predation hazards decrease with decreased exposure time.

In general, sheep have low grazing activity at night, begin grazing at dawn, rest in the middle of the day and graze again in the afternoon, with grazing activity usually being high towards dusk. The morning grazing probably accommodates the hunger developed overnight and the activity late in the day could reflect anticipation of the need to minimize hunger at night.

During grazing the sheep has to seek, prehend, sever, masticate and then swallow the resulting food bolus. This grazing has to be done within a finite time period, as the animal needs time for other activities, including ruminating, resting and walking to and from water and camp areas. The most common constraints on intake, apart from those discussed earlier, are likely to be: (i) limitation of the amount of pasture present per unit area and the structure of the sward, which in turn constrain the amount of feed that can be prehended in the time available for grazing; (ii) physiological responses by the ingestion apparatus to the high workload involved on sparse pastures; and (iii) an untoward response to prehension difficulties on sparse pastures.

The feed-intake response to increasing pasture herbage mass is generally an increase, either linear or curvilinear, until a threshold value is reached, beyond which intake fails to respond to further pasture-mass increase. Accordingly, intake constraint progressively increases as the mass declines below the threshold level. With continuous grazing, threshold values reported by Hodgson (1977) for mixed clover/grass pastures grazed by adult sheep have a mean value (after rejecting one statistical outlier) of 1960 ± 236 kg DM ha^{-1}. With strip-grazing, threshold pasture-mass values with weaner lambs, in terms of daily herbage allowance, have been reported as *c.* 200 g OM kg^{-1} BW for mixed grass/clover swards and *c.* 140 g kg^{-1} BW for predominantly clover swards. Comparable threshold values have also been found for lactating ewes.

Much of the variation in the threshold values, as given above, can probably be explained by variation in sward structure (Allden and Whittaker, 1970). Where grazing time is limited, the amount of feed the sheep can obtain in a bite can be an important determinant of feed intake. The bite size is determined by bite depth, herbage bulk density in the grazed zone and the area of sward covered by the bite, with all being affected by the sward structure. For a pasture with 1500 kg DM ha^{-1}, the average herbage height may be 4–5 cm, but this value will vary, being lower for more prostrate herbage cultivars or higher as plants become more widely spaced in drier environments. Bite depth increases with increase in sward height (see Ungar, 1996), the value with a ryegrass sward increasing from *c.* 3 cm for a leaf length of 5 cm to *c.* 7 cm for a leaf length of 15 cm. The area of the bite can vary appreciably, being equal to about the mouth area with short swards (8–9 cm^2 in adult sheep), but much higher for longer swards from which sheep can gather more leaves into the mouth. Leaf length has direct effects on all three variables and it may be the best single measure for use in predicting bite mass.

Data from studies by Penning *et al.* (1991) show some of the relationships between variables pertinent to pasture-intake constraint (Fig. 2.8). With sward heights of 6 cm and above, daily herbage intake and rate of intake were constant. In this range, bite frequency decreased with increased bite size, indicating that intake rate was affected by the rate of formation of the bolus for swallowing. It is significant that, at the higher values of sward height, the animals could have easily consumed more feed each day simply by extending the time spent grazing. With the 3 cm high sward, bite frequency and the time spent grazing were greater than in the taller swards, but these changes did not compensate for the decreased bite mass; hence both intake rate and daily herbage intake declined appreciably.

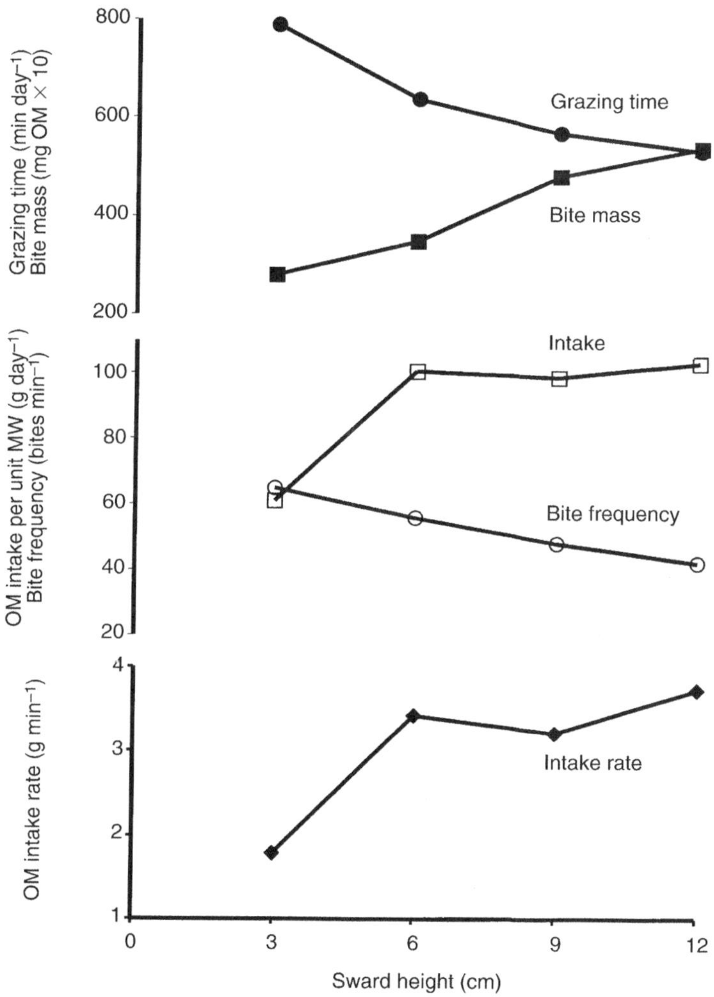

Fig. 2.8. Relationships between sward height and grazing time, bite mass, organic matter (OM) intake per unit metabolic weight (MW), bite frequency and OM intake rate for lactating sheep (*c.* 77 kg BW) grazing spring pasture in which herbage mass was directly related to sward height. The data are from Penning *et al.* (1991).

Three response zones are likely to prevail with respect to herbage-accessibility levels and the sheep's grazing behaviour. First, at high accessibility levels, such as with sward heights of 9 cm and 12 cm in Fig. 2.8 (mass > 4800 kg DM ha^{-1}), sheep eat to maintain an intake that meets requirements for minimizing hunger by adjusting bite rate in relation to bite size. Secondly, as herbage accessibility declines and bite mass decreases, sheep increase time spent grazing and bite rate in a compensatory manner and are able to maintain the daily herbage intake. Thirdly, in the low herbage-accessibility zone bite rate increases, but bite mass and grazing time limitations constrain daily intake.

At high herbage-accessibility levels with high-quality pasture, it is likely that acquisition constraints on intake do not apply, with the quantity of pasture consumed being determined, as with indoor feeding, by the factors indicated in Fig. 2.1. Similarly, the intake advantage of clovers over grasses at these high mass levels with green leafy material is likely to be due to the faster digesta clearance from the rumen rather than any acquisition constraint. However, at lower accessibility levels, a faster rate of intake due to larger bite mass and lower resistance to bolus formation would also contribute significantly to the clover advantage.

With medium- and low-quality pastures, appreciable scope for selection would generally prevail (see Forbes and Mayes, Chapter 3, and O'Reagain and McMeniman, Chapter 12, this volume). Such selection adds complexity to the nature of the relationships influencing constraint on intake. The need to travel to water under dry rangeland conditions will also modulate grazing patterns. Daily walking distances by sheep of up to 25 km have been recorded and sheep having to walk to water have been found to reduce grazing time on the day of walking and increase it on the following day (Hinch *et al.*, 2003).

Sheep are capable of grazing for 13–14 h daily and can accommodate 8.5 h grazing in a single 9.5 h period. However, observations of sheep grazing sparse pastures do not always show long grazing times, values of 7–9 h sometimes being observed. Why grazing time is not an intake constraint in these situations is not understood. The duration of grazing seems too short for muscular fatigue to be implicated. Alternatively, difficulty associated with prehension of the herbage may be involved. Grazing at or near ground level with very short pasture must involve some abrasion of the lips and other parts of the mouth, which in turn could possibly provide inhibitory sensory feedback.

References

Allden, W.G. and Whittaker, I.A.McD. (1970) The determinants of herbage intake by grazing sheep: the interrelationship of factors influencing herbage intake and availability. *Australian Journal of Agricultural Research* 21, 755–766.

Ames, D.R. and Brink, D.R. (1977) Effect of temperature on lamb performance and protein efficiency ratio. *Journal of Animal Science* 44, 136–140.

Arnold, G.W. (1966) Age, pasture conditions and the performance of grazing sheep. *Proceedings of the Australian Society of Animal Production* 6, 213–221.

Barry, T.N. (1981) Protein metabolism in growing lambs fed on fresh ryegrass (*Lolium perenne*)–clover (*Trifolium repens*) pasture *ad lib*. I. Protein and energy deposition in response to abomasal infusion of casein and methionine. *British Journal of Nutrition* 46, 521–532.

Blaxter, K.L. (1989) *Energy Metabolism in Animals and Man*. Cambridge University Press, Cambridge, 96 pp.

Blaxter, K.L., Clapperton, J.L. and Wainman, F.W. (1966) The extent of differences between six British breeds of sheep in their metabolism, feed intake and utilization and resistance to climatic stress. *British Journal of Nutrition* 20, 283–294.

Ciavarella, T.A., Dove, H., Leury, B.J. and Simpson, R.J. (2000) Diet selection by sheep grazing *Phalaris aquatica* L. pastures of differing water-soluble carbohydrate content. *Australian Journal of Agricultural Research* 51, 757–764.

Cruickshank, G.J., Poppi, D.J. and Sykes, A.R. (1992) The intake, digestion and protein degradation of grazed herbage by early-weaned lambs. *British Journal of Nutrition* 68, 349–364.

Dove, H. and Milne, J.A. (1994) Digesta flow and rumen microbial protein production in ewes grazing perennial ryegrass. *Australian Journal of Agricultural Research* 45, 1229–1245.

Dulphy, J.P., Remond, B. and Theriez, M. (1980) Ingestive behaviour and related activities in ruminants. In: Ruckebusch, Y. and Thivend, P. (eds) *Digestive Physiology and Metabolism in Ruminants*. MTP Press, Lancaster, UK, pp. 103–122.

Gherardi, S.G. and Black, J.L. (1989) Influence of post-rumen supply of nutrients on rumen digesta load and voluntary intake of a roughage by sheep. *British Journal of Nutrition* 62, 588–599.

Hight, G.K., Sinclair, D.P. and Lancaster, R.J. (1964) Some effects of shading and of nitrogen fertiliser on the chemical composition of freeze-dried and oven-dried herbage, and on the nutritive value of oven-dried herbage fed to sheep. *New Zealand Journal of Agricultural Research* 11, 286–302.

Hinch, G.N., Lynch, J.J., Nolan, J.V. and Provenza, F.D. (2003) Feeding behaviour and the nutrient environment In: Hinch, G.N., Lynch, J.J. and Nolan, J.V. (eds) *Feeding Behaviour of Farm Animals*. CAB International, Wallingford, UK (in preparation).

Hodgson, J. (1977) Factors limiting the herbage intake by the grazing animal. In: *Proceedings of an International Meeting on Animal Production from Temperate Grassland*. Irish Grassland Society, Dublin, pp. 70–75.

John, A. and Ulyatt, M.J. (1987) Effects of forage maturity and dry matter content on voluntary intake of grass forage. *Proceedings of the New Zealand Society of Animal Production* 47, 17–19.

Kennedy, P.M. and Doyle, P.T. (1993) Particle-size reduction by ruminants – effects of cell wall composition and structure. In: Jung, H.-J.G., Buxton, D.R., Hatfield, R.D. and Ralph, J. (eds) *Forage Cell Wall Structure and Digestibility*. American Society of Agronomy, Madison, Wisconsin, pp. 348–376.

Laredo, M.A. and Minson, D.J. (1973) The voluntary intake, digestibility and retention time by sheep of leaf and stem fractions of five grasses. *Australian Journal of Agricultural Research* 24, 875–888.

Laredo, M.A. and Minson, D.J. (1975) Intake of grass leaf and stem by sheep. *British Journal of Nutrition* 33, 159–170.

Leury, B.J., Siever-Kelly, C., Gatford, K.L., Simpson, R.J. and Dove, H. (1999) Spray-topping annual grass pasture with glyphosate to delay loss of feeding value during summer IV. Diet composition, herbage intake and performance in grazing sheep. *Australian Journal of Agricultural Research* 50, 487–495.

Lloyd Davies, H. (1962) Intake studies in sheep involving high fluid intake. *Proceedings of the Australian Society of Animal Production* 4, 167–171.

Minson, D.J. (1990) *Forage in Ruminant Nutrition*. Academic Press, San Diego, California, 36 pp.

Orr, R.J., Penning, P.D., Harvey, A. and Champion, R.A. (1997) Diurnal patterns of intake rate by sheep grazing monocultures of ryegrass or white clover. *Applied Animal Behaviour Science* 52, 65–77.

Penning, P.D., Parsons, A.J., Orr, R.T. and Treacher, T.T. (1991) Intake and behaviour responses by sheep to changes in sward characteristics under continuous stocking. *Grass and Forage Science* 46, 15–28.

Pittroff, W. and Kothmann, M.M. (1999) Regulation of intake and diet selection by herbivores. In: Jung, H.-J.G. and Fahey, G.C. Jr (eds) *Nutritional Ecology of Herbivores, Proceedings of the Vth International Symposium on the Nutrition of Herbivores*. American Society of Animal Science, Savoy, Illinois, pp. 366–422.

Poppi, D.P., Minson, D.J. and Ternouth, J.H. (1981) Studies of cattle and sheep eating leaf and stem fractions of grasses. I. The voluntary intake, digestibility and retention time in the reticulo-rumen. *Australian Journal of Agricultural Research* 32, 99–108.

Rees, M.C. and Little, D.A. (1980) Differences between sheep and cattle in digestibility, voluntary intake and retention time in the rumen of three tropical grasses. *Journal of Agricultural Science, Cambridge* 94, 483–485.

SCA (1990) *Feeding Standards for Australian Livestock. Ruminants*. Standing Committee on Agriculture and CSIRO, Melbourne, 266 pp.

Thornton, R.F. and Minson, D.J. (1972) The relationship between voluntary intake and mean apparent retention time in the rumen. *Australian Journal of Agricultural Research* 23, 871–877.

Thornton, R.F. and Minson, D.J. (1973) The relationship between apparent retention time in the rumen, voluntary intake, and apparent digestibility of legume and grass diets in sheep. *Australian Journal of Agricultural Research* 24, 889–898.

Underwood, E.J. and Suttle, N.F. (1999) *The Mineral Nutrition of Livestock*, 3rd edn. CAB International, Wallingford, UK.

Ungar, E.D. (1996) Ingestive behaviour. In: Hodgson, J. and Illius, A.W. (eds) *The Ecology and Management of Grazing Systems*. CAB International, Wallingford, UK, pp. 185–218.

Weston, R.H. (1971) Factors limiting the intake of feed by sheep. V. Feed intake and the productive performance of the ruminant lamb in relation to the quantity of crude protein digested in the intestines. *Australian Journal of Agricultural Research* 22, 307–320.

Weston, R.H. (1973) Factors limiting the intake of feed by sheep. VII. The digestion of a medium quality roughage and the effect of post ruminal infusion of casein on its consumption by young sheep. *Australian Journal of Agricultural Research* 24, 387–397.

Weston, R.H. (1996) Some aspects of constraint to forage consumption by ruminants. *Australian Journal of Agricultural Research* 47, 175–197.

Weston, R.H. and Hogan, J.P. (1971) The digestion of pasture plants by sheep. V. Studies with subterranean and berseem clovers. *Australian Journal of Agricultural Research* 22, 139–157.

Weston, R.H. and Poppi, D.P. (1987) Comparative aspects of food intake. In: Hacker, J.B. and Ternouth, J. (eds) *Nutrition of Herbivores*. Academic Press, Sydney, pp. 138–162.

Weston, R.H., Lindsay, J.R., Purser, D.B., Gordon, G.L.R. and Davis, P. (1988) Feed intake and digestion responses in sheep to the addition of inorganic sulfur to a herbage diet of low sulfur content. *Australian Journal of Agricultural Research* 39, 1107–1119.

Wilson, G.F. (1978) Effect of water content of Tama ryegrass on voluntary intake by sheep. *New Zealand Journal of Experimental Agriculture* 6, 53–54.

Wilson, J.R. and Kennedy, P.M. (1996) Plant and animal constraints to voluntary feed intake associated with fibre characteristics and particle breakdown and passage in ruminants. *Australian Journal of Agricultural Research* 47, 199–205.

Young, B.A. (1987) The effect of climate on intake. In: Hacker, J.B. and Ternouth, J. (eds) *Nutrition of Herbivores*. Academic Press, Sydney, pp. 163–190.

3 Food Choice

J.M. Forbes[1] and R.W. Mayes[2]

[1]*Centre for Animal Sciences, Leeds Institute of Biotechnology and Agriculture, University of Leeds, Leeds, UK;* [2]*Macaulay Land Use Research Institute, Craigiebuckler, Aberdeen, UK*

Introduction

This chapter addresses the ability of sheep to make nutritionally wise choices when presented with more than one food. We first consider how sheep identify different foods and then review diet selection when individuals are offered two foods under controlled conditions; then we cover the outdoor grazing situation. Space does not permit extensive citation in support of the concepts presented here, but discussion of results from many earlier studies can be found in Forbes (1995).

There is ample evidence that animals of many species, including ruminants, are capable of making choices between different foods that provide a more balanced diet than would be obtained by eating at random. While sheep are not usually considered as being endowed with much intelligence, there is no doubt that they can make nutritionally wise selection, given appropriate circumstances. The simplest hypothesis of food choice would be that animals eat at random, in which case it might be expected that they would eat equal amounts (weights? volumes?) of each of the foods on offer. It will become clear from the examples given below that this is rarely the case.

If they do not eat at random, then it might be expected that the 'palatability' of each food would determine the proportion eaten. Thus, a food with a sweet flavour would be expected to be preferred to one with a bitter taste. However, 'palatability' is not simply a function of the chemical and physical properties of a food but it also depends on the animal's nutritional history; for example, a bitter food that an animal has had a chance to learn is nutritionally well balanced will be more 'palatable' than a sweet one that it has learned to be nutritionally imbalanced, e.g. toxic. Thus an animal's choice between foods is likely to be influenced by its nutrient requirements as well as characteristics of the foods.

It should be noted, therefore, that there may be large differences between the proportions of two foods eaten during short-term selection tests ('palatability tests'), especially when the animals have no experience of one or both foods, and their long-term choices after they have had a chance to match diet with metabolism. The distinction must also be noted between relative intakes when ample choice is provided (preference) and the absolute intake of a selected diet in a given feeding situation. From a nutritional point of view, the latter is the 'bottom line'.

Detection of Food

Clearly, in order to make choices between foods, sheep must be able to differentiate between them by sight, smell, taste or other sensory characteristics. The sense of vision allows animals to detect food at a considerable distance. Smell is also a sense that allows identification of distant food sources and some species have very sensitive 'noses'. Once food has been identified it may be taken into the mouth and this is when the sense of taste comes into play. As well as taste, food in the mouth also has characteristic physical properties, e.g. texture. Once the food has been fully identified by all the senses, then the animal has to decide whether to swallow it. If the combination of sensory properties has not been experienced before, the animal will proceed cautiously (neophobia); if it has previously experienced unpleasant consequences of eating food with this set of sensory properties, it is likely to reject this food (unless very hungry); otherwise it will proceed to eat.

Vision

Sheep are probably colour-blind but can discriminate between objects of different hue due to brightness. This might be important for grass, as brightness is proportional to protein content of perennial ryegrass at any given stage of development.

Sheep can see food in front of them very clearly and can make quite complex discrimination between shapes. They can be trained to associate non-food objects with food, but this association only develops for foods that the animals have found previously to have pleasant consequences when eaten, not those that have caused discomfort after eating.

Temporary covering of the eyes does not interfere with the preference for herbage species by grazing sheep, suggesting that they use smell, taste and tactile stimuli to a great extent to discriminate between different plant species.

Smell

It is usually difficult to differentiate between animals' appreciation of smell (from volatile components of the food) and taste (from soluble components) as, once the food enters the mouth, both can be sensed (flavour). Removal of the sense of smell by surgical removal of the olfactory bulbs did not affect daily intake of a complete pelleted food or meal pattern, even though it was clear that the sheep had olfactory deficits (McLaughlin *et al.*, 1974). Feeding was less intense, however, with more re-entries into the feeder during meals. An extreme case of smell affecting choice was when sheep were given two bins of food, one tainted with odours of the faeces of a carnivore, and took 95% of their intake from the uncontaminated pellets (Pfister *et al.*, 1990). The animals went as far away as possible from the tainted bins and there was no evidence of habituation to this smell.

Taste

Sheep have a well-developed sense of taste and are sensitive to bitter, sour, salty and sweet solutions. Animals are born with (innate) taste preferences and aversions, which can be modified by experience of food. It can be difficult, therefore, to differentiate responses to taste and the post-ingestive consequences of eating, as the normal type of two-choice preference test confounds the sensory impressions of the foods or liquids offered with post-ingestive factors. By using sheep with oesophageal fistulas, Chapman and Grovum (1982) were able to determine the responses of sheep to only the taste of various additions of sodium chloride or urea to hay, without the confounding effect of learning about the metabolic consequences of eating foods with those tastes. Thus, while salt (sodium chloride) solutions of low concentration (22 g l^{-1}) became aversive if sheep were allowed to swallow them into the rumen, due presumably to the post-absorptive effects of sodium ions, they preferred hay containing up to 200 g kg^{-1} of sodium chloride. However, care must be taken in the interpretation of results from oesophageal-fistulated sheep, as they invariably lose a lot of saliva through the fistula and become sodium-deficient. Their preference for a higher concentration of sodium chloride than intact sheep might therefore be due to their higher requirement to maintain body levels of sodium.

The short-term nature of flavour aversions is demonstrated by the observation that sheep, which initially strongly discriminated against quinine-treated hay, after a few days ate equal amounts of treated and untreated hay (Jones and Forbes, 1984). They had learned by sampling small amounts of the quinine-flavoured food that there were no harmful consequences from eating it. Palatability effects are not important in determining the level at which a single food is eaten after the first few days, even though they can have marked effects on the relative intakes when two foods are on offer. However, if a particular flavour of food becomes associated in the minds of sheep with unpleasant consequences, then they avoid food with that flavour.

Diet Selection under Controlled Conditions

Much of our basic information comes from indoor experiments, often with individually penned sheep. While such methodology might be considered unnatural, it is often only by adopting this type of procedure that we can gain clear information by testing hypotheses in a critical manner.

Animals offered identical food from two containers are expected to eat equal amounts from each. However, this is not always true, as, for example, when one is favoured because it is nearer the source of drinking-water. Foods with the same nutritional properties but different sensory characteristics (flavour, colour) are not usually eaten in equal quantities, as one is innately preferred to the other. Innate preferences should be useful in helping to attract young animals to foods that are nutritious, or at least not toxic. The young of most mammalian species have innate preferences for sweet foods and aversions to bitter ones. However, an animal might eventually come across a sweet food that is toxic or a bitter food that is nutritious, so it should have the flexibility to modify its innate preferences in the light of experience.

Choice according to nutritional requirements

Where two foods differ in the concentration of a nutrient such that one contains more and the other less than optimal, in relation to energy requirements, then the animal's interests are best served by eating the two in such a ratio that the intake of the nutrient in question is optimized. The higher the demand for the nutrient, the greater should be the proportion of the food high in that nutrient. Note that animals can cope with mildly imbalanced diets, but at a metabolic cost; where possible, it should avoid this cost by eating that amount and mixture of foods that minimizes the cost (discomfort) of metabolism.

For example, mature ewes were offered foods with different contents of sulphur – 1.1 and 9.5 g S kg^{-1} – after having been fed on a diet adequate in sulphur (Hills *et al.*, 1998). When given a choice between high- and low-sulphur foods, they initially ate at random, but, within 2 days, increased the proportion of the low-sulphur food so that their daily intake of sulphur was very close to that required. They were avoiding excessive intake of sulphur as well as avoiding a deficient intake. However, sheep previously made sulphur-deficient by feeding on a low-sulphur diet initially ate a high proportion of the high-sulphur food but later reduced the sulphur content chosen until it stabilized at the optimum level. Foods deficient or excessive in sulphur also induced conditioned taste aversions in mature ewes, while those approximately meeting the animals' requirements induced taste preferences (Hills *et al.*, 1999). Figure 3.1 shows that a sheep's preferences for a food declined when that flavour had become associated with a high (mildly toxic) dose of sulphur.

Test substances may be administered by gavage (i.e. stomach-tube), with the intention that the sheep should not identify them by taste, smell or sight. Administration of moderate amounts of protein in this way, followed by

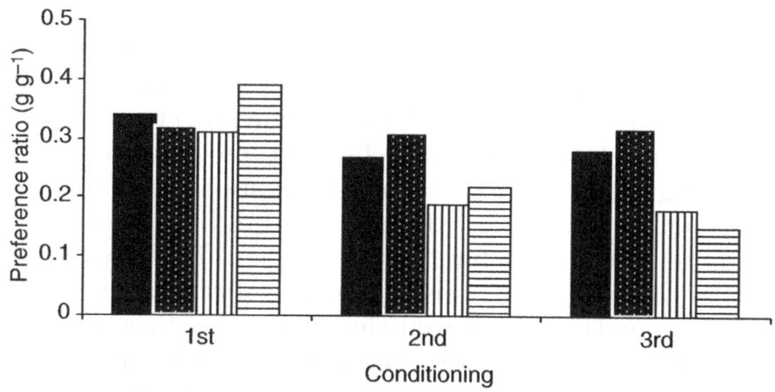

Fig. 3.1. Preference ratios of sheep for food of the flavour associated with doses of 3 g (solid bars), 6 g (dotted), 9 g (vertical) or 12 g (horizontal) sulphur given intraruminally (Hills *et al.*, 1999).

access to food with a novel flavour, eventually led to wether sheep preferring that flavour over another with which the food was flavoured for a short time after gavage of water (Arsenos *et al.*, 2000). The basal diet was relatively low in protein so that it was expected that the gavaged protein (casein) would alleviate a deficiency and the sheep would prefer the flavour associated with the administered protein. This in fact occurred with low to medium doses (8.75 g and 17.5 g), supporting the hypothesis. However, higher doses (35 g and 52.5 g) led to significant aversion towards the flavour associated with the supplementary protein. It was proposed that this was due to an oversupply of protein and a measured excess of ammonia in rumen fluid; concentrations were 280, 332, 533 and 699 mg l^{-1} for the four treatments, i.e. a big increase between the 17.5 g (preferred) and the 35 g (aversive) doses.

These results illustrate a continuum of flavour preferences and aversions created by different amounts of the same nutrient source, which is due, not to the specific nature of the flavour (the same flavour could be preferred or aversive depending on which dose of casein it was paired with), but to the associations between the sensory properties of the food and the metabolic consequences of eating food with that flavour.

It can be seen from these examples how 'nutritional wisdom' can occur, i.e. selecting a mixture of foods that most closely meets the animal's nutrient requirements. However, it is unclear to what extent the animal is choosing in order to supply its body with nutrients as compared with seeking optimal conditions in its rumen.

Choosing to avoid rumen imbalance

Given a choice between finely ground and fibrous foods, ruminants invariably choose a significant proportion of the latter, even though the former might have a much higher proportion of available nutrients (e.g. a concentrate food). An adequate amount of long fibre in the rumen is a prerequisite for normal rumen function and a lack of dietary fibre leads to large fluctuations in rumen pH and an absence of rumination. Which is the more aversive – the low and fluctuating pH or the absence of rumination – is unclear.

To investigate an appetite for fibre, sheep were given a food free of long fibre for 7 days, which reduced rumination to zero (Campion and Leek, 1997). When polyethylene fibre, chopped into 10 mm lengths, was offered, sheep ingested 35 g day^{-1} and rumination was stimulated. In another experiment, sheep were fed on hay and did not select any of the polyethylene fibre, but on switching to the pelleted diet they commenced eating the fibre within 24 h. Surprisingly, when offered a choice between short (3 mm) and long (15 mm) polyethylene fibre, the sheep showed a significant preference for the short. This did not evoke much rumination but the long fibre was quite difficult for the sheep to eat. Finally, when the rumen wall was 'tickled' with a polyethylene fibre 'pompom' introduced via the rumen fistula, voluntary intake of polyethylene fibre was reduced, suggesting that the selection of inert fibre may be a response to a need for physical stimulation of the rumen mechanoreceptors. This does not rule out an additional response to avoid extremes of pH or osmolality as well.

Excessive acid production by the rapid fermentation of concentrate food can be prevented by including a buffer (sodium bicarbonate) in the diet. Such inclusion allowed sheep to eat voluntarily a higher proportion of high-energy food, given in choice with a low-energy food, as it alleviated the low pH post-feeding condition associated particularly with the high-energy food (Cooper *et al.*, 1996).

Physiological state

So far we have dealt with situations in which animals can manipulate the nutrient supply by choosing appropriate amounts and ratios of food. The animal's nutrient requirements often vary over time as well, such as during growth, pregnancy and lactation. It has been observed that growing lambs offered high- and low-protein foods chose a diet well matched to their requirements for growth and, even when one of the foods required up to 30 responses to obtain a reinforcement, the lambs responded accordingly, to maintain this balanced diet (Hou *et al.*, 1991).

Pregnant ewes selected a significantly greater proportion of a food of high crude protein (CP) concentration than non-pregnant ewes, reflecting their enhanced demand for protein (Cooper *et al.*, 1994). Thus, diet selection is not only driven by the composition of the foods on offer, but also by the requirements of the animal, which change in a systematic manner with growth and reproductive cycles.

Learned associations between nutritional and sensory properties of foods

Rarely will the innate preference or aversion for a particular food give an animal the appropriate message about its eventual yield of nutrients after ingestion. Preferences or aversions are developed by individual animals according to their nutritional requirements and the concentration of nutrients in the food(s), as demonstrated above (Arsenos and Kyriazakis, 1999; Hills *et al.*, 1999).

Time-scale

In most conditioned responses it is necessary for the conditioning stimulus to follow the unconditioned stimulus within a few seconds. However, the ingestion of a novel food and the metabolic consequence can be several hours apart, although a shorter delay leads to more rapid learning. In addition, the more severe an aversion the longer it persists. If conditioned taste aversions did not persist, they would have no function; on the other hand, if they persisted for the rest of an animal's life, they would prevent the flexibility necessary when both the animal's requirements and the concentrations of nutrients in food are continually changing.

An integration of factors involved in the control of diet selection into a comprehensive model of food intake and diet selection will be made at the end of the chapter.

The Grazing Situation

Sheep evolved to graze and browse, a state that has not altered throughout the long period of exploitation by humans, so the pastoral situation can be considered to reflect closely the habitat to which they are naturally suited. It is therefore not surprising that the physiological and behavioural processes described earlier, which relate to the ability of these animals to make informed choices about their diet, are generally applicable to grazing and browsing animals. However, it can be expected that energy expended in activities associated with grazing and browsing and, occasionally, the need to maintain body temperature under cold conditions will increase the appetite drive of outdoor sheep and possibly affect their choice of diet.

Sheep can tolerate grazing conditions ranging from pastures of a single species of grass in abundance to heterogeneous scrub or rangeland with limited amounts of poor-quality vegetation from a wide range of plant species (see O'Reagain and McMeniman, Chapter 12, this volume). Thus, particularly under the latter conditions, the choices available to sheep are likely to be much more complex than those of the controlled conditions described earlier. The grazing animal is likely to have many more opportunities to choose what, how much, when and where to eat, all of which may be influenced by a range of constraints.

The high degree of complexity of the factors affecting dietary choice in grazing sheep is one of the many reasons why the amount of research carried out on dietary selection in free-ranging animals, and consequently the level of knowledge about these animals, is less than that about housed animals. Furthermore, the degree of experimental control that can be imposed in a grazing situation is substantially less. Not only can human intervention cause disturbance to free-ranging animals, and hence alter their behaviour, but also the scope for manipulation of food items, in terms of their nutritive value or toxin content, is limited. Perhaps the greatest limitation to progress in the study of diet selection in grazing or browsing animals is the paucity of reliable techniques for assessing diet composition and intake. Because direct quantitative estimation is virtually impossible, there has tended to be a reliance on short-term methods, such as the identification and/or separation of plant species and plant parts in stomach contents, faeces and extrusa from oesophageal-fistulated animals or the use of markers in faeces or extrusa. Identification methods are prone to large errors because, being short-term, they represent 'snapshots' of the animal's diet. Results are operator-dependent and a substantial proportion of the material in the analysed sample may be unidentifiable. In more recent years, plant wax components, especially the alkanes (saturated hydrocarbons), have been used as markers to estimate intake and diet composition (Mayes and Dove, 2000). Intake is estimated from the concentrations in herbage and faeces of an alkane from the herbage, the daily dose rate of a synthetic alkane and the faecal concentration of that alkane. The method has been well validated for intake in a range of herbivores, including sheep (see Mayes and Dove, 2000). Diet composition is estimated by relating the pattern of alkane concentrations in the faeces of grazing animals to the alkane patterns in the plant species on offer. The method has been validated with relatively simple dietary mixtures (Mayes and Dove, 2000) but its reliability for animals grazing complex vegetation environments requires further evaluation.

Preference in the context of diet composition has been defined as the choice of dietary components that an animal will make when there are no constraints on availability of the food components on offer (see Rutter *et al.*, 2000). Because such constraints are usually present, there are relatively few situations where grazing sheep may be free to fully exercise their dietary preferences. However, they will usually select a diet that differs from the vegetation available as potential food. Even on high-quality monospecific grass swards, sheep may select parts of the grass plant in proportions differing from those in the available herbage. Under extensive conditions, where there could be considerable heterogeneity in available food supply, in terms of food-plant species, food quality and spatial distribution, animals will probably select a diet of higher nutritional value than that of the overall average for the vegetation in the area. Because constraining influences on diet choice by the grazing sheep are likely to be least extreme in simple swards with high availability, it is understandable that most experimental studies have been carried out under such conditions.

In meeting its nutritional needs and other requirements for survival, the animal must have an awareness of its environment, obtained from both current and memorized information. It must employ this awareness in conjunction with long-established behaviours, such as those of the feeding process and interactions with other sheep, which may have been innate, learned from its mother or learned by experiment from an early age. Figure 3.2 indicates some of the factors that make food choice in grazing sheep such a complex issue.

Learning and diet choice in grazing sheep

In order to graze or browse, the sheep needs to be able to search for and recognize potential food items and then use appropriate body movements to harvest and process the food in the mouth prior to swallowing. It will also need to know when to cease eating and, some time later, when to ruminate. While some of these so-called 'normal' behaviours may be innate, it is undoubtedly true that others are learned. For example, it has been demonstrated that sheep learned to recognize food items that had been introduced to them at an early age. For example, when allowed to select a ryegrass/white clover diet from alternating strips of the two species in paddocks, lambs aged 23 weeks that had been exposed to clover 4 weeks earlier (at weaning) or 9 weeks earlier (before weaning) spent more time grazing clover than lambs previously exposed to ryegrass (Ramos and Tennessen, 1992). Similar observations have been made with supplementary feeds (see Dove, Chapter 6, this volume).

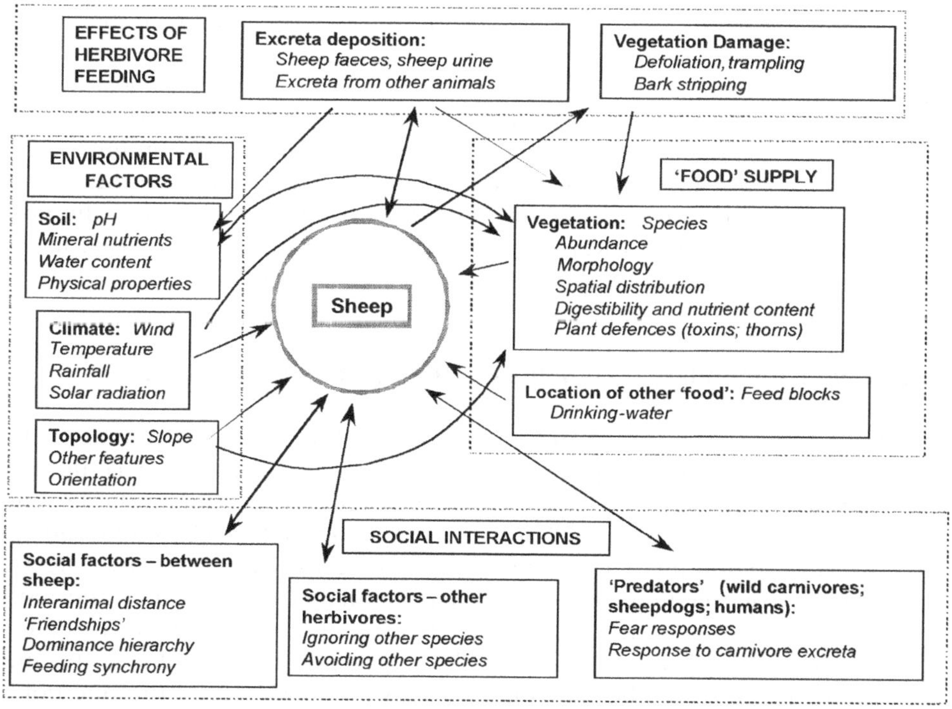

Fig. 3.2. External factors that may directly and indirectly affect the dietary choices and intake of grazing or browsing sheep.

Evidence of grazing sheep making nutritionally wise dietary choices

Because grazing animals ingest plant material rather than dietary ingredients, there is limited scope for dietary manipulation in experimental work to separate sensory properties, such as taste and smell, from nutritional characteristics. Therefore, caution must be exercised in interpreting diet-selection measurements. For example, it has been demonstrated that sheep select more grass-stem material when its water-soluble carbohydrate (WSC) content has been elevated as a result of treatment of the grass with glyphosate (Leury *et al.*, 1999). Similarly, sheep grazing *Phalaris aquatica* pasture selected against grass patches that had been shaded from the sun, in favour of unshaded grass. Shading the grass reduced its WSC content but did not affect N and fibre levels or *in vitro* digestibility (Ciavarella *et al.*, 2000). It could be argued that the selection of material with a higher WSC content could be a nutritionally wise choice, since the sugars provide an energy source for the rumen microbes in synchrony with ruminal breakdown of dietary protein. However, the tendency for sheep and other herbivores to select diets high in soluble sugars may be simply a response to the taste of the sugars.

Ozanne and Howes (1971) observed that Merino sheep showed preference for phosphorus-fertilized plots of grass in the Australian dry season, but, since the phenol content of the grass fell as phosphorus levels increased, it was not possible to establish whether the diet selection response was due to phenol or to phosphorus level. It may be that phenol was being used as a cue or the primary stimulus or was not used at all.

Sheep spent more time grazing on areas of heather (*Calluna vulgaris*) that had been treated with N fertilizer than on unfertilized areas (Duncan *et al.*, 1994). It is likely that the resultant increase in CP content was the stimulus, since heather normally has a low protein level, the digestion of which is compromised by significant levels of tannins. However, the possibility that the animals were responding to alterations in the taste, flavour or levels of secondary compounds cannot be excluded.

Effects of plant secondary metabolites or toxins on dietary choice

While grass is somewhat unusual in having low levels of compounds that may be harmful to sheep, most other plants contain secondary compounds that may be toxic to the microbes of the digestive tract or to the host animal (see Waghorn *et al.*, Chapter 15, this volume). Such compounds are probably acting as defences for the plant against herbivory, by deterring animals from feeding on the plant. Hence dietary choice will be affected. It has been postulated that herbivores develop aversions to plants containing such toxins, with the toxin being the unconditioned stimulus; taste, smell and/or flavour may be the conditioned stimuli. However, the question of how an animal recognizes which plant was responsible for post-ingestive discomfort after eating a mixed diet remains unanswered.

Neutralizing the effects of plant toxins may remove their deterrent effect and hence change dietary choice. Well-known examples include increased selection of high-tannin shrubs after dosing animals with polyethylene glycol (PEG), which, by binding to tannins, removes their antinutritional effects (e.g. Titus *et al.*, 2001). There is also evidence to suggest that, in order to suppress parasite infestation, birds and primates may consume plants containing secondary compounds with anthelmintic properties. It is uncertain whether, given the opportunity, sheep would follow similar strategies; certainly they avoid the smell of faeces and parasitized animals are more selective eaters (Hutchings *et al.*, 1999).

Despite the deterrent effects of plant secondary compounds, large herbivores, including sheep, can ingest substantial quantities of plants containing secondary compounds. Depending upon the particular plant toxin, the sheep and/or the microbial population of its digestive tract may adapt to detoxifying the secondary compound. Such adaptation may, in turn, affect diet choice. Adaptation by the host animal, predominantly through induction of detoxifying enzymes in the liver, can be considered to be a more rapid process than adaptation of the gut microflora. Duncan *et al.* (2000) observed that goats with a rumen microflora adapted to oxalate by daily oral dosing selected a higher dietary proportion of spinach (which contains oxalate) than unadapted goats.

Constraints on intake and diet selection that are external to the animal

The constraints limiting intake are often more closely related to the characteristics of the vegetation on offer, environmental factors and other influences external to the animal than to physiological constraints.

Ease of harvesting

Daily intake can be considered as the product of the short-term intake rate while feeding and the time spent grazing or browsing (see Weston, Chapter 2, this volume). The short-term intake rate, being largely influenced by the type and quantity of vegetation available as a food, is often the major constraint limiting daily intake. On single-species swards, daily intake increases in an asymptotic fashion as herbage mass per unit area increases. This relationship has been defined as the functional response. At low herbage availabilities, which lead to submaximal intakes, it is likely that the short-term rate of intake has been limited because material is more difficult to harvest; the amount of herbage consumed in each bite declines as sward height decreases (Hodgson, 1986). The process of obtaining food under free-ranging conditions involves numerous steps, any one or more affecting the ease by which that food item is obtained. These steps include finding the food, moving to the food, harvesting (biting, nibbling, stripping leaves from twigs, etc.), manipulating the material in the mouth (mastication, adding saliva, bolus formation) and swallowing. The ease of harvesting is likely to be an important factor affecting the choice of diet made by an animal, whether it is the choice of plant part from a single species or selection from a range of different species.

Limitations to intake due to restrictions on the harvesting process are likely to be particularly important in scrub and rangeland areas, where animals have to work hard to select a reasonable diet from woody plants and poor-quality grasses and forbs.

Spatial heterogeneity

The effects of heterogeneity on intake and diet choice are likely to be most profound in situations where there are a large number of different food-plant species that are spatially distributed in a non-random manner. In order to understand how the effects of heterogeneity on intake and diet choice could be studied, the concept of the 'patch' evolved. At its simplest, each patch consists of a different food type – for example, a single tree or bush could represent a patch. A patch could also represent an area of vegetation with a mixture of potential food items that is different from that of the surrounding area. The size of patches and their distribution (degree of aggregation) relative to the size of the animal (sheep) have important impacts on foraging decisions made by the animal. At one extreme, a patch can be considered as small as a single bite and, at the other, as large as a sizeable section of landscape (e.g. the side of a hill). If different food items are mixed at a smaller scale than that of a bite, as they often are in grass/forb pastures, it is considered that animals cannot effectively make choices at that scale. It has been postulated that animals with their teeth set in a narrower jaw (incisor arcade) can select to a higher degree of resolution than animals with wider arcades (Illius *et al.*, 1995). At slightly larger scales, where sheep have to locate accurately the head and mouth to choose preferred food items, selective feeding is likely to be more arduous than in bigger patches where discrimination is easy.

For herbivores in heterogeneous vegetation environments, there will always be a trade-off between the costs of movement to preferred food items and the benefits of ingesting them. Thus, at any point in time, the existing location of an animal in a heterogeneous area will have an effect on its subsequent movements and dietary choices. As a consequence, grazing and/or browsing activity would be expected to be concentrated on patches of preferred vegetation, with less-preferred material in the immediate surroundings also being consumed. Under arid conditions, animals will graze more intensively near water-holes than elsewhere; the water-hole represents a patch containing a preferred food item (water) and attracts animals to the area (see O'Reagain and McMeniman, Chapter 12, this volume). Similarly, the placement of food blocks or a supply of supplementary feed may attract animals to an area having less-preferred plant material, such as heather, which is then heavily grazed.

Other factors affecting dietary choice and intake

Diet choice and intake can be affected by a range of other external factors, including soil, landscape topology, climate and animal excreta and through social interactions with other sheep (in particular, suckling ewes), other herbivores and potential predators, sheepdogs and humans. Most of these factors influence diet selection indirectly; direct effects are relatively few.

Effects on vegetation that indirectly influence dietary choice

Since a grazing sheep has the opportunity to choose only the potential food items that are available to it, anything that affects the nature of available vegetation will influence the diet of the animal. Factors that affect the abundance, morphology, nutritional quality and heterogeneity of available vegetation will indirectly affect dietary choice. Such factors include soil fertility and water status, climate and the topology of the area. Herbivores will also affect the amount and botanical composition of the vegetation, through defoliation and trampling and through the plants' subsequent responses to such damage and to the nutrients supplied from herbivore excreta.

Location of the sheep within a heterogeneous habitat

Spatial heterogeneity in a herbivore's habitat can be a contributory factor in affecting diet composition and intake in a range of ways other than through a direct effect on feeding behaviour and food availability. Within a heterogeneous environment, anything that causes an animal to remain in a particular place or to move to a different location is likely to indirectly influence the diet selected. Because of the tendency for a herbivore to limit its movements, the animal is likely to choose food items present in its immediate vicinity.

In a hill environment, sheep tend to choose sites of differing altitude at different times of the day. They may also seek out sheltered areas under extreme weather conditions. Certain areas may be avoided; for example, they tend not to graze close to vegetation contaminated with sheep excreta or muddy conditions.

Sheep tend to graze at a preferred distance apart from other sheep. If a sheep were to move in order to maintain that distance from its neighbour, its dietary choice might be affected. The location of a group of sheep within an area may be influenced by the avoidance of other groups of sheep or other species, such as cattle. Sheep may also change their location in response to the presence, real or perceived, of predators, sheepdogs or people.

Indirect effect of activities other than foraging

Sheep and other herbivores spend much of their time foraging and there are many situations where intake and possibly diet composition are affected by the amount of time available to exhibit feeding behaviour. Thus, any other activity that a sheep carries out that displaces feeding behaviour could influence the dietary choices made by the animal. Such activities include behavioural responses to other sheep and the effects that predators and sheepdogs have in prompting flocking behaviour and cessation of grazing activity. The presence of other sheep may also initiate foraging behaviour and thus affect intake and diet composition. It is likely that synchrony between sheep in starting and finishing feeding bouts is the result of one animal copying another's activity; such effects have been described as facilitation.

Integration

Seeking to attain minimal total discomfort (MTD)

Very rarely will a single sheep be offered a single food that provides a mixture of nutrients that exactly balances its needs, whether it is indoors or outdoors. Even when two foods are available or two species of herbage and the animal can balance both its energy supply and that of another nutrient, additional nutrients are not likely to be supplied in optimal quantities. Thus, there is a dilemma if one food has a higher concentration of energy than another, but also has a higher concentration of a toxin.

Wang and Provenza (1997) observed that lambs preferred barley to lucerne pellets in the absence of added toxin (LiCl), but, when LiCl was added to the barley in increasing amounts, the preference for barley became an aversion. Natural toxins have similar effects: tannin added to previously preferred food high in readily available carbohydrate reduced lambs' preference, but, when PEG was given, their aversion to the higher-energy foods was significantly less than without the PEG supplement (Titus *et al.*, 2000).

These are very simple, two-dimensional examples of the sort of trade-offs sheep have to make on a daily or hourly basis. There is an optimum rate of supply for each nutrient for an animal in a given physiological state. Exceed that and a surfeit or even a toxicity develops; fail to meet it and the animal is faced with a deficiency of that nutrient. Only when the surfeit or deficiency becomes severe will the animal be unable to cope, but the fact that it can, by adjusting its metabolism, manage mild departures from optimal nutrition does not mean that no discomfort is being generated. As has been shown above, the greater the deviation from optimal supply of a nutrient, the more the sheep becomes averse to that food, even though it can cope if that is the only food on offer. It may cope by eating less to avoid too much toxin or by eating more to increase the supply of a limiting nutrient.

All this brings us to the concept of minimal total discomfort (MTD) (Forbes, 1999; Forbes and Provenza, 2000): 'discomfort' because a departure from optimal supply of a nutrient is avoided if possible; 'total' because the discomforts from numerous sources (nutrient imbalance, social stress, etc.) are postulated to be added together by the central nervous system in order to generate an overall controlling signal (Forbes, 1996); 'minimal' because the animal is postulated to eat that amount of food(s) that minimizes the total discomfort.

If we know the optimal supply of a nutrient for a given animal (that which minimizes discomfort) and the concentrations of that nutrient in the foods on offer, then we can calculate the discomfort generated by eating a range of different daily intakes of the foods in various ratios. There are also food and environmental constraints of relevance, such as the bulkiness of the foods (described, for example, by their neutral-detergent fibre (NDF) content) and the time needed to graze the available foods, described by the rate at which they can be eaten by the sheep in question. We shall use the daily intake of metabolizable energy (ME) and NDF and the rate of intake of sparse pasture as 'resources' in the following example and use optima for growing lambs (20 MJ, 350 g, 10 h day^{-1}, respectively). In the case of NDF and grazing time, it is proposed that it is only when 'supply' exceeds a threshold that discomfort is experienced. The desire always to consume a minimum amount of fibre (see above) is not taken into account in the current model as the foods used have an adequate fibre content. ME supply, on the other hand, generates discomfort, both when in excess of and when lower than requirements. Starting with a likely daily intake of the food (or, in the case of choice, foods) on offer, the supply of each 'resource' is calculated and the deviations from optimal are calculated, expressed as proportions of requirements, squared and added together to give an estimate of total discomfort. For example, if the supply of the three 'resources' were, respectively, 0.8, 1.3 and 1.4 times their optimal values, then the squares of the deviations would be 0.04, 0.09 and 0.16, respectively, giving a total of 0.29.

Intake of each food in turn is increased and decreased, repeating the calculations in each case until the MTD has been reached. Figure 3.3 shows discomforts for a range of intakes of a single food with 10 MJ ME kg^{-1} dry matter (DM) and 600 g NDF kg^{-1}. Let us further assume that the sheep can harvest at 1.5 g DM min^{-1} and that it prefers its grazing time to not exceed 10 h day^{-1}, i.e. grazing time generates a discomfort if it exceeds this total length. (This is a simplification, as the time available for ruminating is important, especially for forage feeds.) In order to harvest 1.2 kg DM day^{-1}, as required for MTD calculated from ME and NDF, the lamb will have to graze for 900 min (15 h), i.e. more than the threshold of 10 h day^{-1}. As a result, the proportional discomfort will be (15 – 10)/10 = 0.5. Adding this into the previous calculations gives an MTD with an intake of 1.0 kg DM day^{-1}.

Application of the MTD concept to diet selection under grazing

It is logical to assume that the concept that an animal will feed so as to seek to attain MTD will apply equally to free-ranging conditions and to housed animals. Although several other factors come into play, such as social inter-

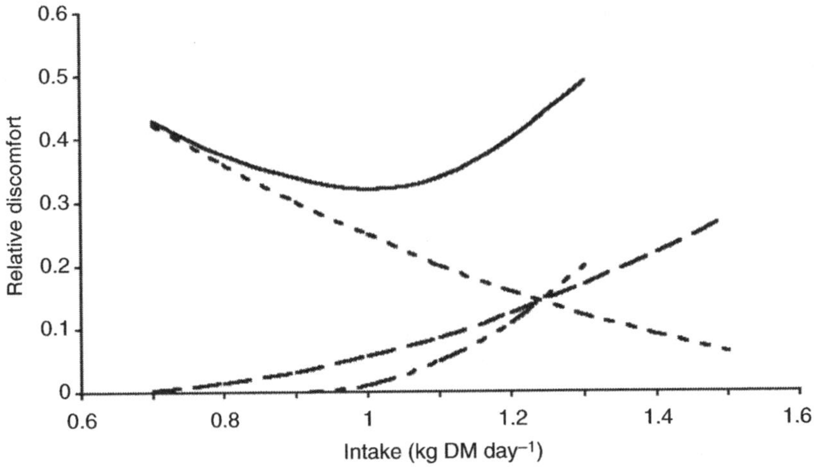

Fig. 3.3. Calculated relative discomforts due to ME (dotted), NDF (dashed) and grazing time (dot–dash), and the total of these (solid), plotted against daily intake of DM for the conditions described in the text, with an eating rate of 1.5 g DM min^{-1}. The predicted level of intake, 1.0 kg day^{-1}, is at the point of minimal total discomfort (Forbes, 2001).

actions with other sheep, risk of predation and inclement weather, our example will build on the single-food situation outlined in the previous section. A sheep with the same specifications as above is grazing an area in which there are two types of herbage. One contains 10 MJ ME kg^{-1} DM and 600 g NDF kg^{-1} and can be harvested at 1 g DM min^{-1}. The other is of poorer nutritional value, with 9 MJ ME kg^{-1} and 650 g NDF kg^{-1}, but can be harvested at a faster rate due to its greater height.

The model was run for rates of eating forage 2 ranging from 1.0 to 2.4 g DM min^{-1} and the output is shown in Fig. 3.4. When the rates at which the two forages are eaten were similar, then only forage 1 was chosen, as this has the higher energy and lower fibre levels. As the rate of eating forage 2 increases, the proportion of forage 1 chosen declines rapidly and the total daily intake increases, because eating forage 2 becomes less time-consuming. However, when the rate of eating forage 2 becomes greater than 1.6 g min^{-1}, there is sufficient time available for the sheep to be able to eat a little of forage 1, which gives a higher yield of energy and less fibre per unit of DM than forage 2. With the increase in ease of harvesting forage 2 comes a reduction in discomfort as the animal's energy supply comes closer to optimal and it is only exceeding its 'desired' grazing time by a small margin.

Note that it is not being claimed that the predictions of this model of choice between herbage types with different characteristics are quantitatively realistic. The purpose of presenting this example is to illustrate how a simple theory of control of intake and diet selection can come up with some complex predictions when several factors are taken into account simultaneously. There is still a great deal to be done in developing this theory, in particular in specifying the relative weights to be placed on the discomfort generated by over- and undersupply of the many resources provided by food(s).

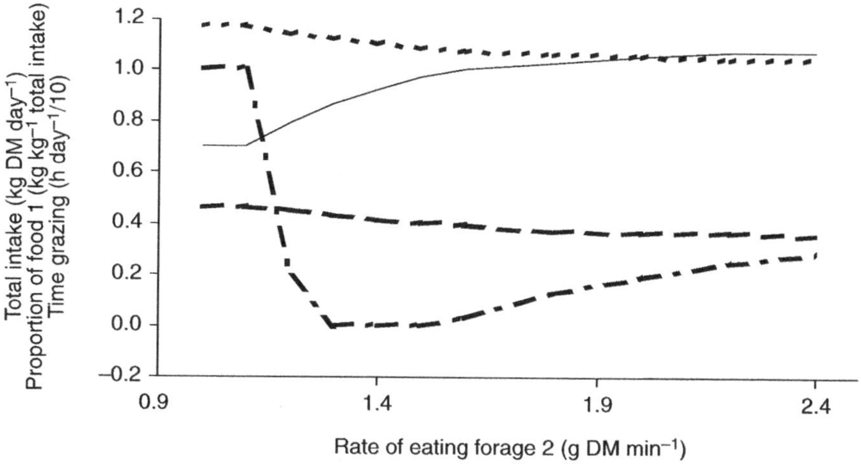

Fig. 3.4. Calculated total intake (kg DM day^{-1}, solid line); proportion of food 1 (kg kg^{-1} total intake, dot–dash); time grazing (h day^{-1}/10, short dashes); and total discomfort (arbitrary units, long dashes) for grazing sheep with a choice between two types of herbage (see text for details), plotted against the rate at which the poorer-quality herbage can be harvested.

Conclusion

We have based our discussion of diet selection on the premise that sheep, like other animals, learn to associate the sensory properties of a food with the metabolic and other internal consequences of eating that food. They have to trade off the various beneficial and harmful consequences in order to achieve what we term MTD. In controlled conditions, with few competing factors, this process works relatively well and the results of diet-selection experiments can usually be interpreted in a sensible manner. However, in the grazing situation, the number of factors capable of inducing discomfort are greater and prediction of how a sheep or a flock will behave becomes more difficult.

If we accept MTD as a reasonable working hypothesis, then we face the challenge of how best to weight the various factors involved in the control of intake and selection. By a series of experiments investigating the importance sheep attach to pairs of factors, it should be possible to build up a matrix of relative weightings that can be applied to MTD calculations. For example, Sibbald *et al.* (2000) monitored sheep for the trade-offs between herbage height and distance from their social group, in determining their grazing behaviour, thereby providing information relevant to MTD calculations. However, they found large differences between individuals in their willingness to graze further from their group in order to harvest a taller sward on which they could achieve a high rate of eating. This highlights the fact that there will always be a significant proportion of variation in behaviour between individuals that cannot be predicted from a knowledge of their physiological state and the composition of the food(s) on offer.

References

Arsenos, G. and Kyriazakis, I. (1999) The continuum between preferences and aversions for flavoured foods in sheep conditioned by administration of casein doses. *Animal Science* 68, 605–616.

Arsenos, G., Hills, J. and Kyriazakis, I. (2000) Conditioned feeding responses in sheep towards flavoured foods associated with casein administration: the role of long delay learning. *Animal Science* 70, 157–169.

Campion, D.P. and Leek, B.F. (1997) Investigation of a 'fibre appetite' in sheep fed a 'long fibre-free' diet. *Applied Animal Behaviour Science* 52, 79–86.

Chapman, H.W. and Grovum, W.L. (1982) Studies on the palatability of salt and urea in sheep. *Proceedings of the Nutrition Society* 41, 73A.

Ciavarella, T.A., Dove, H., Leury, B.J. and Simpson, R.J. (2000) Diet selection by sheep grazing *Phalaris aquatica* L. pastures of differing water-soluble carbohydrate content. *Australian Journal of Agricultural Research* 51, 757–764.

Cooper, S.D.B., Kyriazakis, I. and Oldham, J.D. (1994) The effect of late pregnancy on the diet selections made by ewes. *Livestock Production Science* 40, 263–275.

Cooper, S.D.B., Kyriazakis, I. and Oldham, J.D. (1996) The effects of physical form of feed, carbohydrate source, and inclusion of sodium-bicarbonate on the diet selections of sheep. *Journal of Animal Science* 74, 1240–1251.

Duncan, A.J., Hartley, S.E. and Iason, G.R. (1994) Fine-scale discrimination of forage quality by sheep offered a soybean meal or barley supplement while grazing a nitrogen-fertilized heather (*Calluna vulgaris*) mosaic. *Journal of Agricultural Science, Cambridge* 123, 363–370.

Duncan, A.J., Frutos, P. and Young, S.A. (2000) The effect of rumen adaptation to oxalic acid on selection of oxalic-acid-rich plants by goats. *British Journal of Nutrition* 83, 59–65.

Forbes, J.M. (1995) *Voluntary Food Intake and Diet Selection in Farm Animals*. CAB International, Wallingford, UK, 532 pp.

Forbes, J.M. (1996) Integration of regulatory signals controlling forage intake in ruminants. *Journal of Animal Science* 74, 3029–3053.

Forbes, J.M. (1999) Minimal total discomfort as a concept for the control of food intake and selection. *Appetite* 33, 171.

Forbes, J.M. (2001) Consequences of feeding for future feeding. *Comparative Biochemistry and Physiology* 128, 461–468.

Forbes, J.M. and Provenza, F.D. (2000) Integration of learning and metabolic signals into a theory of dietary choice and food intake. In: Cronje, P. (ed.) *Ruminant Physiology: Digestion, Metabolism, Growth and Reproduction*. CAB International, Wallingford, UK, pp. 3–19.

Hills, J., Nolan, J.V., Hinch, G.N. and Lynch, J.J. (1998) Selection of diets differing in sulphur content by sheep in sulphur adequate or depleted states. *Proceedings of the British Society of Animal Science*, 28.

Hills, J., Kyriazakis, I., Nolan, J.V., Hinch, G.N. and Lynch, J.J. (1999) Conditioned feeding responses in sheep to flavoured foods associated with sulphur doses. *Animal Science* 69, 313–325.

Hodgson, J. (1986) Grazing behaviour and herbage intake. In: Frame, J. (ed.) *BGS Occasional Symposium No. 19*. British Grassland Society, Reading, pp. 51–64.

Hou, X.Z., Lawrence, A.B., Illius, A.W., Anderson, D. and Oldham, J.D. (1991) Operant studies on feed selection in sheep. *Proceedings of the Nutrition Society* 50, 95A.

Hutchings, M.R., Kyriazakis, I., Gordon, I.J. and Jackson, F. (1999) Trade-offs between nutrient intake and faecal avoidance in herbivore foraging decisions: the effect of animal parasitic status, level of feeding motivation and sward nitrogen content. *Journal of Animal Ecology* 68, 310–323.

Illius, A.W., Albon, S.D., Pemberton, J.M., Gordon, I.J. and Clutton-Brock, T.H. (1995) Selection for foraging efficiency during a population crash in Soay sheep. *Journal of Animal Ecology* 64, 481–492.

Jones, R. and Forbes, J.M. (1984) A note on effects of glyphosate and quinine on the palatability of hay for sheep. *Animal Production* 38, 301–303.

Leury, B.J., Siever-Kelly, C., Gatford, K.L., Simpson, R.J. and Dove, H. (1999) Spray-topping annual grass pasture with glyphosate to delay loss of feeding value during summer. IV. Diet composition, herbage intake, and performance in grazing sheep. *Australian Journal of Agricultural Research* 50, 487–495.

Mayes, R.W. and Dove, H. (2000) Measurement of dietary nutrient intake in free-ranging mammalian herbivores. *Nutrition Research Reviews* 13, 107–138.

McLaughlin, C.L., Baldwin, B.A. and Baile, C.A. (1974) Olfactory bulbectomy and feeding behaviour. *Journal of Animal Science* 39, 136.

Ozanne, P.G. and Howes, K.M.W. (1971) Preference of grazing sheep for pasture of high phosphate content. *Australian Journal of Agricultural Research* 22, 941–950.

Pfister, J.A., Muller-Schwarze, D. and Balph, D.F. (1990) Effects of predator fecal odors on feed selection by sheep and cattle. *Journal of Chemical Ecology* 16, 323–329.

Ramos, A. and Tennessen, T. (1992) Effect of previous grazing experience on the grazing behavior of lambs. *Applied Animal Behaviour Science* 33, 43–52.

Rutter, S.M., Orr, R.J. and Rook, A.J. (2000) Dietary preference for grass and white clover in sheep and cattle: an overview. In: Rook, A.J. and Penning, P.D. (eds) *Grazing Management*. British Grassland Society, Reading, pp. 73–78.

Sibbald, A.M., Smith, D.J.F. and Hooper, R.J. (2000) Individual differences in sociability and their consequences for foraging in sheep. *Proceedings of the British Society of Animal Science*, 129.

Titus, C.H., Provenza, F.D., Perevolotsky, A. and Silanikove, N. (2000) Preferences for foods varying in macronutrients and tannins by lambs supplemented with polyethylene glycol. *Journal of Animal Science* 78, 1443–1449.

Titus, C.H., Provenza, F.D., Perevolotsky, A., Silanikove, N. and Rogosic, J. (2001) Supplemental polyethylene glycol influences preferences of goats browsing blackbrush. *Journal of Range Management* 54, 161–165.

Wang, J. and Provenza, F.D. (1997) Dynamics of preference by sheep offered foods varying in flavors, nutrients, and a toxin. *Journal of Chemical Ecology* 23, 275–288.

4 Microbial Ecology of the Ovine Rumen

R.I. MACKIE,[1] C.S. MCSWEENEY[2] AND A.V. KLIEVE[3]

[1]Department of Animal Sciences, University of Illinois, Urbana, Illinois, USA; [2]CSIRO Livestock Industries, Long Pocket Laboratory, Indooroopilly, Queensland , Australia; [3]Agency for Food and Fibre Sciences, Animal Research Institute, Moorooka, Queensland, Australia

Introduction

In 1843, Gruby and Delafond claimed to be the first to describe living 'animalcules' in the rumen (four species) and horse caecum (seven species), since Leeuwenhoek's observations in 1685 of three species in frog faeces. However, the importance of intestinal bacteria in digestion dates from 1913, when Osborne and Mendel noted coprophagy in rats kept for a long time on purified diets. The role of bacteria in the fermentation of plant materials became well known in 1863 as a result of the genius of Pasteur. It was inferred by Zuntz in 1879 that rumen microbes fermented fibre anaerobically and thus formed acids and gas. He postulated that the acidic fermentation products were absorbed and oxidized by the host. By 1940, the time was ripe for a more widespread appreciation of rumen microbial activities and an animal physiology unit was set up at Cambridge. This group, under the leadership of Sir Joseph Barcroft, recognized that fermentation was the basic mechanism involved and demonstrated quantitatively the uptake of short-chain fatty acids (SCFA) across the rumen wall into circulating blood.

As a result of these and many other investigations on rumen function, it is now firmly established that the ruminant animal and the rumen microbial population exist in a reciprocally beneficial relationship, termed mutualism, in which plant material consumed by the mammalian host is digested and fermented by the rumen microbes to form chiefly SCFA, carbon dioxide and methane. The gases are voided by the ruminant and the acids absorbed and oxidized. The microbes provide the host not only with a source of energy, but also with proteins, vitamins and other nutrients essential for cell maintenance and production. Favourable conditions provided by the host permit the growth of large numbers of diverse microbes. The microbial population in the rumen and other gut compartments, such as the caecum and colon, is thus characterized by high density, wide diversity and the complexity of interactions that occur. Hungate (1960) was the first to study rumen microbial ecology and described the steps required to provide a complete ecological description and analysis of any complex ecosystem. First, the numbers and types of organisms present must be described, involving enumeration, identification and classification. Secondly, their activities must be measured. Finally, the extent to which these activities are performed in the environment must be determined, involving quantitative measurements of the entire complex as well as the component parts.

Interested readers are referred to a number of books and references therein that provide detailed descriptions and information on topics covered in brief in the following chapter. Chronologically these are R.E. Hungate's (1966) classic book *The Rumen and its Microbes*, *Microbial Ecology of the Gut* (Clarke and Bauchop, 1977), *The Rumen Microbial Ecosystem* (Hobson and Stewart, 1997) and *Gastrointestinal Microbiology* (Mackie *et al.*, 1997).

Components of the Ecosystem

Description of the components

The individual components of the ruminal ecosystem can be broadly divided into host-related factors, dietary factors and the microbiota itself. These three components interact in a dynamic equilibrium and a disturbance in one of these factors leads to an alteration or perturbation of the other components.

Host factors

The rumen has evolved as an adaptation that allows retention and digestion of ingested food, followed by absorption and metabolism of digestion products, while feeding and other activities continue. The ruminant host provides a means of selecting and gathering feed, comminution or reduction in particle size of ingested feed by chewing and rumination, mixing by rumen contractions and movements, temperature and pH control (bicarbonate and phosphate in saliva) and provision of nutrients, such as urea (recycled in saliva and through the rumen wall) and phosphate. The host also removes inhibitory acidic end-products of digestion (by absorption) and fermentation gases (by eructation), as well as the passage of undigested dietary residues out of the rumen. Ruminants have at least one structural difference (the reticulo-omasal orifice for selective retention of larger undigested feed particles) and one physiological difference (rumination) that set them apart from all other fore-stomach fermenters and suggest a more recent evolution.

An early step in the study of the ecology of any microbial ecosystem is the enumeration and isolation of component bacteria. This requires the formulation of suitable media, based on a detailed analysis of the physical and chemical conditions in the intestinal tract, and also of diet composition. The microbial environment in the rumen has been closely defined and, allowing for variation in the quality and quantity of feed ingested, serves as a model for other gut ecosystems. A summary of the chemical, physical and microbiological characteristics is provided in Mackie *et al.* (2001).

Dietary factors

One of the chief factors influencing rumen fermentation is the variation in feed composition. Carbohydrates are the most important source of energy for rumen microbes. The types of carbohydrates most common in forages are soluble carbohydrates, starch and the insoluble cell-wall components of plants. Sugars and other soluble carbohydrates, which may constitute 30% of the dry matter in forage, are rapidly metabolized. However, too much readily fermentable carbohydrate in the diet can lower the digestibility of fibre. Starch is digested rapidly in the rumen but more slowly than sugars. Increased acidity and higher proportions of propionate often accompany increased fermentation rates, although in some cases butyrate is increased. The rumen protozoa are at an advantage in the microbial competition for starch in the rumen and rapidly engulf large numbers of starch granules, removing them from the available fermentation pool. Various feed treatments, such as grinding and pelleting, affect the rates at which bacteria and protozoa attack starch. Heat treatment of grains also influences fermentation rate and the acetate : propionate ratio. Plant cell-wall material, with the exception of pectin, is fermented slowly, resulting in high proportions of acetate. Microbial digestion of the major plant cell-wall components is a complex enzymatic process, mediated by the combined activities of bacteria, fungi and, maybe, protozoa. The lignin content of herbage varies between 4 and 12% and, in general, the higher the lignin content the lower the digestibility.

Protein breakdown in the rumen is correlated with solubility. Production of short-branched (isobutyric, isovaleric and 2-methyl butyric acid) and straight-chain (valeric acid) SCFA, which are required for the growth of cellulolytic bacteria from deamination of amino acids, is important in poor-quality diets. Fats added to diets limit the digestibility of forage fibre. Addition of fats has been shown to reduce methane production. Other important examples of the effects of variation in feed composition are comparisons between legume and grass forages and between hay and concentrate diets, which influence the composition and activities of the rumen microbial population. Digestion in the rumen is discussed in more detail by Annison *et al.* (Chapter 5, this volume).

The quantity of feed consumed can also play a major role in the activities of the rumen microbiota. Two examples of this factor are lactic acidosis (see below) as a result of grain overfeeding and the influence of feeding level (up to three times the maintenance level during lactation) on the activities of rumen bacteria and protozoa.

The use of feed additives has been an area of active research for many years. The most important and widely used feed additives in ruminant diets are ionophore antibiotics, but feed enzymes, probiotics (live microbial feed supplements), buffering agents, methane inhibitors and many other additives are used in a variety of feeding situations. Details are provided in the section on manipulation of rumen fermentation and the review of Nagaraja *et al.* (1997).

Microbiota

The microbial community inhabiting the rumen is represented by all major groups of microbes. This complex, mixed microbial culture, which comprises strictly anaerobic bacteria, ciliate and flagellate protozoa, anaerobic chytridiomycete fungi and bacteriophages, can be considered the most metabolically adaptable and rapidly renewable organ of the body, which plays a vital role in the normal nutritional, physiological and protective functions of the ruminant animal. The rumen, the most intensively studied gut ecosystem, contains large numbers of bacteria (up to 10^{11} viable cells ml^{-1}, comprising 200 phenotypically different species), ciliate protozoa (10^4–10^6 ml^{-1} spread over 25 genera), anaerobic fungi (zoospore population densities of 10^3–10^5 ml^{-1}, divided into five genera) and bacteriophages (10^7–10^9 particles ml^{-1}). However, despite this vast amount of knowledge, the basic prerequisites for ecological studies – namely, enumeration and identification of all community members – have tremendous limitations. The two major problems faced by microbial ecologists studying the gastrointestinal ecosystem are the inevitable bias introduced by techniques based on enumeration and characterization from cultures and the lack of a phylogenetically based classification scheme. It is estimated that 10% or less of the total viable bacteria in the rumen of forage-fed animals can be cultivated. Modern molecular ecology techniques based on sequence comparisons of nucleic acids (DNA and RNA) can be used to overcome these limitations and advance our understanding of the ecology, diversity, structure–function and evolutionary relationships in the rumen and other gastrointestinal compartments (Mackie *et al.*, 1997). This approach is likely to provide not simply increased understanding but a complete description of the gut ecosystem for the first time.

Microbial interactions

Microorganisms are most often studied in pure culture, which provides detailed knowledge regarding their growth and metabolism. However, these studies fail to take into account that microbes live in communities and the fundamental importance of the influence that they have on each other. Only with a knowledge of both the properties of individual species and populations and the interactions that occur between them will it be possible to gain some understanding of the structure and function of complex microbial communities. The rumen provides many examples of competitive and non-competitive interactions (Hobson and Stewart, 1997; Mackie *et al.*, 1997). Degradation of organic matter, in general, and plant cell-wall material, in particular, is an excellent example of microbial interactions, where stepwise degradation of the substrate is carried out in a characteristic and sequential pattern by a range of organisms with a high degree of specialization. The nature of interspecies interactions and the extent of mutual dependence vary enormously, ranging from simple cross-feeding of essential nutrients, vitamins or carbon and energy sources to very specialized total dependence. The best-known of these interactions in the rumen is the removal of electrons formed during fermentation, often in the form of molecular hydrogen, by methanogenic bacteria and possibly hydrogen-oxidizing acetogens. Through this mechanism of interspecies hydrogen transfer, thermodynamically unfavourable reactions can proceed through coupling to exergonic reactions.

The influence of ciliate protozoa on the activity and size of bacterial populations in the rumen has been studied for many years. This provides an excellent example of the inverse relationship between predator and prey. However, the observation that fungal zoospores increase in number after defaunation is more recent, providing evidence for a role of protozoa in determining the size of fungal populations. Further research is required to elucidate the exact nature of these predatory interactions, which have been demonstrated by electron microscopy, enumeration and substrate disappearance. However, it is likely that hydrogen transfer is a significant component of the symbiosis between ciliates and methanogens.

Various antagonistic interactions that occur between microrganisms in the gastrointestinal tract are thought to be important in controlling proliferation of enteric bacteria and in providing a primary line of defence for the host. Our knowledge of this phenomenon, termed competitive exclusion or colonization resistance, is still rudimentary. However, considerable attention has been focused on bacteriocins in lactic acid bacteria, although not in an ecological sense. Thus our knowledge of the ecological and economic significance of antagonistic microbial interactions in animals is scant. Bacteriocin-like inhibitory substances have been detected in several genera of rumen bacteria, including *Streptococcus bovis*, staphylococci isolated from preruminant calves and lambs, *Enterococcus faecium*, *Ruminococcus albus* and *Butyrivibrio fibrisolvens*. To date, only two bacteriocins from *B. fibrisolvens* (butyrivibriocin) and one from *S. bovis* (bovicin) have been purified, characterized and confirmed as bacteriocins. These antagonistic compounds are likely to play an important role in inter- and intraspecific competition in the rumen.

The Microbiota

The rumen ecosystem comprises a complex of dense microbial communities of bacteria, archaea, ciliate protozoa, anaerobic fungi and bacteriophages (summarized in Table 4.1). The fermentation effected by this complex microbiota is responsible for the conversion of plant feedstuffs to compounds that can be utilized by the animal. Hence, the fermentations and interactions of

Table 4.1. Summary of primary metabolic activities attributable to typical and predominant examples of the ruminal microbiota.

Microbial grouping	Major substrates metabolized	Products of metabolism
Bacteria		
Fibrobacter succinogenes	Cellulose	Acetic acid, succinic acid
Ruminococcus spp.	Cellulose	Acetic acid, succinic acid, ethanol, CO_2 and H_2
Prevotella ruminicola	Hemicelluloses, starches, mono- and disaccharides	Acetic acid, succinic acid, formic acid
Butyrivibrio fibrisolvens	Cellulose (only some strains), hemicelluloses, starches, mono- and disaccharides	Butyric acid, acetic acid, formic acid, CO_2 and H_2
Selenomonas ruminantium	Starches, mono- and disaccharides, lactic acid (one subspecies only)	Acetic acid, propionic acid, lactic acid, CO_2 and H_2
Streptococcus bovis	Starches, mono- and disaccharides	Lactic acid and CO_2
Megasphaera elsdenii	Lactic acid	Caproic acid, butyric acid, CO_2 and H_2
Clostridium aminophilum	Peptides and amino acids	Branched-chain fatty acids
Archaea (methanogens)	Carbon dioxide and hydrogen	Methane
Ciliate protozoa		
Isotrichidae (six species)	Mono- and disaccharides	Acetic acid, butyric acid, CO_2 and H_2
Large-sized genera of Entodiniomorphidae (38 species)	Cellulose and hemicelluloses	Acetic acid, butyric acid, CO_2 and H_2
Entodinium (17 species)	Starches	Acetic acid, butyric acid, CO_2 and H_2
Chytridiomycete fungi (five genera)	All colonize fibrous plant material and metabolize cellulose, hemicellulose and sugars	Lactic acid, acetic acid, formic acid, CO_2 and H_2

the microbes are central to ruminant digestion and nutrition. At birth, the digestive tract of ruminants, in common with other mammals, is devoid of bacteria. Colonization begins during and shortly after birth and is via the oral route. Establishment of the microbial communities requires contact with an adult animal, usually the mother, and the rumen environment must be suitable for the microbes to establish a population (Hobson and Stewart, 1997).

Bacteria

Bacteria are the most numerous and important of the microbes in the rumen. They are present at densities of up to 10^{11} cells ml^{-1} (Hungate, 1966) and are capable of undertaking all the necessary biochemical transformations to convert plant material into products of nutritional value to the host ruminant. The bacteria are, in the main, obligate anaerobes. Classic microscopic observation and culturing techniques have revealed a great diversity in terms of size, shape and form of bacteria living in the rumen (Hungate, 1966; Hobson and Stewart, 1997). Both Gram-positive and Gram-negative bacteria occur and range in diameter from less than 0.1 μm (mycoplasmas) to greater than 50 μm (*Oscillospira*). Shapes include cocci, rods, crescents and spirals. These cells can also be motile or not and vary greatly in growth habit, ranging from single cells to duplex cells, short chains, long chains, clumps, tetrad groupings and large sheetlike structures. The diversity of rumen bacteria in terms of size, shape and growth habit is well illustrated by Ogimoto and Imai (1981).

Prior to the advent of molecular biology and the use of DNA sequencing as a taxonomic tool, the differentiation between bacterial taxa was largely based on a combination of morphological and biochemical characteristics (Hungate, 1966; Hobson and Stewart, 1997) and could be applied only to culturable bacteria. On this basis, 200 or so species of culturable bacteria were known to be present in the rumen, with some 20 species occurring at densities above 10^7 cells ml^{-1} of rumen fluid; about 30 species are regarded as normal rumen inhabitants (Bryant, 1959).

The bacterial species present and their relative densities within the rumen ecosystem fluctuate markedly in response to feed composition and dietary changes. Hungate (1966) found that the rumen bacteria of animals on hay or forage rations are composed mainly of Gram-negative organisms, while animals on grain diets have increased numbers of Gram-positive organisms. The common culturable bacteria are often grouped within functional substrate-utilizing groups. Cellulose, the most stable structural polysaccharide in plants, is degraded by only a few species of rumen bacteria: *Fibrobacter succinogenes*, *Ruminococcus flavefaciens*, *R. albus* and some strains of *B. fibrisolvens*. These species are very important, as a lack of breakdown of cellulose will impede access of other bacteria to their required substrates. The hemicelluloses, glucomannans and pectins are also degraded by the cellulolytic bacteria, but a larger number of non-cellulolytic bacteria are able to ferment these substrates. The predominant culturable species involved are *Prevotella ruminicola*, *Eubacterium ruminantium* and *B. fibrisolvens*. *Lachnospira multiparus* and *S. bovis* are pectinolytic. Common starch degraders are *P. ruminicola*, *Ruminobacter amylophilus*, *Selenomonas ruminantium*, *Succinomonas amylophilus* and *S. bovis*. Many of the rumen bacteria also utilize the fermentation products of other bacteria (e.g. lactate utilization by *Megasphaera elsdenii*), intermediate metabolic substrates, proteins and lipids.

With the advent of molecular biological techniques, based on DNA sequencing, it became possible to elucidate bacteria that had not been cultured and to determine genetic similarity between bacteria. These techniques have dramatically increased our knowledge of the diversity and complexity of ruminal bacterial communities in two major directions: (i) the uncultured diversity of bacteria present in ruminal contents; and (ii) the genetic diversity within culturable bacterial assemblages previously thought to constitute a 'species'.

Recent phylogenetic analyses of cloned 16S rRNA genes of rumen bacteria indicate the degree of uncultured bacterial diversity present in the rumen. Whitford *et al.* (1998) examined 84 cloned sequences from dairy cattle and deduced that 53 represented novel species and genera of bacteria. A recent study in cattle using direct retrieval of 16S rDNA sequences in a culture-independent manner showed that only 6% (ten of 161) of sequences could be identified directly by comparison with the sequence database (Tajima *et al.*, 1999). In general, results show high diversity, large proportions of operational taxonomic units represented by single clones and large proportions of clones distantly related to deposited sequences and so far uncultivated.

In addition to the discovery of many novel bacterial 16S rDNA sequences, considerable genetic diversity has been found within cultivable species. Of the common cultivable species, *P. ruminicola* (Wood *et al.*, 1998), *B. fibrisolvens* (Forster *et al.*, 1997), *F. succinogenes* (Ogata *et al.*, 1997) and the genus *Ruminococcus* (Krause *et al.*, 1999a) have been found to be genetically heterogeneous, comprising a variety of genetically distinct species and even genera.

It would appear that considerably more work will be required if we are to obtain a complete understanding of the bacteria that inhabit the rumen in the future.

Archaea

The major group of organisms inhabiting the rumen within the domain Archaea are the methanogens. In the rumen, methanogens synthesize methane mainly from CO_2 and H_2 (Hobson and Stewart, 1997). A variety of species have been cultured and these belong to three distinct families, Methanobacteriaceae, Methanomicrobiaceae and Methanoplanaceae. It was concluded that *Methanobrevibacter ruminantium* and *Methanosarcina* isolates were likely to be the most significant contributors to ruminal methanogenesis, based on archaea that can be cultured.

Concerns over global warming and the release of greenhouse gases, such as carbon dioxide and methane, into the atmosphere have created renewed interest in ruminal methanogens. Ruminal methanogenesis is a significant source of atmospheric methane, particularly in Australia, New Zealand and many developing nations. In Australia, for example, it is estimated that methane from enteric fermentation in ruminants accounts for 12% of total greenhouse gas emissions while in New Zealand this figure is 46%. A number of studies using culture-independent, DNA sequence-based techniques have investigated the ruminal archaea (Lloyd *et al.*, 1996; Lin *et al.*, 1997; Tokura *et al.*, 1999). Lin *et al.* (1997) found that the archaea, while functionally a very significant section of the rumen microbiota, were numerically inferior to the bacteria and eucarya, accounting for 0.5–3% of total microbes. They also noted a ruminant host preference for ruminal methanogens, with Methanobacteriales predominating in cattle and goats while Methanomicrobiales were predominant in sheep.

Not all methanogens occur freely in the rumen liquor. Ciliate protozoa provide a habitat for up to 20% of rumen methanogens. These methanogens can exist as endosymbionts or attached to the pellicle. Lloyd *et al.* (1996), using fluorescent *in situ* hybridization, were able to determine rates of colonization by bacteria and archaea in a range of ciliate protozoal species within the sheep rumen. In general, fewer Isotrichidae contained endosymbionts than Entodiniomorphidae and less than 3% of *Daytricha ruminantium* contained endosymbionts. *Polyplastron multivesiculatum* contained many bacteria but no archaea. Many larger Entodiniomorphidae, with the exception of *Eudiplodinium maggii*, contained both bacteria and archaea. Another study investigating the archaea of ciliate protozoans in the sheep rumen (Tokura *et al.*, 1999) found that DNA sequences with similarities to *Methanobrevibacter smithii* predominated, while *M. ruminantium* appeared to be absent.

Protozoa

Protozoans, particularly the ciliates, are the largest and most conspicuous of the rumen microbiota. They are obligate anaerobes, motile, eucaryotic microbes and were first discovered as early as 1843. Both ciliate and flagellate protozoans occur in the rumen, although in recent times some microbes that had been thought to be flagellate protozoa were subsequently identified as the zoospore stage in the life cycle of ruminal chytridiomycete fungi (covered in the section following). The ciliates are regarded as the more numerous and important of the two. Ruminal ciliates belong to a range of subclasses, orders and families within the class Kinetofragminophorea (Dehority, 1993). However, those likely to be encountered in the ovine rumen will almost certainly belong to either the family Isotrichidae (order Trichostomatida) or family Ophryoscolecidae (order Entodiniomorphida). The protozoans of the family Ophryoscolecidae are the major rumen ciliates, with more than 100 described species.

Entodiniomorphid protozoa are described and assigned to a taxon on the basis of morphological characteristics. Basically, the major characters are the number of ciliary zones (one or two) on an otherwise naked and rigid pellicle, the size and shape of the macronucleus and where it is positioned in relation to the micronucleus, number and position of vacuoles, number and position of skeletal plates and presence or absence of caudal spines (Fig. 4.1). Numerous descriptions, which include detailed line drawings and photographs, of the genera and species within this family are available (Ogimoto and Imai, 1981; Hobson and Stewart, 1997). Although many of the Ophryoscolecidae are well described and documented, there is still considerable debate on the taxonomy of these protozoans, particularly at the species level, largely due to the variable nature of key characters, such as caudal spines.

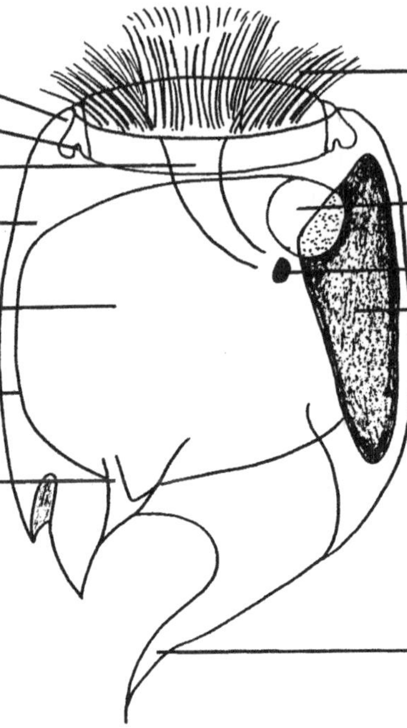

Fig. 4.1. Line drawing of typical entodiniomorph protozoan from the rumen, *Entodinium caudatum*, with caudal spine (mean length × width, 35 μm × 28 μm). Features of cell morphology useful for taxonomic purposes are included.

Ciliates of the family Isotrichidae are far less complex taxonomically than the Ophryoscolecidae, with only the three species *Isotricha intestinalis*, *Isotricha prostoma* and *Dasytricha ruminantium* being commonly encountered. Despite there being few common species of isotrich ciliates, they are numerous and often account for 30% or more of total ciliates in the rumen. *Isotricha* spp. and *D. ruminantium* have a flexible cell wall and their entire surface is covered by cilia; *D. ruminantium* is smaller than the other species (Dehority, 1993).

Recent genetic studies, based on the DNA sequence of small subunit rRNA genes (Wright *et al.*, 1997) and internally transcribed spacer regions (Wright, 1999), have shed some light on the genetic relatedness and evolutionary divergence of the rumen ciliates. Wright *et al.* (1997) determined from their analysis that *Isotricha* and *Dasytricha* always paired in the same clade (or branch of the phylogenetic tree) with the entodiniomorphid ciliates to form a monophyletic grouping of ruminal ciliates (the trichostomes). This conclusion has been supported with the analysis of more DNA sequences from species within the Ophryoscolecidae. In a study of isolates of *I. prostoma* from distinct geographical areas (northern America and Australia), Wright (1999) found no genetic variation based on the DNA sequence of spacer regions, which were 100% conserved.

The entodiniomorphid protozoa ferment two different carbohydrate substrates. The larger species, *E. maggii*, *Epidinium ecaudatum caudatum* and *Ostracodinium obtusum bilobum*, have high cellulolytic activities and rapidly colonize fibrous material that is introduced into the rumen. The smaller *Entodinium* spp. are mainly starch digesters and appear to have little or no cellulolytic activity. All of the entodiniomorphid protozoa prey on rumen bacteria, and *Entodinium bursa* and *P. multivesiculatum* also prey on other protozoa. The major substrates for the holotrich protozoa are soluble sugars. The holotrichs also prey on rumen bacteria.

Fungi

Chytridiomycete fungi are the major fungal inhabitants of the gastrointestinal tract of herbivores. These organisms are obligate anaerobes, saprotrophic on ingested feedstuffs, and may contribute significantly to the ability of the animal to utilize plant material through the digestion and fermentation of plant structural polysaccharides. They are only found inhabiting the gastrointestinal tract of herbivores, and are believed to have evolved from aquatic *Chytridiomycetes* (Hobson and Stewart, 1997). They were first recorded from the rumen, but until comparatively recently were confused with flagellate protozoa. Orpin (1974) examined the diurnal fluctuations in numbers of these 'flagellates', and was successful in cultivating the organisms and unravelling the life cycle to show the resemblances to aquatic chytridiomycetes.

Currently, the gut-inhabiting *Chytridiomycetes* comprise five genera within the family *Neocallimastigaceae* in the order *Neocallimastigales*. The first organism to be formally described was *Neocallimastix frontalis*, a species with polyflagellate zoospores and a monocentric thallus. Two other genera of monocentric fungi are morphologically distinct from *Neocallimastix*. *Piromyces* has a similar rhizoidal and sporangial development to *Neocallimastix* but is characterized by uniflagellate zoospores. *Caecomyces* also has uniflagellate zoospores but has a rhizoidal development quite distinct from the other monocentric genera. The normal rhizoidal system is absent and appears to have been replaced by a bulbous type of rhizoid, comprising up to seven spherical bodies (Hobson and Stewart, 1997).

Recently, in addition to the fungi with monocentric thalli, fungi possessing more than one sporangium per thallus (polycentric thalli) were isolated from ruminants. Two genera, *Orpinomyces* and *Anaeromyces*, are currently recognized. Species of *Orpinomyces* are characterized by an extensive rhizoidal system with numerous sporangia and polyflagellate zoospores. *Anaeromyces* are characterized by monoflagellate zoospores and ellipsoidal to fusiform sporangia.

Comparative sequence analysis of 18S-like rRNA genes from the rumen chytrids has shown that they form a cohesive group that are more closely related to the true fungi than to other eukaryotes (Li and Heath, 1993). Isozymes have also been used to identify the relationships between 23 anaerobic rumen fungi and seven aerobic chytrids. The anaerobic rumen fungi formed a monophyletic group that was distinct from the aerobic chytrids.

The generalized life history of gut-inhabiting anaerobic chytridiomycetes is well known (Fig. 4.2) and has been reviewed on a number of occasions (Hobson and Stewart, 1997). Motile zoospores attach to freshly ingested plant material and encyst. Germination follows, and rhizoidal growth ramifies through the plant material, digesting it for the nutrition of the fungus. In monocentric genera, a single zoosporangium arises and, within the zoosporangium, zoospores develop and mature. Release of zoospores to complete the life cycle is dependent on plant material entering the rumen, and the peak population density of zoospores occurs from 15 min to 1 h after once-daily feeding, depending on the genera of fungi present.

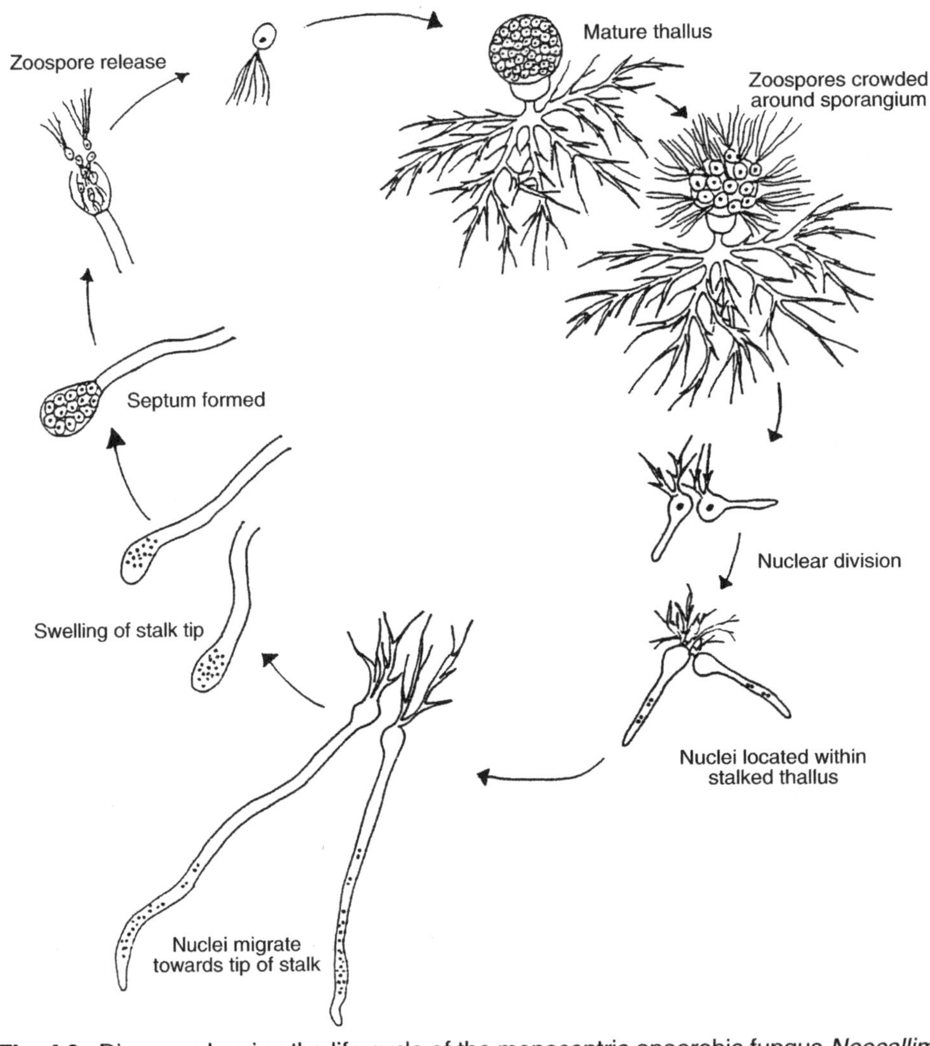

Fig. 4.2. Diagram showing the life cycle of the monocentric anaerobic fungus *Neocallimastix* commonly found in the rumen. Resting sporangia are not included in the diagram but are most probably responsible for survival in the environment outside the intestinal tract.

A further stage in the life cycle of the anaerobic chytrids has been postulated (Davies *et al.*, 1993): a survival stage (cyst or resistant zoosporangium) that is tolerant of oxygen. It was found that survival rates were much higher in samples of fungal populations taken from postgastric regions of the alimentary tract, particularly from the large intestine and faeces, rather than samples taken from pregastric regions. Viable organisms were cultured from faeces up to 252 days after storage at ambient room temperature.

Bacteriophages

Large numbers of bacterial viruses – bacteriophages – are present in the rumen. Bacteriophages are obligate pathogens of bacteria and are ubiquitous in the rumen ecosystem. Bacteriophages lyse their bacterial hosts within the rumen and are a factor involved in protein recycling within the rumen, a process identified as reducing the efficiency of feed utilization. However, their presence may not be entirely detrimental to the ecosystem and it has been argued (Swain *et al.*, 1996) that bacteriophages may also be involved in the maintenance of a balanced ecosystem and may play a role in recycling limiting nutrients within the rumen.

Early reports provided detailed accounts of the numbers and morphological diversity of bacteriophages observed in the rumen. More than 10^9 bacteriophage particles ml^{-1} of ruminal contents and between 26 and 40 morphologically distinct types, within more than 20 morphologically different bacteria, have been reported. Bacteriophages have been classified into three viral families (*Myoviridae*, *Siphoviridae* and *Podoviridae*). Most recently, in an effort to enable the accurate and reproducible enumeration of bacteriophages in the rumen, Klieve and Swain (1993) developed a DNA-based method of enumeration, which confirmed phage densities of 10^9–10^{10} particles ml^{-1} of rumen fluid.

Both classic lytic bacteriophages and temperate bacteriophages occur in the rumen. The former infect and then lyse bacteria, whereas the latter infect bacteria and either lyse the cells or integrate their DNA into the bacterial chromosome. Thereafter these bacteriophages exist from one generation to another as an integral part of the bacteria. Many of the bacteriophages that have been isolated on rumen bacteria are lytic to their hosts, but temperate bacteriophages have been recorded from several rumen bacterial species. Klieve *et al.* (1989) concluded that temperate bacteriophages were widespread among the rumen bacteria and reported that 25% of culturable rumen bacterial isolates contain temperate bacteriophages that could be induced to enter vegetative growth and lyse the host with mitomycin C. As not all bacteriophages respond to a single inducing agent, the true numbers of temperate bacteriophages in rumen bacteria is likely to be much greater than 25%.

In addition to high numbers and diversity, the bacteriophage populations in the rumen have been found to be highly dynamic. Swain *et al.* (1996) found that no two animals had identical bacteriophage populations, even when penned together and consuming the same ration. This suggested that considerable individual diversity in bacteriophage populations occurred between animals. Despite these individual differences, total bacteriophage DNA was similar for animals within groups and varied between groups of animals, suggesting that nutritional and environmental factors may influence overall phage activity in the rumen. In sheep fed once daily, a distinct diurnal variation in the bacteriophage population was observed (Swain *et al.*, 1996). In a survey of the total bacteriophage numbers present in the rumen contents of beef cattle, dairy cattle and sheep offered diets of fresh forage, dry forage or grain, with and without a variety of supplements (Klieve *et al.*, 1998), animals on dry feed had 30–50% fewer bacteriophages than those on green pasture; animals in feedlots had fewer again (10% of those at pasture). This trend appeared to be unaffected by animal species or the feeding of supplements. These authors concluded that the extent of bacteriophage activity could be influenced by diet, suggesting that, if the factors involved could be found, it might be possible to reduce bacteriophage-mediated bacterial lysis through dietary manipulation.

Although considerable progress towards a better understanding of bacteriophages in the rumen has been made in recent times, our knowledge of their interactions with bacterial populations, the factors controlling population dynamics and their impact on animal nutrition remains limited.

Stability of the Ecosystem

Ruminal disorders

When ruminants are offered diets containing a high proportion of cereal grain, the pH of the rumen contents often falls to very low levels. This decreases the efficiency of conversion of feed to SCFA and microbial protein for animal production. The drop in pH is often associated with the accumulation of lactic acid, which can lead to acute lactic acidosis (Hobson and Stewart, 1997).

S. bovis has been implicated as the main causative agent in the syndrome, as it is capable of rapid growth on starch-based substrates, with the production of lactic acid as the primary fermentation end-product (Hobson and Stewart, 1997). It has been generally hypothesized that the rapid growth by *S. bovis* exceeds the rate that can be attained by lactic acid-utilizing bacteria and other starch-utilizing bacteria, which might compete with *S. bovis* for substrate (Hobson and Stewart, 1997). This results in an overgrowth by the faster-growing *S. bovis* and the accumulation of lactic acid, with the concomitant drop in pH leading to acidotic ruminal conditions and reduced efficiency of feed utilization. This mechanism is summarized in Fig. 4.3.

On the basis of this hypothesis, it is a widely practised management strategy to introduce ruminants to grain over an extended period, with the proportion of grain in the diet increasing over that period. This is thought

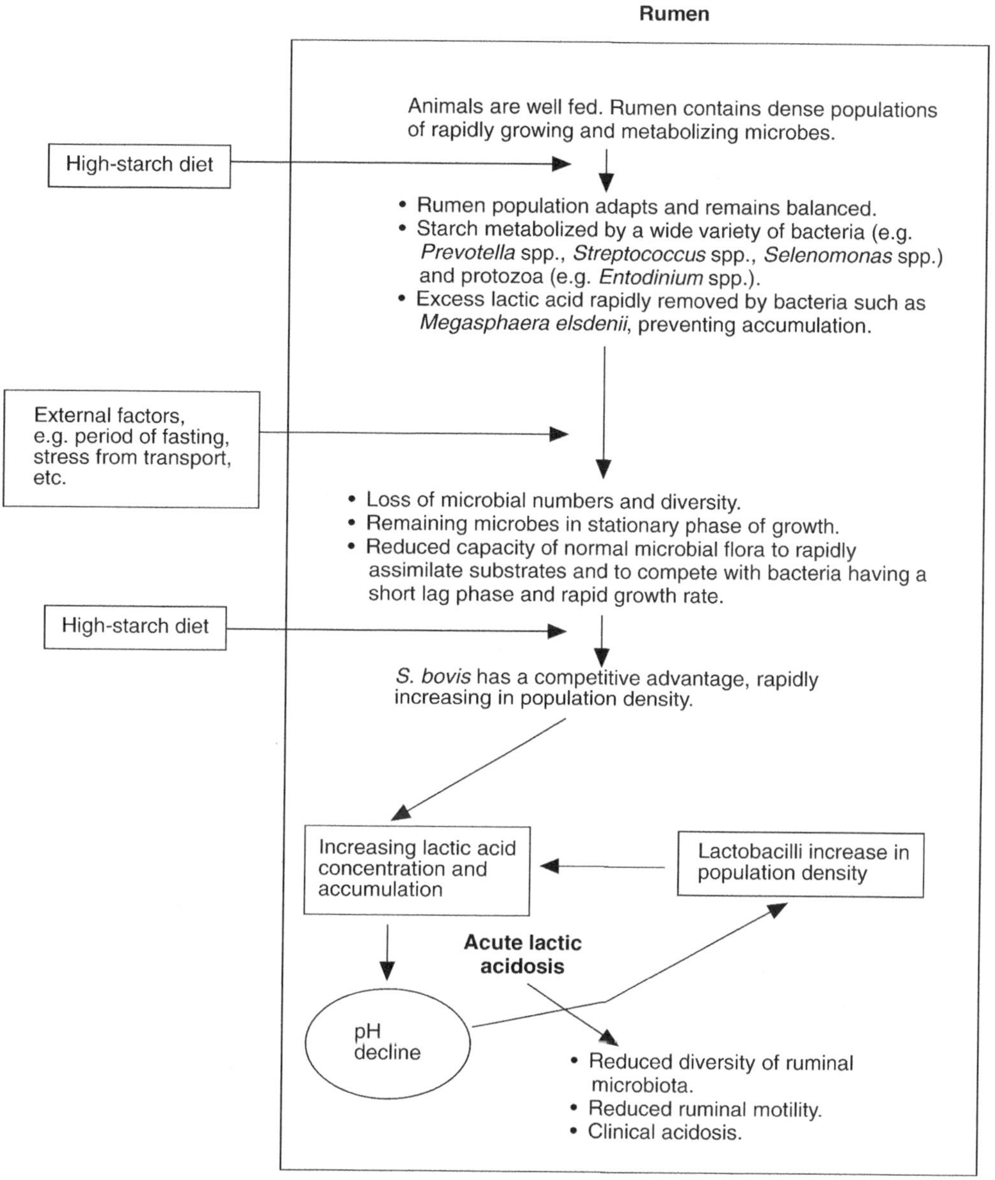

Fig. 4.3. Development of acute ruminal lactic acidosis on high-starch diets.

to allow time for the resident populations of bacteria that utilize lactic acid and others that ferment starch to keep up with the growth of *S. bovis* and to prevent acidosis from occurring. Alternative preventive biocontrol measures have been suggested and these include the inoculation of ruminants probiotically with lactate-utilizing bacteria, such as *M. elsdenii* and *S. ruminantium*, and alternative starch-degrading bacteria, and the control of the growth of *S. bovis* with antibiotics or bacteriophages (Owens *et al.*, 1998).

However, it appears that the use of bacteriophages may be limited, due to the narrow, strain-specific, host range of the bacteriophages isolated to date (Klieve *et al.*, 1999).

With the exception of probiotically introduced bacteria to control acidosis, most other alternative strategies are directed at the removal or reduction in the size of the *S. bovis* population. From both *in vitro* and *in vivo* work, it would appear that the presence of *S. bovis* and the rapid introduction to a starch-based diet alone are insufficient to trigger an episode of lactic acidosis. It would appear that other factors – perhaps a period of feed deprivation – are required to predispose the rumen and allow *S. bovis* to outcompete other, normally dominant bacteria.

Detoxification by rumen microbes

Forage plants often contain antinutritive or secondary compounds that can seriously restrict their value as animal feeds. These secondary metabolites are thought to have a defensive role that ensures survival of the plant, by protecting them against insect predation or by restricting grazing by herbivores. There are many examples of plants being toxic to non-ruminant but not ruminant animals, because ruminal microbial activity transforms or degrades these compounds into less toxic or harmless products (Hobson and Stewart, 1997; Mackie *et al.*, 1997).

Ruminal adaptation to plant toxins

Apart from degrading polysaccharides, nitrogenous compounds, lipids and nucleic acids, the ruminal ecosystem has the ability to adapt and increase its capacity to metabolize minor components, such as plant secondary compounds. The size of the population of toxin-degrading microorganisms in the unadapted rumen is determined primarily by its ability to derive energy for growth from the normal feed constituents. The population is likely to increase in size when a toxic substrate can be exploited as an additional source of energy. Also, the toxin-degrading population can be selected for by providing a diet that contains preferred nutrients and substrates that are cometabolized with the toxin. Induction of enzyme(s) may also influence the rate of detoxification and this can be manipulated by feeding non-toxic analogues of the secondary compound. The degradative pathway for a toxin often involves a consortium of microorganisms, since the enzymes involved may not be present in one organism. Even when a single species of ruminal bacterium is capable of degrading a toxin, there are probably several distinct strains of the species present in the rumen.

The best example of the commercial exploitation of ruminal detoxification for production purposes is the use of the ruminal bacterium *Synergistes jonesii* to detoxify the mimosine (Fig. 4.4) from tropical browse legume *Leucaena leucocephala* (Jones and Megarrity, 1986). This tree is

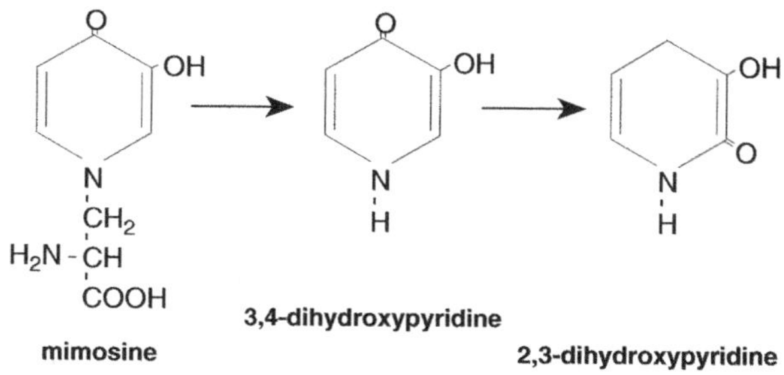

Fig. 4.4. Detoxification of mimosine to 3,4-dihydroxypyridine and 2,3-dihydroxypridine by *Synergistes jonesii.* This is followed by ring cleavage and subsequent metabolism to volatile fatty acids and ammonia.

widely used as a supplement but is toxic to ruminants in some parts of the world. However, tolerance to mimosine by animals in different geographical regions led to the proposal that detoxification was related to the presence or absence of rumen microbes capable of degrading mimosine. Support for this hypothesis was provided by transferring mimosine-degrading activity to Australian ruminants from goats adapted to *Leucaena* in Indonesia and Hawaii. This work has provided the precedent for exploiting the diverse and dynamic population of rumen microorganisms as a solution to the antinutritive properties of many forages. The ecology of *S. jonesii* is remarkable in that the organism appears to be transferable between cattle, sheep and goats and can establish in the rumen after being cultured in the laboratory (Mackie *et al.*, 1997). Several attempts to colonize the rumen with different genera of laboratory strains of bacteria have failed and thus the microbial ecology of mimosine detoxification may be exceptional (see Krause *et al.*, 1999b; McSweeney *et al.*, 1999).

Ruminal metabolism of toxins associated with fodder plants

A summary of cases of ruminal detoxification in which there has been chemical confirmation of the degradation or biotransformation of toxin and in which the microbes have been (in part or fully) identified or characterized is presented in Table 4.2. At this stage it is not known whether or not the detoxifying microorganisms are specific to a ruminant species (cattle, sheep or goats).

Manipulation of the rumen ecosystem

The gut ecosystem of ruminants can be manipulated to improve production efficiency, product quality and microbial food safety. Modification strategies that are used commercially or are the focus of recent research include feeding antimicrobial compounds, probiotics and inoculants of natural and genetically modified organisms (GMOs).

Table 4.2. Microbial detoxification mechanisms in the rumen (referenced in Hobson and Stewart, 1997; Mackie *et al.*, 1997).

Compound	Modification/activity	Microorganisms involved
Nitrogenous compounds		
Non-protein amino acids		
Mimosine	Ring cleavage of 3,4-dihydroxypyridine	*Synergistes jonesii*
Lathrogens		
Diaminobutyric acid	Modification not determined	Unidentified isolates
Oxalyldiaminopropionic acid		
Aliphatic nitro compounds		
3-nitro-1-propionic acid	Reduction of the nitro group and deamination to β-alanine	*Megasphaera elsdenii*, *Coprococcus* spp.,
3-nitro-1-propanol	Reduction to 3-amino-1-propanol	*Selenomonas* spp.
Nitrate–nitrite	Reduction of nitrate to nitrite	*Selenomonas* spp.
	Reduction of nitrite to ammonia	No isolates identified
Phenolics		
Hydrolysable tannin	Ester hydrolysis	*Selenomonas ruminantium*, *Streptococcus* spp.
Trihydroxybenzenoids (e.g. gallate)	Dehydroxylation	*Eubacterium oxidoreducens*
	Ring cleavage	*Streptococcus bovis*, *Syntrophoccus bovis*, *Coprococcus* spp.
Ferulic and *p*-coumaric acid	Dehydroxylation	Unknown
Flavonoid glycosides	Glycoside hydrolysis	*Selenomonas* spp., *Butyrivibrio* spp.
	Heterocyclic ring cleavage	*Peptococcus* spp., *Eubacterium oxidoreducens*, *Butyrivibrio* spp.
Condensed and hydrolysable tannin	Tannin tolerance	*Streptococcus gallolyticus*, *Streptococcus bovis*, *Clostridium* spp., *Prevotella ruminicola*, *Selenomonas ruminantium*
Phyto-oestrogens		
Isoflavones		
Formononetin, daidzein, genistein, biochanin, coumestrol	Demethylation Heterocyclic ring cleavage	No isolates identified
Oxalate	Metabolized to formate	*Oxalobacter formigenes*

Table 4.2. *Continued.*

Compound	Modification/activity	Microorganisms involved
Pyrrolizidine alkaloids		
Heliotrine	Ester hydrolysis of carbon side-chain Reduction of 1,2 double bond of the heterocyclic ring	*Peptococcus heliotrinereducens*
Mycotoxins		
Trichothecenes T-2 toxin, HT-2 toxin Deoxynivalenol, diacetoxyscirpenol, ochratoxin	De-epoxidation De-esterification Isovaleryl de-esterification	*Butyrivibrio fibrisolvens* *Selenomonas ruminantium*

Antimicrobial agents and microbial feed additives

Several excellent reviews on antimicrobial agents and microbial feed additives for ruminants have already been undertaken (Nagaraja *et al.*, 1997). However, the use of these feed additives is currently limited in sheep production systems compared with cattle.

Ionophore antibiotics are the most commonly used antimicrobial agent in ruminant production, and improvements in feed conversion efficiency and growth are attributed mainly to changes in microbial fermentation. Monensin has gained wide acceptance, particularly in cattle production, but other ionophores in use include lasalocid, laidlomycin, lysocellin, narasin, salinomycin and tetronasin. In general terms, ionophore antibiotics disturb the flow of cations across the cell membrane of Gram-positive bacteria, thus producing a bacteriostatic effect, which alters rumen microbial populations and fermentation patterns. The primary changes in rumen function due to ionophore feeding are: (i) increased propionate and decreased methane production; (ii) decreased proteolysis and deamination of amino acids; and (iii) decreased lactic acid production and froth development. These ruminal effects improve productivity through increased efficiency of energy and nitrogen metabolism in ruminal disorders associated with grain feeding. Monensin has produced improvements in microbial protein synthesis and nitrogen digestion in sheep fed concentrate diets and these responses are also associated with decreased rumen protozoa.

Inclusion of strains of *Saccharomyces cerevisiae* and *Aspergillus oryzae* in the diet of sheep has stimulated the total and cellulolytic bacterial numbers in the rumen and resulted in increased rates of digestion, but this has not consistently translated into production responses on a range of diets (Jouany *et al.*, 1998).

Inoculants of natural ruminant microorganisms

The introduction of naturally occurring organisms into the ruminant gut has been investigated for protection from plant toxicity and decreased susceptibility to rumen acidosis (discussed in previous sections), for improving fibre digestion and for controlling the shedding of pathogenic gut bacteria.

Highly fibrolytic *Ruminococcus* strains have been evaluated for ability to colonize the rumen and enhance fibre digestion when used as inoculants (Krause *et al.*, 2001a). Tracking systems based on strain-specific 16S rDNA sequences indicate that inoculated *Ruminococcus* strains did not persist for longer than 3 weeks before reaching undetectable levels. However, these trials demonstrated that some improvement in digestibility of cellulose may be possible when highly fibrolytic bacteria are dosed into ruminants, but changes were small and they do not necessarily translate into an increase in forage digestion.

Gut bacteria such as *Escherichia coli* O157:H7, which is carried by ruminants and causes haemorrhagic colitis and haemolytic–uraemic syndrome in humans, have caused concern recently, due to an increase in frequency of human illness. One approach to dealing with this problem has been to isolate from ruminants non-pathogenic *E. coli*, which, when administered as probiotics, appear to reduce the level of carriage of *E. coli* O157:H7 (Zhao *et al.*, 1998).

Inoculants of recombinant ruminal microorganisms

Enhancing or introducing a foreign metabolic function to the rumen by genetic manipulation holds significant potential, but few GMOs have been tested in animals. The most successful project involving recombinant ruminal bacteria involves reducing toxicity from forage plants that contain fluoroacetate. A gene encoding a dehalogenase for fluoroacetate from the soil bacterium *Moraxella* species has been introduced into *B. fibrisolvens* OB156 and AR14. The modified organisms detoxified fluoroacetate and survived in the rumen of sheep for 5 months without loss of the gene (Gregg *et al.*, 1994). However, these experiments demonstrated that the population of GMOs differed between animals and fluctuated substantially within an animal from day to day.

A major research effort has recently been directed at constructing recombinant ruminal bacteria with enhanced fibre-degrading capacity. *B. fibrisolvens* H17c was transformed with a plasmid containing a xylanase gene from *Neocallimastix patriciarum* (Xue *et al.*, 1997). Although this GMO had enhanced xylan-degrading capacity, it failed to establish in the rumen (Krause *et al.*, 2001b). Attempts to introduce cellulases (CelA and CelD) from *N. patriciarum* and *R. albus* and an acetylxylan esterase from *N. patriciarum* into *B. fibrisolvens* using the same strategy have not been successful.

Even though there has been a substantial research effort during the last decade, there are still major technical difficulties restricting the utility of recombinant technology for the rumen (McSweeney *et al.*, 1999). Rapid progress is being impeded by a lack of transformation systems for different genera and species of bacteria (Flint, 1994), insufficient control of gene expression and efficiency of enzyme production and secretion, genetic instability and the poor competitive fitness of GMOs.

The fluoroacetate-degrading GMO demonstrates that the approach is technically feasible, but environmental and regulatory concerns must be addressed if this technology is to be adopted. The spread of recombinant organisms from the target host animal to other herbivores and their impact on dietary preference and grazing behaviour is of primary concern.

Future Directions

The use of molecular ecology techniques will revolutionize our approach to microbial ecology in the gastrointestinal tract and will provide not simply increased understanding, but a complete description of the gut ecosystem. Rather than replacing the classical culture-based system, the new molecular techniques can be used in combination with the classical approach to improve cultivation, speciation and evaluation of biodiversity. Development and application of these procedures and techniques will result in greater insight into the community structure and activity of gut microbial communities, in relation to functional interactions between different bacteria and spatial and temporal relationships between different microbes and between microbes and feed particles, as well as between the indigenous microbes and the host animal. This will link the distribution and identity of microbes in their natural environment with their genetic potential and *in situ* activities. This is the ultimate goal of the microbial ecologist.

Future developments in rumen microbial ecology, diversity and metabolism will be greatly influenced by the application of genomics – the mapping and sequencing of genomes and analysis of gene and genome function – especially the tools of comparative and functional genomics. At present, genome sequencing of two major rumen fibre-degrading bacteria (*F. succinogenes* S85 and *R. albus* 8) is being carried out by the North American Consortium for Genomics of Fibrolytic Rumen Bacteria. Despite these anticipated advances, animal agriculture is under increasing pressure and public scrutiny to make animal production and animal products safe and sustainable. This will drive future developments in: (i) eliminating the use of growth-promoting antibiotics; (ii) the strategic application of probiotics to enhance adaptation and control ruminal disorders; (iii) reducing shedding and carcass contamination by food-borne pathogens using preharvest technologies and strategies; and (iv) controlling the transmission of neurological spongiform encephalopathies by regulating by-product feeding.

References

Bryant, M.P. (1959) Bacterial species in the rumen. *Bacteriological Reviews* 23, 125–153.

Clarke, R.T.J. and Bauchop, T. (1977) *Microbial Ecology of the Gut*. Academic Press, New York, 410 pp.

Davies, R.D., Theodorou, M.K., Lawrence, M.I.G. and Trinci, A.P.J. (1993) Distribution of anaerobic fungi in the digestive tract of cattle and their survival in faeces. *Journal of General Microbiology* 139, 1395–1400.

Dehority, B.A. (1993) *Laboratory Manual for Classification and Morphology of Rumen Ciliate Protozoa*. CRC Press, Boca Raton, Florida, 120 pp.

Flint, H.J. (1994) Molecular genetics of obligate anaerobes from the rumen. *Microbiology Letters* 121, 259–268.

Forster, R.J., Gong, J. and Teather, R.M. (1997) Group-specific 16S rRNA hybridization probes for determinative and community structure studies of *Butyrivibrio fibrisolvens* in the rumen. *Applied and Environmental Microbiology* 63, 1256–1260.

Gregg, K., Cooper, C.L., Schafer, D.J., Sharpe, H., Beard, C.E., Allen, J. and Xu, J. (1994) Detoxification of the plant toxin fluoroacetate by a genetically modified rumen bacterium. *Bio/Technology* 12, 1361–1365.

Hobson, P.N. and Stewart, C.S. (1997) *The Rumen Microbial Ecosystem*. Chapman & Hall, New York, 719 pp.

Hungate, R.E. (1960) Symposium: selected topics in microbial ecology. I. Microbial ecology of the rumen. *Bacteriology Reviews* 24, 353–364.

Hungate, R.E. (1966) *The Rumen and its Microbes*. Academic Press, New York, 533 pp.

Jones, R.J. and Megarrity, R.G. (1986) Successful transfer of DHP-degrading bacteria from Hawaiian goats to Australian ruminants to overcome the toxicity of *Leucaena*. *Australian Veterinary Journal* 63, 259–262.

Jouany, J.P., Mathieu, F., Senaud, J., Bohatier, J., Bertin, G. and Mercier, M. (1998) Effect of *Saccharomyces cerevisiae* and *Aspergillus oryzae* on the digestion of nitrogen in the rumen of defaunated and refaunated sheep. *Animal Feed Science and Technology* 75, 1–13.

Klieve, A.V. and Swain, R.A. (1993) Estimating ruminal bacteriophage numbers using pulsed field gel electrophoresis and laser densitometry. *Applied and Environmental Microbiology* 59, 2299–2303.

Klieve, A.V., Hudman, J.F. and Bauchop, T. (1989) Inducible bacteriophages from ruminal bacteria. *Applied and Environmental Microbiology* 55, 1630–1634.

Klieve, A.V., Holroyd, R.G., Turner, A.F. and Lindsay, J.A. (1998) Rumen bacterial and protozoal populations in cattle being relocated in tropical Queensland. *Australian Journal of Agricultural Research* 49, 1153–1159.

Klieve, A.V., Heck, G.L., Prance, M.A. and Shu, Q. (1999) Genetic homogeneity and phage susceptibility of ruminal strains of *Streptococcus bovis* isolated in Australia. *Letters in Applied Microbiology* 29, 108–112.

Krause, D.O., Dalrymple, B.D., Smith, W.J., Mackie, R.I. and McSweeney, C.S. (1999a) 16S rDNA sequencing of *Ruminococcus albus* and *Ruminocccus flavefaciens*: design of a signature probe and its application in adult sheep. *Microbiology* 145, 1797–1807.

Krause, D.O., Smith, W.J., Ryan, F.M.E., Mackie, R.I. and McSweeney, C.S. (1999b) Use of 16S rRNA based techniques to investigate the ecological succession of microbial populations in the immature lamb rumen: tracking of specific strains of inoculated *Ruminococcus* and interactions with other microbial populations *in vivo*. *Microbial Ecology* 38, 365–376.

Krause, D.O., Bunch, R.J., Conlan, L.L., Kennedy, P.M., Smith, W.J., Mackie, R.I. and McSweeney, C.S. (2001a) Effect of continuous dosing of highly fibrolytic strains of *Ruminococcus* to adult sheep: assessment of populations using 16S rRNA based methodology and measurement of physiological parameters of fibre digestion. *Microbiolology* 147, 1719–1729.

Krause, D.O., Bunch, R.J., Dalrymple, B.D., Gobius, K.S., Smith, W.J., Xue, G.-P. and McSweeney, C.S. (2001b) *In vitro* and *in vivo* characterization of *Butyrivibrio fibrisolvens* H17c containing a xylanase construct derived from *Neocallimastix patriciarum*. *Journal of Applied Microbiology* 90, 388–396.

Li, J. and Heath, I.B. (1993) Chytridiomycetous gut fungi, oft overlooked contributors to herbivore digestion. *Canadian Journal of Microbiology* 39, 1003–1013.

Lin, C., Raskin, L. and Stahl, D.A. (1997) Microbial community structure in gastrointestinal tracts of domestic animals: comparative analyses using rRNA-targeted oligonucleotide probes. *FEMS Microbiology Ecology* 22, 281–294.

Lloyd, D., Williams, A.G., Amann, R., Hayes, A.J., Durrant, L. and Ralphs, J.R. (1996) Intracellular prokaryotes in rumen ciliate protozoa: detection by confocal laser scanning microscopy after *in situ* hybridisation with fluorescent 16S rRNA probes. *European Journal of Protistology* 32, 523–531.

Mackie, R.I., White, B.A. and Isaacson, R.E. (1997) *Gastrointestinal Microbiology*, Vols 1 (658 pp.) and 2 (680 pp.). Chapman & Hall, New York.

Mackie, R.I., McSweeney, C.S. and Aminov, R.I. (2001) Rumen. In: *Encyclopedia of Life Sciences*. MacMillan Reference, London. (www.els.net)

McSweeney, C.S., Dalrymple, B.P., Gobius, K.S., Kennedy, P.M., Krause, D.O., Mackie, R.I. and Xue, G.-P. (1999) The application of rumen biotechnology to improve the nutritive value of fibrous feedstuffs: pre- and post-ingestion. *Livestock Production Science* 59, 265–283.

Nagaraja, T.G., Newbold, C.J. and Wallace, R.J. (1997) Manipulation of rumen fermentation. In: Hobson, P.N. and Stewart, C.S. (eds) *The Rumen Microbial Ecosystem*. Chapman & Hall, New York, pp. 523–632.

Ogata, K., Aminov, R.I., Nagamine, T., Sugiura, M., Tajima, K., Mitsumori, M., Sekizaki, T., Kudo, H., Minato, H. and Benno, Y. (1997) Construction of a *Fibrobacter succinogenes* genomic map and demonstration of diversity at the genomic level. *Current Microbiology* 35, 22–27.

Ogimoto, K. and Imai, S. (1981) *Atlas of Rumen Microbiology*. Japan Scientific Societies Press, Tokyo, 230 pp.

Orpin, C.G. (1974) The rumen flagellate *Callimastix frontalis*: does sequestration occur? *Journal of General Microbiology* 84, 395–398.

Owens, F.N., Secrist, D.S., Hill, W.J. and Gill, D.R. (1998) Acidosis in cattle: a review. *Journal of Animal Science* 76, 275–286.

Swain, R.A., Nolan, J.V. and Klieve, A.V. (1996) Natural variability and diurnal fluctuations within the bacteriophage population of the rumen. *Applied and Environmental Microbiology* 62, 994–997.

Tajima, K., Aminov, R.I., Nagamine, T., Ogata, K., Nakamura, M. and Benno, Y. (1999) Molecular bacterial diversity of the rumen as determined by sequence analysis of 16S rDNA libraries. *FEMS Microbiology Ecology* 27, 159–169.

Tokura, M., Chagan, I., Ushida, K. and Kojima, Y. (1999) Phylogenetic study of methanogens associated with rumen ciliates. *Current Microbiology* 39, 123–128.

Whitford, M.F., Forster, R.J., Beard, C.E., Gong, J. and Teather, R.M. (1998) Phylogenetic analysis of rumen bacteria by comparative sequence analysis of cloned 16S rRNA genes. *Anaerobe* 4, 153–163.

Wood, J., Scott, K.P., Avgustin, G., Newbold, C.J. and Flint, H.J. (1998) Estimation of the relative abundance of different *Bacteroides* and *Prevotella* ribotypes in gut samples by restriction enzyme profiling of PCR-amplified 16S rRNA gene sequences. *Applied and Environmental Microbiology* 64, 3683–3689.

Wright, A.D.G. (1999) Analysis of intraspecific sequence variation among eight isolates of the rumen symbiont, *Isotricha prostoma* (Ciliophora), from two continents. *Journal of Eukaryotic Microbiology* 46, 445–446.

Wright, A.D.G., Dehority, B.A. and Lynn, D.H. (1997) Phylogeny of the rumen ciliates *Entodinium*, *Epidinium* and *Polyplastron* (Litostomatea: Entodiniomorphida) inferred from small subunit ribosomal RNA sequences. *Journal of Eukaryotic Microbiology* 44, 61–67.

Xue, G.-P., Johnson, J.S., Bransgrove, K.L., Gregg, K., Beard, C.E., Dalrymple, B.P., Gobius, K.S. and Aylward, J.H. (1997) Improvement of expression and secretion of a fungal xylanase in the rumen bacterium *Butyrivibrio fibrisolvens* OB156 by manipulation of promoter and signal sequences. *Journal of Biotechnology* 54, 139–148.

Zhao, T., Doyle, M.P., Harmon, B.G., Brown, C.A., Mueller, P.O.E. and Parks, K. (1998) Reduction of carriage of enterohemorrhagic *Escherichia coli* O157:H7 in cattle by inoculation with probiotic bacteria. *Journal of Clinical Microbiology* 36, 641–647.

5 Digestion and Metabolism

E.F. Annison,[1] D.B. Lindsay[2] and J.V. Nolan[3]

[1]*Faculty of Veterinary Science, University of Sydney, Camden, New South Wales, Australia;* [2]*66 Lantree Crescent, Trumpington, Cambridge, UK;* [3]*School of Rural Science and Agriculture, University of New England, Armidale, New South Wales, Australia*

Introduction

In sheep and other ruminants, the exposure of ingested food to the metabolic activities of ruminal bacteria, protozoa and fungi (see Mackie *et al.*, Chapter 4, this volume) has profound implications for the digestion and metabolism of food.

Plant carbohydrates, usually the major sources of energy in ruminant diets, are largely fermented to short-chain fatty acids (SCFA). These consist mainly of acetate, propionate and butyrate and are readily absorbed from the rumen and metabolized in tissues to support maintenance and production. The degradation of β-linked glucose polymers (cellulose and hemicellulose) from plant cell walls is of obvious nutritional benefit, since these materials are not hydrolysed by the endogenous enzymes of the host animal. In contrast, the ready fermentation of starch and other α-linked glucose polymers, which are potential sources of glucose if they reach the small intestine (SI), implies that only small amounts of glucose are absorbed from the SI (see p. 106).

Complex dietary lipids are rapidly hydrolysed in the rumen by bacterial lipases, with the production of free fatty acids. These are largely unsaturated and undergo extensive biohydrogenation, which accounts for the relative hardness of ruminant carcass fat, and for the difficulty in changing the degree of unsaturation of the fatty acids of carcass fat and milk fat by dietary manipulation.

The fate of dietary protein in the rumen is a further striking example of the impact of rumen microorganisms on digestion and metabolism. Whereas in non-ruminants the quality of dietary protein largely depends on its amino acid(s) (AA) composition and digestibility, in ruminants dietary protein is substantially, but rarely completely, degraded by microbial activity, with the formation of ammonia. Part of this ammonia, together with peptides and free AA produced during its formation, are utilized by ruminal microorganisms for protein synthesis, the energy for cell growth being provided by the anaerobic fermentation of organic matter. The remainder of the ammonia produced in the rumen is absorbed, and a varying proportion returned to the rumen as urea in saliva. This urea is rapidly broken down to ammonia to become available as a nitrogen source for autotrophic microorganisms. These processes mean that the AA reaching the SI are largely provided by undegraded food protein and microbial protein (see p. 108). The postruminal digestion of protein and, indeed, the utilization of absorbed AA in tissues are qualitatively similar in ruminants and non-ruminants.

The integration of ruminal and tissue metabolism in the utilization of feed by sheep is summarized in Fig. 5.1.

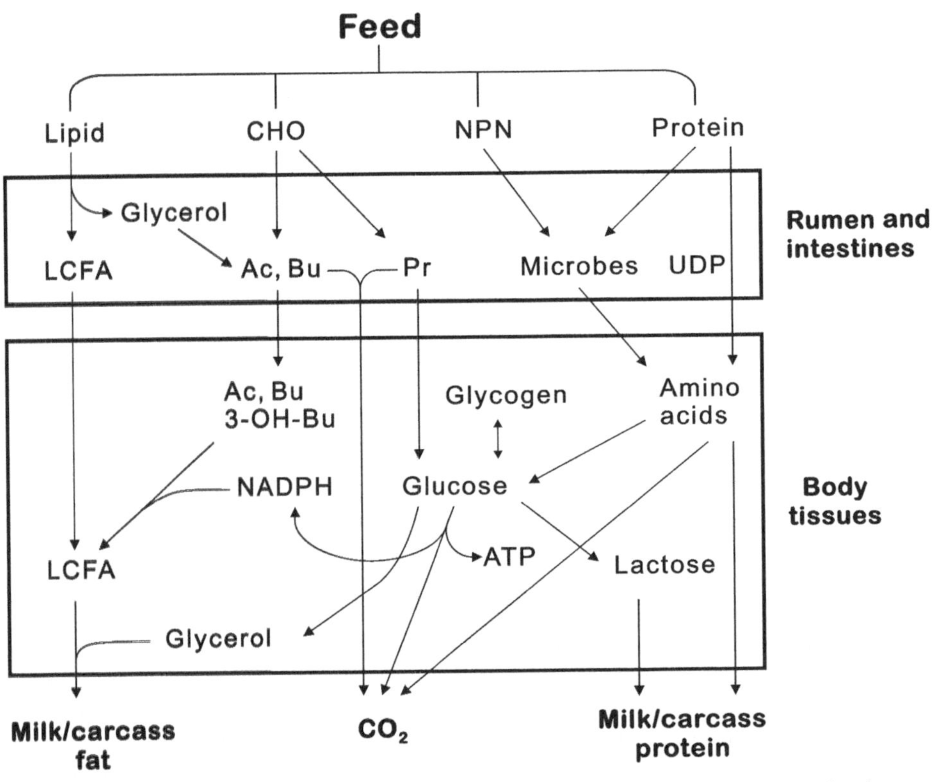

Fig. 5.1. A summary of the digestion and metabolism of feed components into simpler intermediates and oxidation or resynthesis of the latter into materials in animal products. The top box represents fermentation in the rumen and hind-gut, and digestion and absorption of simpler products from the gut; the lower box represents metabolism of absorbed short- and long-chain fatty acids, glucose and amino acids in host tissues where oxygen is present. CHO, carbohydrate; NPN, non-protein nitrogen; LCFA, long-chain fatty acids; Ac, acetate; Bu, butyrate; Pr, propionate; UDP, undegraded dietary protein; NADPH, nicotinamide adenine dinucleotide phosphate; ATP, adenosine triphosphate.

Digestion and Metabolism in the Rumen

The maintenance of a healthy rumen ecosystem is a prerequisite of ruminant nutrition, because the digestion of the cellulose/hemicelluloses, the major sources of energy in forage-based ruminant diets, depends on the activities of the microflora. In this context, active microbial growth can only occur if adequate amounts of energy substrates, nitrogen sources and other minerals and growth factors are simultaneously present in the medium: this condition has been referred to as 'synchrony of nutrient supply'. The greatest threat to the stability of the ecosystem is increased rumen acidity, since rumen pH has a major influence on the type and number of microflora. In particular, below pH 6.0 the growth of cellulolytic bacteria is inhibited, and rates of cellulose/hemicellulose digestion fall. In practice, major changes in diet should be gradually introduced over 7–10 days to allow the rumen microflora to adapt to the new substrates.

Carbohydrate digestion

Plant carbohydrates can be loosely grouped into storage carbohydrates and polysaccharides, which form part of the cell-wall structure (Table 5.1). Structural polysaccharides can be either covalently linked or not linked to lignin. The former group, which include cellulose and hemicellulose, are insoluble and only partially digested in the rumen. The latter group (pectins, β-glucans) are readily fermented in the rumen but, like cellulose and hemicellulose, do not give rise to lactic acid. Their fermentation is inhibited by low pH.

Insoluble structural polysaccharides

Cellulose is the major structural component of the forage cell wall. Its close physical and, to a lesser extent, chemical association with other cell-wall components (Table 5.1) results in a complex and heterogeneous structure, which makes chemical analysis a formidable task. Indeed, the difficulty in defining the composition of forages has bedevilled attempts to predict their nutritive value from their composition, as perceptively discussed by Van Soest (1994).

The microbial degradation of complex polysaccharides in the rumen is accomplished by the cooperative efforts of a range of cellulolytic and non-cellulolytic microorganisms (Flint and Forsberg, 1995). Synergy between consortia of microorganisms, involving sequential hydrolysis and end-product utilization, has been demonstrated in studies using co-cultures of cellulolytic fungi or bacteria and non-cellulolytic species. Plant materials entering the rumen are rapidly colonized with bacteria and fungi, and close contact of microorganism and substrate facilitates the ready uptake by microflora of the products released by enzymic activity.

Table 5.1. Characteristics of forage carbohydrates.

Class	Component	Structure	Remarks
Insoluble structural polysaccharides	Cellulose	β1–4-glucan in intimate association with hemicellulose, lignin, cutin and silica	Rumen digestion involves the combined effects of a range of cellulolytic and non-cellulolytic organisms
	Hemicellulose	Heterogeneous mixture; common factor is xylan core polymer linked to arabinose and uronic acid	Soluble in acid and alkali
Soluble structural polysaccharides	Pectins	Complex mix of polysaccharides rich in galacturonic acid	Classified chemically by solubility in hot neutral solutions of EDTA
	β-glucans	β1–4-glucose polymers with random β1–4 linkages	Low in grasses, high in lupins and some cereals (oats, barley); limited solubility in water, forming viscous gums
Storage mono-, oligo- and polysaccharides	Starch	α1–4-linked glucose polymers with varying proportions of amylose (linear) and amylopectin (branched)	Degree of branching determines ease of gelatinization and digestion
	Fructans	Fructosans (levans) of grasses are β2–6-linked glucose polymers; inulins of vegetables have β2–1 linkages	Major storage carbohydrates of grasses
	Water-soluble carbohydrates	Include mono-, di-, oligo- and polysaccharides soluble in water	Contribute to storage polymer synthesis

EDTA, ethylenediamine tetra-acetic acid.

The nutritional significance of cellulose utilization has led to an interest in the genetic modification of rumen microorganisms to enhance cellulose fermentation (Russell and Wilson, 1988). A major problem with the enhancement of cellulase/hemicellulase activity in specific organisms is that, as outlined above, the degradation of complex polysaccharides in the rumen involves a consortium of microorganisms. In the short term, the modification of cellulolytic bacteria to improve their tolerance of lower rumen pH may be a more achievable objective (Russell and Wilson, 1988).

The digestibility of cellulose-rich fibrous feeds can be increased by treatment with alkaline reagents to rupture lignin–carbohydrate bonds (Van Soest, 1994). Sodium hydroxide has been used extensively, but in developing countries, where vast amounts of straw are fed to ruminants, ammonia is the preferred alkaline source. Ensiling straw with urea at high moisture levels provides an attractive, low-cost means of treatment. The liberated ammonia, in addition to its role in delignification, contributes to rumen ammonia, which is often a rate-limiting nutrient for microbial growth in forage-fed animals (Preston and Leng, 1987).

Soluble structural polysaccharides

Both pectins and β-glucans are readily fermented in the rumen. The β-glucan content of grasses is low, but the relatively high levels in lupins and some cereal grains, particularly oats and barley, may have antinutritive effects in some non-ruminant species, attributed to the formation of viscous digesta in the SI.

Storage carbohydrates

STARCH. The structure of starch is complex, and the proportions of amylose and amylopectin (Table 5.1), which vary considerably in the cereals commonly used in animal feeds, influence the ease of gelatinization of starch in response to heating under moist conditions. Gelatinization causes loss of hydrogen-bonded internal structures, and the amorphous product is more susceptible to amylase attack. Amylose is more resistant than amylopectin both to gelatinization and to the reassociation of starch molecules in gelatinized starch, termed retrogradation, which gives rise to a form of starch resistant to enzyme attack in the SI.

Methods of processing to increase the digestibility of cereal grains fall into three main groups: those designed to break the pericarp and expose the starch-rich endosperm to enzymic attack, processes that gelatinize the starch and processes involving soaking and partial germination. The first include crushing, grinding, cracking, rolling and crimping, and extrusion and pelleting, although it must be borne in mind that the heat produced by friction in pelleting and extrusion may cause some gelatinization in moist grains.

Unlike cattle, sheep are able to utilize unprocessed grain reasonably well, because they chew it into small fragments, exposing the endosperm to microbial attack. When cereal grains are finely ground before inclusion in ruminant diets, considerable amounts of starch escape ruminal digestion, presumably because the particles are of the size and density that allow them to flow from the rumen before significant microbial attack (Huntington, 1997). Published data on the digestibility of the starch content of maize, sorghum, barley, wheat and oats in the rumen and in the whole alimentary tract have been summarized by Rowe and Pethick (1994).

The increased acidity in the rumen which may occur with starch-rich diets is due to increased production of lactic acid. Both D- and L-lactic acid are produced in the rumen, but the D-isomer, which is cleared more slowly from the circulation, is mainly responsible for lactic acidosis, which, if severe, may cause sickness and death (Mackie *et al.*, Chapter 4, this volume).

The bacteria mainly responsible for lactic acid production in the rumen are *Streptococcus bovis* and *Lactobacillus* spp. The antibiotic virginiamycin can control the proliferation of these bacteria in the rumen and prevent lactic acid accumulation, even when animals are fed high-starch diets without prior adaptation (Rowe and Pethick, 1994).

WATER-SOLUBLE CARBOHYDRATES (WSC). Carbohydrates soluble in cold water include monosaccharides, disaccharides, oligosaccharides and some polysaccharides. A number of free sugars are present in forages at levels too low to be of nutritional significance, but sucrose is the primary sugar for energy transport and, in some plants, energy storage. Sucrose contributes to fructan synthesis (see below). Temperate grasses store fructans in leaves and stems and starch in the seed, whereas tropical plants store only starch. The sugar content of forages is greatly influenced not only by ambient temperatures, but also by light intensity, which regulates photosynthesis. High temperatures promote increased metabolic activity at the expense of sugar content. These factors account for the marked diurnal fluctuations in the sugar content of pasture plants.

FRUCTANS. The glucose chains in both forms of fructans (Table 5.1) begin with a sucrose molecule. The fructan content of grasses is increased at low environmental temperatures and, in perennial ryegrass, may account for as much as 30% of dry matter (DM) (Van Soest, 1994).

Short-chain fatty acid metabolism

The SCFA, which comprise mainly acetate, propionate and butyrate, with small amounts of straight-chain and branched-chain higher acids, are produced in the rumen as end-products of microbial fermentation. The energy generated is utilized for the maintenance and growth of the microbial population. The SCFA account for between 50 and 70% of digestible energy intake.

In adequately fed ruminants, the molar proportions of individual rumen SCFA largely reflect the nature of the diet. High-roughage diets result in increased proportions of acetate, whereas herbage with high levels of WSC or concentrate-based diets result in increased proportions of propionate. Increases in the ratio of rumen acetate to propionate in sheep reduce both the efficiency of use of metabolizable energy (ME) (see SCA, 1990) and microbial protein production. Reasons for the less efficient use of acetate from high-roughage diets are discussed in a later section (p. 112). Microbial protein production can be directly related to rumen propionate concentration (e.g. Dove and Milne, 1994; Trevaskis *et al.*, 2001), and it has been suggested that at rumen acetate : propionate ratios above 3 : 1, the supply of readily available energy limits microbial protein synthesis (Corbett, 1987).

Formation of SCFA

Dietary carbohydrates are degraded to their constituent hexoses and pentoses before being fermented to SCFA via pyruvate (France and Siddons, 1993). The initial conversion of pentoses to hexoses implies that dietary carbohydrate metabolism largely proceeds via hexose, which is metabolized to pyruvate almost exclusively by the Embden–Meyerhof glycolytic pathway. The formation of both acetate and butyrate involves acetyl-coenzyme A (CoA), while propionate production occurs mainly via succinate, although an alternate pathway involving acrylate has been identified. The reductive capacity generated by the conversion of hexose to acetate and butyrate is largely channelled into the formation of propionate from pyruvate and the reduction of CO_2 to methane (Fig. 5.2).

Absorption and metabolism of SCFA in the rumen wall

There is convincing evidence that SCFA transport from the rumen is primarily a passive permeation process, with a linear relationship between concentration and net absorption. Rates of SCFA absorption are influenced by rumen pH, however, since undissociated forms of the acids are absorbed more rapidly than fatty acid anions. At pH 6.0, for example, which is at the lower end of the normal range of rumen pH, only about 5% of acetic acid in the rumen is undissociated, but this value rises to about 25% at pH 5.0. Another factor that influences SCFA absorption is their metabolism by the rumen epithelium. Although only a small amount of absorbed acetate is lost, a considerable proportion of butyrate and significant amounts of propionate are metabolized during passage from the rumen. These metabolic activities, which help to main-

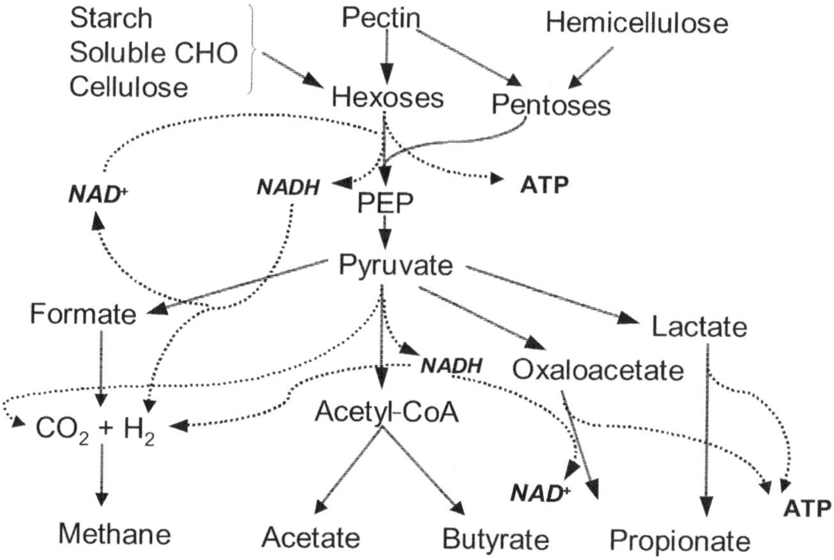

Fig. 5.2. The pathways by which plant constituents are fermented by anaerobic microorganisms in the rumen and converted to short-chain fatty acids and gases (CO_2, CH_4 and H_2). ATP and NADH are generated within the microbial cells by this fermentation process. The ATP is used for cell maintenance and formation of new polymers (cell growth); the reducing power of NADH is used in the formation of propionate and methane, thereby regenerating NAD^+, which enables the continued conversion of hexose to pyruvate by the glycolytic pathway. CHO, carbohydrate; PEP, phosphoenolpyruvate.

tain concentration gradients between rumen fluid and the portal system, inevitably influence rates of SCFA absorption. The conversion of absorbed butyrate to 3-hydroxybutyrate in the rumen epithelium is largely completed in the liver, and little butyrate enters the general circulation. In a similar fashion, propionate entering the portal system is almost completely removed by the liver to constitute the major contributor to hepatic gluconeogenesis.

Lipid digestion and metabolism

The complex mixture of lipids (phospho- and glycosylglycerides, waxes, pigments and cutin) in forages is usually present at levels of 30–40 g kg^{-1} (DM basis). Cereal grains vary widely in lipid content: about 20 g kg^{-1} in wheat to as much as 70 g kg^{-1} in oats. In herbage the lipid occurs mainly as mono- and digalacto-1,2-diacylglycerides, whereas in cereal grains most of the lipid is in the form of triacylglycerides (TAG). Both classes of lipids contain high proportions of C18 unsaturated fatty acids: linolenic acid predominates in galactolipids and linoleic acid in cereal lipids.

In the rumen, all classes of lipids are rapidly hydrolysed by bacterial lipases, with the liberation of free long-chain fatty acids (LCFA), a high proportion of which are unsaturated. For sheep on forage diets, intakes of LCFA are low – about 12–16 g day^{-1}. These fatty acids are adsorbed on to the surface of finely divided food particles, where they undergo extensive biohydrogenation, with the production of a range of *cis* and *trans* positional isomers of octadecenoic acid. The extent of ruminal biohydrogenation of dietary linolenic and linoleic acids is 85–100% and 70–95% respectively, the lower value for linoleic acid being attributed to the uptake of this acid by bacteria (Bauchart *et al.*, 1990).

The first step in the biohydrogenation of linoleic acid in the rumen is isomerization to *cis*-9-, *trans*-11-octadecenoic acid, known as conjugated linoleic acid (CLA), which is a mixture of eight possible positional isomers. Most of the CLA is hydrogenated to stearic acid, but small amounts escape hydrogenation and reach the SI, where CLA is absorbed and incorporated into adipose tissue and milk fat, together with other fatty acids absorbed from the SI. Current interest in CLA stems from reports that it exhibits a range of biological activities, which include inhibition of carcinogenesis and the reduction of carcass fat deposition and milk fat production (see Dunshea and Ostrowska, 1999). The significance of CLA in sheep production is as yet unknown. There is no evidence of LCFA absorption from the rumen, omasum or abomasum.

The inhibitory action of dietary fat on forage digestibility when present in the diet at levels above 5–6% is caused by the antimicrobial activity of the surface-active LCFA liberated by the lipolysis of lipids in the rumen. These effects can be overcome by the inclusion of calcium hydroxide in the diet, which immobilizes LCFA as calcium salts. A process for the protection of unsaturated fat from biohydrogenation was developed by Scott *et al.*

(1970). The feeding of protected fat makes it possible to increase the degree of unsaturation of both carcass fat and milk fat. The LCFA produced by lipolysis leave the rumen adsorbed on to particulate matter and become available for absorption from the SI.

Protein digestion and nitrogen metabolism

The microbes in the rumen ferment and modify the majority of feed proteins and non-protein nitrogen (NPN) just as extensively as they modify feed carbohydrates. Nitrogenous feed materials that are digested by these microbes are considered to be ruminally degradable crude protein (RDP), which is the source of N from which microbial protein is synthesized by microorganisms. This microbial protein is the main source of digestible protein for the animal. A variable fraction of the dietary true protein, however, either remains undegraded or is only partially degraded. This fraction passes to the lower gut and augments the microbial protein available for intestinal digestion. In the context of dietary management and feeding standards, this fraction is often referred to as 'escape protein', 'bypass protein' or 'undegraded dietary protein' (UDP).

RDP sources are degraded by plant or microbial proteases first to peptides, then amino acids and finally, by decarboxylation and/or deamination, to ammonia and SCFA. These fermentation intermediates, along with dietary NPN sources, such as amines or urea, may be assimilated to varying degrees by rumen microbes and used to form enzyme and structural proteins, which represent about 40% of the microbial DM.

Catabolic processes (e.g. carbohydrate and protein degradation) and anabolic processes (new protein, polysaccharide and nucleic acid formation) in microbes usually occur simultaneously but to different degrees in different species. The overall effect is usually to alter the profile of protein and NPN in the microbial products in the digesta flowing out of the rumen from that in the diet, so that the potential value of high-quality feed protein is often downgraded whereas NPN sources are upgraded to true protein in the microbial biomass. The latter protein has a high biological value and is a good source of both non-essential and essential AA. The sulphur-containing AA methionine and cysteine (S-AA) are particularly important for wool growth, but their concentration in bacterial proteins may be limiting for optimal production (see Hynd and Masters, Chapter 8, this volume).

The crude-protein concentration in pasture DM may range from 3% in dry, mature roughage (some hays and straws) to over 30% in heavily fertilized grass, where 25–30% of the total N may be present as NPN in forms such as nitrate, ammonia and amides and amines. Legumes, such as white clover, contain up to 24% crude protein in the DM. In leaves, the chloroplasts contain about 75% of the total protein and about 50% of this is a single soluble protein – the photosynthetic enzyme ribulose bisphosphate carboxylase. Proteins are also found in plant cell walls and membranes, and in the mitochondria and nuclei of the cells. Free AA are present in plant cells as intermediates in protein synthesis, as agents in translocation and as the immediate products of assimilation of organic nitrogen by roots. At times, nitrate may be an important non-protein, non-AA N constituent, especially when its rate of reduction to ammonia in plant cells is less than its rate of uptake by the roots (Mangan, 1982).

In general, as plants mature, their fibre content increases and crude-protein content decreases. Moreover, when plants are dried naturally or during haymaking, their proteins tend to be denatured and their solubility and degradability in the rumen reduced. The proportion of UDP in the total crude protein increases accordingly. Heating and solvents used to extract oil from the seeds of cotton, sunflower, canola, coconut and oil-palm also alter the structure of naturally occurring proteins and affect the value of the resulting meals as protein supplements for ruminants, by altering the degradability of these proteins in the rumen. Naturally, in addition to its intrinsic degradability, the time for which any feed protein is subject to attack by plant or microbial enzymes (proteases and peptidases) will also be a major determinant of the extent to which that protein is degraded in the rumen. The turnover rate of feed materials in the rumen, which usually ranges from 2 to 8% h^{-1}, is affected by feed intake, type of feed and other factors.

When formulating diets for sheep or other ruminants, it is helpful to have information about the degradability of dietary protein sources, i.e. the UDP status of the diet. *In vitro* techniques based on protein solubility in rumen fluid or in solutions of commercial enzyme preparations or the so-called *in sacco* technique have been used, despite their limitations, to rank different protein sources. With the *in sacco* technique, test protein sources are placed in bags made of standardized nylon mesh and their disappearance over time is recorded when the bags are placed in the rumen. The results are usually then linked with putative rumen retention times to enable prediction of the proportion of the protein degraded.

After an animal ingests a protein-rich diet, rumen digesta may contain up to 4 g N l^{-1}. Initially, for the reasons given above, the majority of this N is often present as true protein. Degradation of proteins is initiated by plant proteases. Once in the rumen, protein may be adsorbed on to the surface of microbes. Proteolytic enzymes released in the vicinity of the adsorption site then degrade the proteins to peptides. Smaller peptides may appear in rumen fluid or be assimilated locally by the bacteria and further degraded by intracellular deaminases to SCFA and ammonia. These end-products of protein fermentation may be reused within the bacterium in which they were formed or released into the rumen fluid. During periods of rapid degradation of feed protein, rumen peptide and ammonia concentrations tend to increase in the 2–4 h after feeding, with peak concentrations of ammonia rising above 0.4 g N l^{-1}. However, during these periods, peptides and ammonia may also be assimilated by other microbes for growth and protein synthesis, which occur most rapidly when the microbes are simultaneously well supplied with energy-yielding substrates, essential minerals and other growth factors. Trevaskis *et al.* (2001) have stressed the benefits, for synthesis, of synchronizing the availability of fermentable carbohydrate with the N sources. Mean values for the amounts of microbial protein synthesized and available to the animal as digestible true protein are shown in Table 5.2. Assimilation counteracts the build-up in concentrations of peptides and ammonia and lowers the potential peak value after feeding, with the exact nature of the concentration vs. time curve being dependent on the feed protein degradability and the microbial growth conditions.

Some of the ammonia in rumen fluid that is not assimilated by microbes is absorbed via the rumen wall into the bloodstream, at a rate that is determined by its un-ionized concentration in rumen fluid, while a smaller fraction passes out of the rumen in digesta moving to the lower digestive tract. In practical circumstances, when there is rapid production of ammonia in the rumen, e.g. if animals ingest excessive amounts of urea-containing supplements, and especially when pH is relatively high, uptake of ammonia can cause severe ammonia intoxication and deaths of large numbers of animals.

The majority of rumen bacteria have the capacity to assimilate and utilize ammonia as the sole N source when peptides or AA are present in negligible concentrations, although some of the faster-growing species appear to gain a competitive advantage in the rumen when they have access to preformed peptides or AA. Thus, when the natural diet is N-deficient and microbial growth in the rumen is limited only by N availability, supplementation with any source of ammonia may improve rumen microbial activity and growth. In these situations, urea is an effective supplement, provided animals do not ingest excessive amounts (see above). Urea formed in the liver, which enters the rumen in saliva or by diffusion across the rumen wall, is also available to support microbial growth in the rumen in the same way. So-called 'urea recycling' and reuse of N in the rumen for protein synthesis ('protein conservation') enable ruminant animals to survive on diets of relatively low protein content.

Table 5.2. The synthesis of microbial crude protein (MCP) in relation to the intake of fermentable ME (FME), i.e. total ME intake less ME from lipid and UDP, and the level of feeding expressed as multiples of the level for maintenance (M) (AFRC, 1993).

	Level of feeding		
	1M	2M	3M
MCP[a] (g MJ^{-1} FME)	8.8	10.0	10.9
Digestible true protein (g MJ^{-1} FME)	5.6	6.4	7.0

[a]With herbage diets, these values vary with time of year, being directly related to propionate production resulting from the WSC concentration (Dove and Milne, 1994).

Methane production

Methane produced by anaerobic fermentation in the rumen represents an appreciable energy loss, particularly when low-quality roughages are fed (see Kirchgessner *et al.*, 1995). Methane production by ruminants is of considerable current interest in view of the contribution of atmospheric methane to global warming. Attempts to channel the energy normally associated with methanogenesis into assimilable nutrients by the use of additives have been largely unsuccessful. Ionophores, such as monensin, which are widely used in ruminant diets to improve the efficiency of feed utilization, channel the hydrogen involved in methanogenesis into propionate production for the first few days of treatment, but the effects are not sustained (Kirchgessner *et al.*, 1995).

Digestion in the Small Intestine and Absorption of Products

Carbohydrates

Although microorganisms may contain up to 38% DM as α-linked glucose polymers, 6–10% is more typical. In animals given forage diets, this polysaccharide is likely to be their only potential source of glucose. Dietary starch may be significant for sheep when grain is used as a supplement. Substantial variation in the extent of digestion in the rumen was originally reported, depending on the type of grain used. A number of studies with sheep have shown that digestion in the rumen averaged 88 ± 1.4% and in the SI, 7.7 ± 2% (mean starch intake 400 g day^{-1}). For cattle (mean intake 2100 g day^{-1}) the values were, for rumen, 79 ± 3.2% and, for SI, 18.8%.

Starch digestion in the SI is determined by several factors: amylase activity (pancreatic and in the brush-border cells of the mucosa); duodenal pH; oligosaccharidase activity; rate of passage; and rate of absorption of glucose produced.

Amylase has a pH optimum of 6.8, and enzyme activity in the pancreas is 100-fold greater than in the mucosa. Maltase activity (pH optimum 5.8) is two to three orders of magnitude lower and isomaltase is lower still. Amylase activity from the pancreas can be greatly increased by increasing the energy or protein content of the diet. It is now thought – at least for cattle – that amylase activity is likely to be the limiting factor for starch digestion in the SI.

Glucose transport across the enterocyte is predominantly by the $NaHCO_3$/glucose transporter (SGLT1), with exit by the facilitated transporter GLUT2; but there can be a modest amount by paracellular diffusion, which is appreciably greater at high glucose concentrations (Shirazi-Beechey *et al.*, 1995). SGLT1 activity is high in lambs, but declines sharply on weaning; however, it may be reinduced, with a lag period of 3–4 days (probably requiring the production of new enterocytes following the presence of free glucose in the lumen).

Lipids

Some 85% of the lipids entering the SI is in the form of largely saturated LCFA adsorbed on to small feed particles, a consequence of the lipolysis of dietary fats and extensive biohydrogenation of liberated LCFA in the rumen (p. 102). The remaining 15% or so of lipids reaching the SI consist mainly of phospholipids derived from microbial cell membranes. These phospholipids contain a range of odd-numbered carbon-chain fatty acids, mainly C15 and C17, and branched-chain fatty acids. The formation of these LCFA, and of the wide range of isomers of octadecenoic acid during biohydrogenation in the rumen, account for the extraordinarily complex mixture of LCFA present at low levels in ruminant carcass and milk fat.

As in non-ruminants, the key feature of fat absorption from the SI is micelle formation, which depends on the presence of bile salts and an amphiphilic material. In non-ruminants, monoacylglycerides, derived from the partial hydrolysis of dietary TAG, meet this requirement. In the virtual absence of glycerides in ruminant digesta, the role of amphiphile in micelle formation is provided by lysolecithin, derived from the phospholipase-catalysed hydrolysis of lecithin, which enters the SI in bile and pancreatic juice. The latter secretion is the main source of phospholipase.

Micellar fat interacts with the brush border of the intestinal epithelium, with the diffusion of fatty acids and lysolecithin into intestinal cells. The third component of micellar fat, the bile salts, return to the SI where they continue to form micelles before absorption from the ileum, transport to the liver and reincorporation into bile. Absorbed fatty acids are re-esterified to glycerol-3-phosphate to form TAG within small-intestinal cells. These TAG become associated with apolipoproteins, cholesterol and phospholipids to form lipoprotein particles that are secreted from the cells into lymph, which enters the peripheral circulation. These lipoprotein particles are analogous to chylomicrons, but are much smaller and more appropriately classified as very low-density lipoproteins (Drackley, 2000). Fatty acid digestibility in ruminants, which is somewhat lower than in non-ruminants, is similar for C16 and C18 fatty acids (average 79 and 77%, respectively) and is slightly higher for unsaturated than for saturated fatty acids (Doreau and Chilliard, 1997).

Proteins

As a generalization, protein-bound AA entering the SI will be efficiently absorbed as digesta pass through the SI. However, AA N is also secreted into the gut lumen in the form of digestive enzymes and mucus and in sloughed intestinal cells and the net (or apparent) absorption coefficient is lower than 90%. Moreover, the materials with which AA are associated (including lignin and plant cell-wall materials) and the processing or treatment of feeds before they are ingested can affect the overall availability of AA for absorption. A method referred to as the 'mobile nylon bag' method has been used to compare the relative intestinal digestibilities of concentrate (e.g. cereal grains) and roughage materials (grass and silage), and coefficients vary from about 90 to 60% (Tamminga *et al.*, 1990).

Absorption of free AA has long been considered to be the main mode of uptake of AA from the gut, but it is now accepted that uptake of small peptides may often be the predominant mode of AA uptake (Webb and Matthews, 1998).

Microbial protein and UDP are not absorbed intact (except in the neonate when immunoglobular proteins from milk are taken up and provide passive immunity). Rather, they must first be cleaved to di- or tripeptides or hydrolysed further to individual AA before they can be absorbed. Protein digestion begins in the abomasum through the action of gastric proteases, including pepsin and lysozymes. The latter catalyse the hydrolysis of specific glycosidic bonds in mucopolysaccharides found in some bacterial cell walls. In sheep and other ruminants, bacteria usually represent the animal's major source of dietary protein and they should therefore be efficiently digested. Ruminants seem to have evolved with special lysozymes that exhibit activity in the abomasum against the mucopolysaccharides in bacterial cell walls. These lysozymes have lower pH optima and are more resistant to pepsin than lysozymes of other species.

Microbial protein and UDP are partially degraded to medium-length and small peptides in the abomasum and SI by pancreatic proteases. A family of peptidases that are integral membrane proteins is present in the brush border of the small intestine. These continue the hydrolysis of oligopeptides to di- and tripeptides and free AA on the outside surface of the enterocyte, where they become available for absorption.

Di- and tripeptides are taken up by enterocytes via a transporter, which is energized by a transmembrane H^+ gradient via a single H^+-peptide cotransport system (Webb and Matthews, 1998). A transporter (PEPT1) has recently been cloned and its primary structure elucidated. The characteristic of H^+ coupling makes PEPT1 (and a related transporter, PEPT2) unique among the transporters thus far identified in mammalian cells. PEPT1 is expressed only in the brush-border membrane. It displays broader substrate specificity and accepts most charged and neutral di- and tripeptides, but has little affinity for tetra- or higher peptides.

Regulation of AA and di–tripeptide transport depends on the substrate concentration at the mucosal membrane: higher substrate concentrations lead to higher absorption rates. Di- and tripeptides are more efficiently absorbed than free AA, whereas the latter are better absorbed than oligopeptides.

Absorption of free AA requires energy and depends on a transepithelial electrochemical gradient. Absorptive enterocytes have sodium-dependent transporters for acidic, basic and neutral AA. These transporters first bind sodium, which alters their configuration, enabling them to bind AA. The loaded transporters then change orientation, so that the bound AA and sodium ions are carried into and released within the cell cytosol. The transporter is then reorientated, resiting its sodium receptor on the cell surface.

Only a small fraction of the peptides that are absorbed apparently enters the blood in the same form. Once inside the enterocytes, peptides are mostly degraded to AA and, along with absorbed free AA, are exported across the basolateral membrane into the blood by facilitated diffusion. For di- and tripeptides, on the other hand, there is a separate carrier-mediated peptide-transport system energized by an active anion-exchange process.

Digestion and Metabolism in the Large Intestine

As in the rumen, there is microbial activity in the large intestine (caecum, colon and rectum) and the relative magnitude of this activity can be gauged from the extent of production of SCFA and methane, which is usually about 10–15% of that produced in the rumen. By the time dietary components reach the large intestine, they will have been subjected to extensive microbial and animal enzymatic digestion, leaving little scope for their further digestion. Protein (probably endogenous in origin) is an important substrate, however. Ammonia is generated from fermentation of this protein and also from urea, which diffuses into the gut from the blood, and is either assimilated by the microbes or absorbed, along with the methane and SCFA. It is, however, unlikely that microbial protein or its constituent AA can be absorbed from the large intestine of ruminants, and this protein is excreted in the faeces.

Metabolism in the Whole Animal

Introduction

Undoubtedly, the most striking feature characterizing ruminants is the production of SCFA in the rumen and large intestine. There is little glucose absorbed from the gut, so it has to be synthesized in the liver (gluconeogenesis). Dietary propionate provides the main carbon source. Dietary butyrate is extensively oxidized in the rumen wall, with production of acetoacetate and 3-hydroxybutyrate. The liver has little effect on these, apart from some conversion of acetoacetate to 3-hydroxybutyrate. The result is a mild ketonaemia. The low pasture content of LCFA means there is not much to absorb (about 12–16 g day^{-1}). Acetate is the main carbon source for LCFA synthesis and, since little acetate is removed by the liver, there is minimal LCFA (or triacylglyceride) synthesis there, most occurring in adipose tissue. The ruminal degradation of dietary protein results in substantial ammonia absorption. This accounts for most of the urea produced by the liver. The dependence on microbial protein means that the supply of S-AA may be limiting for productive purposes.

As a result of the digestion of microbes, nucleic acids are released, and from them nucleases (which are present in relatively high concentration in the ruminant intestine) release purines, pyrimidines and phosphate. After absorption, phosphate is recycled to the rumen via saliva, while some purine is reutilized by the liver through well-developed salvage pathways, although most is excreted in urine (mainly as allantoin). In addition to the important conservation of phosphate, other characteristics of ruminant mineral metabolism include a large dietary input of potassium, a limited intake of sodium and absorption of magnesium by the foregut. The more or less continuous nature of fermentation results in a continuous absorption of minerals, which may lead to a 'blunting' effect of homoeostatic mechanisms controlling calcium.

Carbohydrate metabolism

Glucose formation

Although glucose is normally absorbed from the gut of ruminants in negligible amounts, glucose entry rate into the circulation is quite comparable to that of other animals. There is a linear relation between entry rate and ME intake, such that the entry rate increases by about 10 g glucose day^{-1} MJ^{-1} of ME whether the sheep are dry, pregnant or lactating. This result implies that about 16% of ME appears as glucose.

Almost all the glucose is derived by gluconeogenesis in the liver and, to a much lesser extent, the kidneys. The precursors are: ruminal propionate, whose absorption accounts for about 13–15% of ME; lactate, isobutyrate, valerate and glycerol, whose total is probably around 5–7% ME; and glycogenic AA. Only for alanine and glutamine is there evidence from isotopic studies of significant contribution from AA. For AA, lactate and glycerol, there are significant endogenous contributions, which make it difficult to assess quantitatively their (dietary) contribution to gluconeogenesis in fed animals. However, it seems that, normally, propionate accounts for most (60–70%) of the glucose produced by gluconeogenesis.

While the main fate of propionate is conversion to glucose, significant amounts of ruminal propionate are lost by oxidation in the rumen and, after passage to the omasum and abomasum, oxidation in the mucosal cells. Smaller amounts are also utilized by conversion to lactate in rumen epithelium. In addition, small amounts of propionate may be used in the formation of odd-chain-numbered fatty acids. On some diets, when large amounts of propionate are available, this may produce undesirable amounts of 'soft fat'. The liver efficiently extracts propionate (> 70%), so that peripheral propionate concentrations are always very low and there is negligible utilization by muscle or, probably, by adipose tissue.

Glucose utilization

After accounting for the contribution of glucose to respiratory CO_2 and the synthesis of glycerol, the fate of between 13 and 50% of the glucose flux is not established. The most likely use is to supply carbon for non-essential AA in protein synthesis. The only positive evidence for this comes from studies in rats (Shipley *et al.*, 1974), where protein was the major tissue component containing ^{14}C after injection of ^{14}C-glucose. In addition, it is known that the plasma flux of aspartate is much less than the amounts required for protein synthesis, implying that some additional synthesis is required.

Perhaps related to this is the question of why glucose is needed in the quantities synthesized. In lactation it is known to be specifically required for the formation of lactose, which is the driving force for milk secretion. In pregnancy, glucose is specifically needed for fetal development, perhaps because the machinery for oxidation of fatty acids develops relatively late in fetal development. There may also be a specific requirement in the testis, perhaps for rete fluid formation, although the amount required is small. However, outside broadly 'reproductive' requirements, the known need is for the brain. Here the indication is clear – there is an absolute requirement because the sheep brain appears able to use no other source. The uptake is just that required (assuming total oxidation) to match the oxygen consumption. Unlike the human brain, the sheep brain has no capacity to use alternative sources, such as ketones, although it is capable of extracting glucose at much lower concentrations than can non-ruminant animals. However, glucose requirement for this need is not great – about 8–10 mg min^{-1}, which is around 10% of the typical glucose entry rate.

While there are no other known requirements for glucose, one possibility is that it is required for optimal growth. The transport of glucose into muscle cells is known to require specific proteins. One (GLUT4) is insulin-sensitive. In mice produced so that this protein is not expressed, it is found that growth is restricted by 15–20%. There is also some evidence that in young lambs, glucose increased growth even when protein was no longer limiting. There is thus at least circumstantial evidence that a significant part of the need for glucose may relate to its requirement for growth, at least in muscle.

Lipid metabolism

Short-chain fatty acid metabolism

The non-glycogenic components are acetic, butyric and isovaleric acids. In sheep, some 15–18% of ME intake is absorbed as acetate, some of which is oxidized in the gut wall; there are indications that this might be as much as 30% of the acetate absorbed. In addition, there is limited conversion of acetate to ketones in rumen epithelium – less than 5% of the rate for butyrate. Little absorbed acetate is then removed by the liver, which is more usually a net producer of acetate. Acetate is produced by a number of tissues, but the liver is perhaps quantitatively the most important source of endogenous acetate. The major fate of acetate is immediate oxidation by peripheral tissues, especially muscle, where oxidation is linearly related to blood acetate concentration. Overall, about 80% of the acetate plasma flux can be accounted for as CO_2; since there is no means of storage of acetate, this means that oxidation occurs during or immediately after feeding. However, appreciable amounts of acetate may be used for the synthesis of LCFA. This does not occur to any appreciable extent in the liver – the major site seems to be adipose tissue. Isotope studies have indicated that around 5–12% of the acetate entry rate is utilized in this way (equivalent to 5–10 g fat deposited 24 h^{-1}). Small amounts may also be used for the synthesis of cholesterol. This occurs predominantly in adipose tissue. A major nutritional problem has been that on poor-quality diets, acetate is used less efficiently. This has been explained as due to a need for adequate glycogenic components – particularly glucose – to make available adequate nicotinamide adenine dinucleotide phosphate (NADPH), which is required for the synthesis of fat but is only available in an adequate amount via the pentose phosphate pathway for the oxidation of glucose. In view of the extensive oxidation of acetate, however, it seems also possible that carbohydrate may be needed to meet the need for an adequate supply of intermediates in the tricarboxylic acid cycle. Such intermediates can be met from either glucose or glycogenic AA; but perhaps, when protein synthesis is stimulated, such supply may become limiting.

Butyrate, the other significant non-glycogenic SCFA produced in rumen fermentation, is extensively metabolized in the rumen wall. In sheep, about 2% ME is absorbed as butyrate and about 7% ME as acetoacetate and 3-hydroxybutyrate – predominantly as the latter. Control of ketogenesis in rumen epithelium is not fully understood. In contrast to events in the liver, glucose stimulates ketogenesis, in part, at least, by providing reducing power, which keeps the ratio of 3-hydroxybutyrate/acetoacetate high. It has been suggested that ruminal ketogenesis is to some extent a detoxification, since butyrate has potent effects on cells, including inhibition of DNA synthesis and of cell division. Isovalerates, which are present and absorbed from the rumen in much smaller amounts than butyrate, are also partly converted to ketones, although the proportion produced as acetoacetate is much higher.

In sheep generally, and especially in ewes, there is also a significant hepatic production of 3-hydroxybutyrate (although usually an uptake of acetoacetate). However, in fasting and particularly in undernourished pregnant ewes, the rate of 3-hydroxybutyrate production in the liver may be doubled, with an appreciable output of acetoacetate. The blood concentration may increase much more (five- to tenfold, implying a limit to peripheral utilization), with a resultant acidosis. Hepatic ketones can be produced from butyrate, but the main sources are non-esterified long-chain fatty acids (NEFA) taken up by the liver. Ketone production is then determined by the rate at which the fatty acids enter mitochondria and the rate of their subsequent oxidation. These processes are inhibited if fatty acid synthesis is stimulated and also by the use of propionate for gluconeogenesis. The biochemical basis of these processes is now fairly well understood (Zammit, 1990).

Long-chain fatty acid metabolism

A modified form of the model of NEFA transport in sheep, proposed by Pethick and Dunshea (1993) and strengthened by recent studies by Freetly and Ferrell (2000), is shown in Fig. 5.3. The model suggests that most LCFA is absorbed as TAG and the sheep liver appears to have limited ability to secrete TAG (about 4–5 g day^{-1}; double this in pregnant animals). The turnover of NEFA (from gut, adipose tissue and plasma triacylglycerides) is about 35 g day^{-1} and increases fourfold or more in fasting. Less than half is oxidized to CO_2, accounting for about 10% of energy requirements. The most striking feature is a rough equivalence between the amount of LCFA being absorbed and that oxidized. Most of the NEFA turnover seems to involve recycling of fatty acids between plasma TAG and adipose tissue.

Of the specific fatty acids, the essential fatty acid, linoleic, is minimally oxidized. This occurs in part because most of the plasma linoleic acid is found in cholesterol esters and phospholipids, which are not used directly as energy sources. In addition, it has recently been shown that the transfer of linoleic acid into mitochondria – the initial step before oxidation – is more readily inhibited in sheep than in rats (and probably other non-ruminant) tissues. This selective protection ensures that sheep have no essential fatty acid deficiency, although most of the dietary linoleic acid is destroyed by biohydrogenation in the rumen.

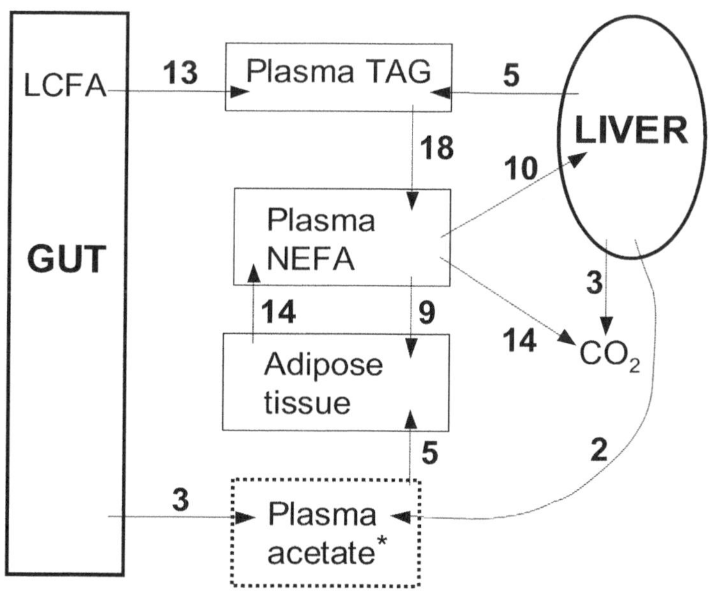

Fig. 5.3. A model of acetate, non-esterified fatty acid (NEFA) and triacylglycerol (TAG) metabolism in a sheep (45 kg) given enough roughage to allow it to just maintain live weight. *The acetate compartment shown includes only that acetate involved in NEFA synthesis; the values assigned to acetate influxes from the gut and liver are arbitrary. LCFA, long-chain fatty acids.

Amino acid and peptide metabolism

Transport and uptake by tissues

There is extensive protein synthesis in the portal-drained viscera (PDV) (the intestines, spleen, pancreas and stomach). In pigs and probably ruminants also, though less than 6% of body weight, the PDV contribute 20–35% of whole-body protein synthesis (Lobley *et al.*, 1980). It has generally been considered that, after release from the PDV, free AA are transported in the blood to body organs and are the main substrates for tissue protein synthesis. Interorgan transport of AA is thought to occur mainly by way of plasma, although red blood cells may at times carry AA such as methionine in concentrations exceeding the contemporary concentrations in plasma (Mackle *et al.*, 2000).

Current evidence strongly suggests that there is also a net appearance of peptide-bound AA in portal and possibly mesenteric blood, despite some uncertainties concerning the analytical techniques used to determine peptide concentrations (Webb, 2000). In addition, peripheral tissues have the ability to assimilate and use small peptides as sources of AA (Webb, 2000). It has been shown, using labelled peptides, that the lactating mammary gland of goats has the ability to utilize AA of peptide origin for milk protein synthesis: the extent to which this actually occurs is as yet unclear (Blackwell *et al.*, 1994). Pierzynowski *et al.* (1997) used a skin perfusion technique to investigate the effect of dipeptide infusion with met–leu and lys–leu (one side patch) or saline (other side patch) on mohair growth of angora goats. The dipeptides were not detected in the blood leaving the perfusion site, indicating that they were hydrolysed at the perfusion site. Moreover, greasy and clean mohair production from the dipeptide-perfused region were increased by the dipeptide perfusion, probably because the infused peptides provided AA that were limiting for protein synthesis, although it is possible that the dipeptides acted as growth promoters.

Intracellular amino acid metabolism

Plants and fungi can synthesize all 20 AA, but animals (from single-celled rumen protozoa to mammalian species) can manufacture the side-chains of only about ten to 12 of them. Mammals must therefore obtain these so-called essential AA by absorption from the gut. In the case of sheep and other ruminants, digestion of microbial protein (derived from the rumen flora) is the major source of these essential AA, i.e. leucine, isoleucine, lysine, methionine, phenylalanine, threonine, tryptophan and valine. Cells in the various organs of sheep obtain AA from the blood (as small peptides or AA – see above) or synthesize non-essential AA in order to maintain adequate intracellular concentrations for protein synthesis.

Viewing the whole animal, any mismatch between the supply of and demand for AA to enable synthesis of particular proteins by cells in general may result in a suboptimal rate of synthesis of protein. In this event, there will be a first-limiting AA (often methionine, lysine or threonine), while the other AA will be present in amounts that are in excess of current requirements but cannot be stored for later use. The concept of 'first-limiting nutrient' is an important one in metabolism and can be applied to most biosyntheses.

The excess AA are catabolized but, although the carbon backbones can be oxidized within the cell and used to generate ATP, the amino groups are potentially a source of ammonia, which is potentially toxic to cells. Toxicity is avoided because the amino groups are transferred within the cells of peripheral organs on to pyruvate (to form alanine) or on to glutamate (to form glutamine). The alanine and glutamine are exported into the bloodstream and act as carriers, delivering the amino-N to the liver, where it is used in the formation of urea. Most of this urea is normally excreted via the kidney, but at times it may be returned to the gut and reused by microorganisms to the animal's advantage, as discussed above. It is appropriate to note at this point that ammonia absorbed from the rumen or lower digestive tract is also potentially toxic, but toxicity is usually averted because this ammonia is removed from the portal blood by the liver and converted to urea.

As well as being substrates for protein formation in cells, some AA (e.g. glycine and glutamate – the so-called glucogenic AA) can be degraded intracellularly, in organs such as the liver, to materials that can be used in gluconeogenesis; others (e.g. leucine and lysine, the ketogenic AA) are converted to materials that can give rise to acetyl-CoA and ketone bodies; and several (e.g. threonine, isoleucine) can contribute to both functions. All AA carbon skeletons can enter the central metabolic pathways and contribute to ATP generation or, if not used in this role, can contribute to fatty acid synthesis and storage.

Partitioning of amino acids

While all organs in the body can be regarded as dependent on the plasma or blood cells as sources of AA, some organs may extract certain AA more efficiently than others, and the drain of AA to the muscle or mammary gland or skin will vary with stage of maturity or physiological state of the animal. Moreover, there may be interactions within some organs for the competing requirements of the biochemical processes for AA to be used to meet the demands for protein synthesis, as compared with glucose or fat synthesis, which will depend on the relative amounts of digestible energy substrates and nutrients. Thus the utilization efficiencies of individual AA for use in feeding systems such as those recommended by the Standing Committee on Agriculture (SCA, 1990) or the Agricultural and Food Research Council (AFRC, 1993) will most probably differ according to the prevailing conditions and therefore will be difficult to quantify with confidence.

Conclusion

Quantitative data on both the digestibility of feedstuffs and the metabolic fate of absorbed nutrients are needed to underpin systems of feeding standards (e.g. SCA, 1990) or computer-based models designed to predict production responses to defined diets. The most important tool in the measurement of digestibility is an appropriate dietary marker (see Faichney, 1986). A major advance in the difficult task of measuring the digestibility of herbage in grazing animals has been the clever use of endogenous indigestible plant alkanes as marker substances (see Coleman and Henry, Chapter 1, this volume).

Isotopically labelled nutrients have proved invaluable in delineating metabolic pathways and in providing data on the rates of turnover and oxidation of the major energy sources both in whole animals and in defined tissues (Annison, 1991). A most exciting advance in sheep metabolism, however, is genetic modification to modulate existing metabolic pathways or, indeed, to introduce new pathways to increase the efficiency of growth and wool production (Ward, 2001).

References

AFRC (1993) *Energy and Protein Requirements of Ruminants: an Advisory Manual Prepared by the AFRC Technical Committee on Responses to Nutrients*. CAB International, Wallingford, UK, 159 pp.

Annison, E.F. (1991) Measurement of metabolism in whole animals and their tissues – overview. *Proceedings of the Nutrition Society of Australia* 16, 146–153.

Backwell, F.R.C., Bequette, B.J., Wilson, D., Calder, A.G., Metcalf, J.A., Wray-Cahen, D., MacRae, J.C., Beever, D.E. and Lobley, G.E. (1994) The utilization of dipeptides by the caprine mammary gland for milk protein synthesis. *American Journal of Physiology* 276, R1-R6.

Bauchart, D.F., Legay-Carmier, F., Doreau, M. and Gaillard, B. (1990) Lipid metabolism of liquid-associated and solid-adherent bacteria in rumen contents of dairy cows offered lipid supplemented diets. *British Journal of Nutrition* 63, 563–578.

Corbett, J.L. (1987) Energy and protein utilization by grazing animals. In: Wheeler, J.L., Pearson, C.J. and Robards, G.E. (eds) *Temperate Pastures*. Australian Wool Corporation/CSIRO, Melbourne, pp. 341–355.

Doreau, M. and Chilliard, Y. (1997) Digestion and metabolism of dietary fat in farm animals. *British Journal of Nutrition* 78 (Suppl. 1), S15-S35.

Dove, H. and Milne, J.A. (1994) Digesta flow and rumen microbial protein production in ewes grazing perennial ryegrass. *Australian Journal of Agricultural Research* 45, 1229–1245.

Drackley, J.K. (2000) Lipid metabolism. In: D'Mello, J.P.F. (ed.) *Farm Animal Metabolism and Nutrition*. CAB International, Wallingford, UK, pp. 97–120.

Dunshea, F.R. and Ostrowska, E. (1999) Conjugated linoleic acid – snake oil or wonder fat? In: Corbett, J.L. (ed.) *Recent Advances in Animal Nutrition in Australia*, Vol. 12. University of New England, Armidale, Australia, pp. 159–166.

Faichney, G.J. (1986) The kinetics of particulate matter in the rumen. In: Milligan, L.P., Grovum, W.L. and Dobson, A. (eds) *Control of Digestion and Metabolism in Ruminants (International Symposium on Ruminant Physiology 6)*. Prentice-Hall, Englewood Cliffs, New Jersey, pp. 173–195.

Flint, H.J. and Forsberg, C.W. (1995) Polysaccharide degradation in the rumen: biochemistry and genetics. In: Englehardt, W.V., Leonard-Marek, S., Breves, G. and Giesecke, D. (eds) *Ruminant Physiology: Digestion, Metabolism, Growth and Reproduction*. Ferdinand Enke Verlag, Stuttgart, pp. 43–63.

France, J. and Siddons, R.C. (1993) Volatile fatty acid production. In: Forbes, J.M. and France, J. (eds) *Quantitative Aspects of Ruminant Digestion and Metabolism.* CAB International, Wallingford, UK, pp. 107–121.

Freetly, H.C. and Ferrell, C.L. (2000) Net flux of non-esterified fatty acids, cholesterol, triacylglycerol and glycerol across the portal-drained viscera and liver of pregnant ewes. *Journal of Animal Science* 78, 1380–1385.

Huntington, G.B. (1997) Starch utilization by ruminants: from basics to the bunk. *Journal of Animal Science* 75, 852–867.

Kirchgessner, M., Windisch, W. and Muller, H.L. (1995) Nutritional factors for the quantification of methane production. In: Englehardt, W.V., Leonard-Marek, S., Breves, G. and Giesecke, D. (eds) *Ruminant Physiology: Digestion, Metabolism, Growth and Reproduction*. Ferdinand Enke Verlag, Stuttgart, pp. 333–345.

Lobley, G.E., Milne, V., Lovie, J.M., Reeds, P.J. and Pennie, K. (1980) Whole body and tissue protein synthesis in cattle. *British Journal of Nutrition* 43, 491–502.

Mackle, T.R., Dwyer, D.A., Ingvartsep, K.L., Chouinard, P.Y., Ross, D.A. and Bauman, D.E. (2000) Evaluation of whole blood and plasma in the interorgan supply of free amino acids for the mammary gland of lactating dairy cows. *Journal of Dairy Science* 83, 1300–1309.

Mangan, J.L. (1982) The nitrogenous constituents of fresh forage. In: Thomson, D.J., Beever, D.E. and Gunn, R.G. (eds) *Forage Protein in Animal Production.* Occasional Publication No. 6, British Society of Animal Production, Thames Ditton, pp. 25–40.

Pethick, D.W. and Dunshea, F.R. (1993) Fat metabolism and turnover. In: Forbes, J.M. and France, J. (eds) *Ruminant Digestion and Metabolism*. CAB International, Wallingford, UK, pp. 291–312.

Pierzynowski, S.G., Puchala, R. and Sahlu, T. (1997) Effects of dipeptides administered to a perfused area of the skin in Angora goats. *Journal of Animal Science* 75, 3052–3056.

Preston, T.R. and Leng, R.A. (1987) *Matching Ruminant Production in the Tropics and Sub-Tropics*. Penambul Books, Armidale, Australia, 49 pp.

Rowe, J.B. and Pethick, D.W. (1994) Starch digestion in ruminants – problems, solutions and opportunities. *Proceedings of the Nutrition Society of Australia* 18, 40–52.

Russell, J.B. and Wilson, D.B. (1988) Potential opportunities and problems for genetically altered rumen microorganisms. *Journal of Nutrition* 118, 271–279.

SCA (1990) *Feeding Standards for Australian Livestock. Ruminants*. Standing Committee on Agriculture, CSIRO, Melbourne, 266 pp.

Scott, T.W., Cook, L.J., Ferguson, K.A., McDonald, I.W., Buchanan, R.A. and Loftus Hills, G. (1970) Production of poly-unsaturated milk fat in domestic ruminants. *Australian Journal of Science* 32, 291–293.

Shipley, R.A., Gibbons, A.P. and Chudzik, E.B. (1974) *In vivo* disposal kinetics of blood glucose carbon to hepatic and non-hepatic products in normal and diabetic rats. *Canadian Journal of Physiology and Pharmacology* 52, 798–807.

Shirazi-Beechey, S.P., Wood, I.S., Dyer, J., Scott, D. and King, T.P. (1995) Intestinal sugar transport in ruminants. In: Englehardt, W.V., Leonard-Marek, S., Breves, G. and Giesecke, D. (eds) *Ruminant Physiology: Digestion, Metabolism, Growth and Reproduction*. Ferdinand Enke Verlag, Stuttgart, pp. 117–134.

Tamminga, S., van Vuuren, A.M., van der Koelen, C.J., Ketelaar, R.S. and van der Togt, P.L. (1990) Ruminal behaviour of structural carbohydrates, non-structural carbohydrates and crude protein from concentrate ingredients in dairy cows. *Netherlands Journal of Agricultural Science* 38, 513–526.

Trevaskis, L.M., Fulkerson, W.J. and Gooden, J.M. (2001) Provision of certain carbohydrate-based supplements to pasture-fed sheep, as well as time of harvesting of the pasture, influences pH, ammonia concentration and microbial protein synthesis in the rumen. *Australian Journal of Experimental Agriculture* 41, 21–27.

Van Soest, P.J. (1994) *Nutritional Ecology of the Ruminant*. Cornell University Press, Ithaca, New York, 374 pp.

Ward, K.A. (2001) The manipulation of intermediary metabolism by transgenic technology to alter nutrient requirements in animals. In: Balnave, D. (ed.) *Proceedings of the Australian Poultry Science Symposium* 13. University of Sydney, New South Wales, pp. 18–21.

Webb, K.E. (2000) Tissue, cellular and molecular aspects of peptide absorption and utilization. In: Cronje, P.B. (ed.) *Ruminant Physiology: Digestion, Metabolism, Growth and Reproduction*. CAB International, Wallingford, UK, pp. 117–130.

Webb, K.E. and Matthews, J.C. (1998) Peptide absorption and its significance in ruminant protein metabolism. In: Grimbel, G. and Backwell, C. (eds) *Peptides in Mammalian Protein Metabolism: Tissue Utilization and Clinical Targeting*. Portland Press, London, pp. 1–10.

Zammit, V.A. (1990) Ketogenesis in the liver of ruminants – adaptations to a challenge. *Journal of Agricultural Science, Cambridge* 115, 155–162.

6 Principles of Supplementary Feeding in Sheep-grazing Systems

H. Dove

CSIRO Plant Industry, GPO Box 1600, Canberra, Australian Capital Territory, Australia

Introduction

In sheep-grazing systems in both temperate and rangeland environments, there are times of the year when animals will require supplementation because the nutrient supply from grazing does not meet their demands for nutrients. The particular needs of sheep grazing in rangelands are discussed by O'Reagain and McMeniman in Chapter 12, this volume; the present chapter will deal mainly with supplementation in more temperate environments. Even under these more favoured conditions, climatic variability or the requirements for profitable sheep production (for example, the overall stocking rate) are such that at least some classes of animal will often need supplements (Plate 6.1).

Supplementary feeds used in the various grazing industries include not only feed purchased off-farm, but also feed grown on-farm (e.g. wheat) or formulated on-farm from a mixture of grown and purchased commodities. As a result, it is difficult to obtain accurate data about the amount of supplementary feed actually used in the grazing industries and especially the sheep industry. If the Australian situation is taken as an example, there are minimal imports of feed grains and pulses for livestock use, so that the availability of domestically produced feed can be approximated to feed usage in the animal industries (see Hafi and Rodriguez, 2000). On this basis, the estimated annual usage of feed grains within the Australian sheep industry is of the order of 400,000–450,000 t. To this must be added an approximately equal quantity of roughage supplement (hay, chaff), since this represents about 45% of the total domestic feed usage (Hafi and Rodriguez, 2000). At a weighted average price of A\$130 t^{-1} across all supplements (Hafi and Rodriguez, 2000), this translates to an annual supplementary feed bill of A\$100–120 million in the Australian sheep industry.

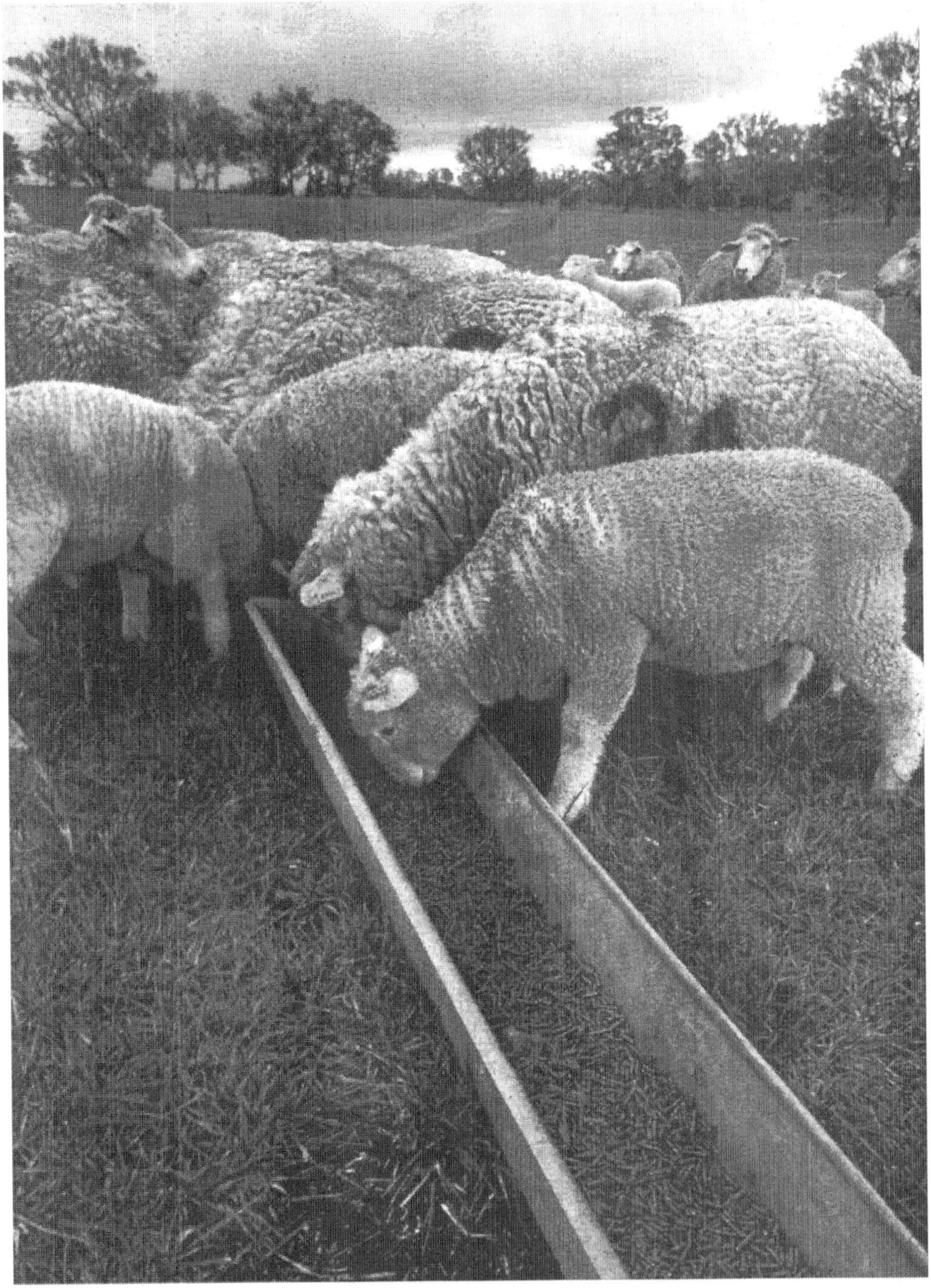

Plate 6.1. Border Leicester × Merino ewes and their Dorset Horn-sired lambs consuming a supplement of pelleted sunflower meal in early spring near Canberra, Australia. The pasture is based on phalaris (*Phalaris aquatica*) and subterranean clover (*Trifolium subterraneum*).

In grazing enterprises, the cost of supplementary feeding is therefore one of the major discretionary expenditures faced by farmers and, equally importantly, is also a major contributor to the so-called 'down-side risk' in farm income. This is the increased year-to-year variability in farm income generated by the costs of extra supplementary feeding in bad seasons, which, because stocking rates are frequently suboptimal, is often not compensated for by the extra income generated in good years. Increases in the efficiency of supplementary feeding are thus of economic importance and will have a major effect on farm income.

The Supplement Response

A supplement has been defined, at the simplest level, as 'something added to remedy a deficiency' (Doyle, 1987). However, the frequency of erratic responses to or complete failures of supplementary feeding suggests that often, in the grazing situation, there is something more complex going on than simply overcoming a deficiency. This should come as no surprise. The interaction of the ruminant with its grazed pasture represents the meeting point of two extremely complex ecosystems: the sward itself, responding to soil nutrients and water, to climatic variables and to the grazing process; and the animal, with its complex control of diet selection and intake, and its nutrient demands both for production and for the support of its resident population of rumen microorganisms (see Weston, Chapter 2; Forbes and Mayes, Chapter 3; Mackie *et al.*, Chapter 4, this volume). The introduction of a supplement into this complex interaction may 'remedy a deficiency', but in the process it may also have positive effects 'through increased forage intake or increased digestion of forage' or negative effects resulting in 'depressed intake and/or decreased digestion of major constituents of the forage' (Doyle, 1987). The nutritional mechanisms generating these positive and negative effects have to be understood (or at least appreciated) in order to unravel the response of the animals to supplements and thus increase the efficiency with which supplements are used.

In general terms, we can consider at least three reasons for offering sheep supplementary feeds, as outlined in Fig. 6.1. There are, for example, circumstances in which the supplement is given in order to negate the effects of something that is already present in the diet. For instance, the high content of condensed tannins in browse species, such as *Acacia* spp., can severely limit intake and performance by sheep (e.g. Degen *et al.*, 2000). Supplementation with the polymer polyethylene glycol under these circumstances can form a complex between the condensed tannins and the polyethylene glycol and overcome their negative effects. These situations arise mainly in rangelands or under browse conditions and are discussed further in other chapters in this volume (Forbes and Mayes, Chapter 3; O'Reagain and McMeniman, Chapter 12, this volume).

	Reason for feeding	Example	Effect on intake of diet
	Negate effects of a substance in diet	Polyethylene glycol to overcome tannin effects	Usually increased
Supplement	Overcome a frank deficiency	Deficiency of vitamin, mineral, rumen-degradable N	Intake increased (complementation)
	Contribute to energy, protein supplies	Increase ME and/or increase amino acid supply as either microbial protein, UDP or both	Intake decreased to variable extent (substitution)

Fig. 6.1. Major reasons for supplementary feeding in grazing systems.

More usually, the supplement is offered either to overcome the frank deficiency of a key nutrient (e.g. the supply of nitrogen (N) to the rumen, or of micronutrients, such as trace elements or vitamins) or to improve total nutrient supply or the efficiency of utilization of nutrients, in order that animals will either survive better or produce more. In this context, 'total nutrient supply' can refer to increased intakes of metabolizable energy (ME), metabolizable protein (MP) or both. Similarly, the increased supply of MP can be due to increased microbial protein synthesis, increased supply of undegraded dietary protein (UDP) or both.

It is therefore frequently difficult to unravel exactly which nutrients are responsible for the response to the supplement; this chapter will thus concentrate on the nutritional interactions that underpin supplement responses under these varying circumstances. Supplementation to negate the effects of an existing component of the diet is relatively uncommon and will not be discussed further, while supplementation with trace elements and vitamins is discussed by Lee *et al.* in Chapter 13, this volume (see, in particular, their Table 13.3). Unfortunately, the discussion of supplementary feeding responses and particularly our understanding of the interaction between supplement and herbage intakes are made complicated by the fact that, at most, we usually only know three things: the amount and quality of the pasture on offer (and that infrequently); the amount and quality of the supplement offered to a group of animals; and the production response of individual animals. The key variables of supplement intake and herbage intake by individual animals are often those about which we know least. A challenge to researchers in recent years has been to obtain estimates of these, in order to explain individual responses to total nutrient supply.

Methods for estimating supplement intake in grazing animals have been reviewed recently by Mayes and Dove (2000). Most are based on the concept of 'labelling' the supplement in some way and then monitoring the concentration of the label in a body pool, such as faeces, blood plasma or total body water. The size of the pool in which the label accumulates also has to be quantified in some way. For example, Kahn (1994) labelled supplement with lithium chloride and then measured the concentration of lithium in blood plasma. Other authors have labelled supplement with faecal markers, such as chromic oxide (e.g. Dove and Coombe, 1992), or markers that accumulate in body water, such as tritiated water in some form (e.g. Dove and Coombe, 1992). All these techniques have been validated under controlled conditions and provide estimates of supplement intake that do not differ from known intakes (see Mayes and Dove, 2000).

As discussed in a previous chapter (see Forbes and Mayes, Chapter 3, this volume), in recent years, the hydrocarbons (alkanes) of plant wax have been used to estimate diet selection and herbage intake in grazing animals. This method can be extended to the estimation of both herbage and supplement intake (see Mayes and Dove, 2000). This approach has promise because natural labels are used, and these involve no toxicity/aversion problems with animals (cf. lithium) or environmental hazards (cf. the radioactivity of tritium). Moreover, herbage and supplement intake can be computed from the same analyses. Hopefully, the field use of such techniques will allow a better understanding of the interaction between herbage and supplement intakes in grazing animals.

Interactions between Herbage and Supplement Intakes

When animals consuming roughage also eat supplements, this alters the total amount of digesta in the rumen (fill), the amount of dry matter (DM) in the rumen (load), the rate of digestion of cell-wall constituents, the pH and the ammonia concentration in the rumen, the rate of synthesis of microbial protein, the rate of outflow of liquid and particulate material from the rumen and the amount of energy and amino acids available at the tissue level. All of these have the potential to influence the intake of the basal roughage. At the extreme (e.g. pH and ammonia concentration) there can also be pathological consequences, as described in more detail by Mackie *et al.* (Chapter 4, this volume).

Under most grazing situations, we can define three basic outcomes when sheep (or other grazing ruminants) are offered supplements.

1. Supplementation: strictly speaking, this only occurs when the supplement is eaten and the intake of pasture is not reduced. This is usually the desired outcome of the manager, but is a rare event.
2. Substitution: most or all of the supplement is consumed and, as a result, pasture intake is reduced. 'Substitution rate' is then defined as the reduction in pasture intake per unit increase in supplement intake; if a daily

supplement intake of 250 g DM reduces pasture intake by 150 g DM, then the substitution rate is 60%. Substitution is what usually happens when supplements are given to grazing sheep, and there are times when the reduction in pasture intake may be enough to counteract the effects of the supplement.

3. Complementation: the consumption of the supplement actually increases pasture intake. This usually occurs in situations where the supplement makes good a frank deficiency of a nutrient (e.g. a mineral or rumen-degradable protein (RDP)). Deficiencies in most of the minerals required by the sheep will result in reductions in feed intake, with the extent of reduction varying with the mineral concerned (see Weston, Chapter 2, this volume). It follows that supplementation with the mineral will overcome the constraint on intake and increase feed consumption. An analogous situation is commonly encountered when sheep grazing low-quality roughages are given protein supplements that make good a deficiency in RDP.

Appreciating that these can be the outcomes is helpful, but the real need is to know why and especially to use this understanding to predict the likely outcomes of supplementary feeding, so that this can be done more efficiently and profitably. This is the purpose of the remainder of the chapter.

Substitution

There is an extensive scientific literature, dating back over half a century, indicating that when ruminants consume energy-rich supplements, they are likely to reduce their intake of the herbage component of the diet; early studies in this area are well summarized by Allden (1981). The fact that research in this area still continues indicates, first, the complexity of the processes involved and, secondly, the difficulty of extending results from pen studies to the grazing situation, in which it is much more difficult to quantify both herbage and supplement intakes.

In general terms, the extent of substitution between supplement and herbage will depend on the following factors, though it is still not easy to use these generalized responses to quantify the expected response to the supplement.

1. Substitution is likely to be greater when more pasture is available. For example, in early work Langlands (1969) fed five levels of wheat supplements to sheep grazing herbage ranging in availability from 760 to 4788 kg DM ha^{-1}. Relationships were estimated between herbage intakes (relative to unsupplemented sheep) and supplement intake, from which it is possible to calculate the levels of substitution occurring at the different herbage availabilities (Table 6.1). When only 760 kg DM ha^{-1} of herbage was available, the calculated level of substitution was 38.0%, but this rose markedly until, at a herbage availability of 4788 kg DM ha^{-1}, calculated substitution between herbage and supplement was 66.7%. An important point to note is

Table 6.1. Effect of the amount of pasture available on the rate of substitution between pasture and supplement in Merino sheep offered supplements of wheat grain (0, 100, 200, 300 and 400 g day^{-1}).

Total pasture[a]	Green pasture[a]	Substitution (total)
760	650	38.0
1303	833	41.9
1357	949	42.2
3528	2087	57.7
4788	1934	66.7

[a]Availabilities of total and green pasture in kg DM ha^{-1}. Rates of substitution calculated from regression relationships in Langlands (1969), relating herbage intake (relative to unsupplemented sheep) and supplement intake at the different pasture availabilities.

that substitution can occur even when pastures are sparse; even at the lowest pasture availability, substitution was still 38%. This may be an effect of grazing behaviour, with the sheep showing a disinclination to graze when supplement is freely available. Freer *et al.* (1985) postulated a similar mechanism to explain the difference in substitution between weaned lambs grazing mature pasture or consuming hay in yards.

2. The quality of the pasture on offer affects the degree of substitution, which appears to be greater when herbage quality is high (see Allden, 1981). Milne *et al.* (1981) reported effects of herbage availability on the level of substitution between herbage and grain supplement in grazing ewes, which were similar to the earlier results of Langlands (1969), except that substitution levels were much higher (e.g. 88% at a herbage availability of 750 kg organic matter (OM) ha^{-1}). This can probably be related to the difference in the digestibility of the herbage on offer in the two studies (58–75% in Langlands (1969); 83% in Milne *et al.* (1981)). However, the interaction between the nature of the supplement and the quality of the herbage is not simple. Supplements that contain high levels of starch (e.g. wheat or barley) can depress the rate of digestion of cell-wall material in the rumen. This has been described as the 'associative effect'; the mechanisms involved have been reviewed recently by Dixon and Stockdale (1999). The provision of large quantities of starch perturbs rumen microbial ecology in the direction of amylolytic organisms rather than cellulolytic organisms and, if the perturbation is sufficient, the rate of digestion of cell-wall constituents will be decreased. As a consequence, rumen outflow will slow and intake of the roughage component will decrease. However, Dixon and Stockdale (1999) have stressed two further points. First, the reduction in whole-tract digestibility may not be as great as the reduction in cell-wall digestibility in the rumen, indicating that there are compensating increases in digestibility elsewhere in the tract. Secondly, the degree of substitution occurring with high-starch supplements is frequently larger than the extent of depression in cell-wall digestibility, indicating that other factors are involved in causing the substitution between roughage and supplement. Since the level of substitution is influenced by both the amount and the quality of the pasture, obtaining information about these is a key element for successful supplementary feeding.

3. Substitution is usually greater when high-quality supplements are fed. In part, this can be attributed to associative effects between high-quality supplements, such as grains, and the roughage component of the diet. However, the effect is also apparent with high-quality, non-starchy supplements, such as lupins or oilseed meals.

4. The substitution rate may be greater when more supplement is fed, though this is not a universal finding. An example is shown in Table 6.2, derived from the data reported by Freer *et al.* (1988), for yarded lambs offered supplements of 2 : 1 oat-grain : sunflower meal and a basal ration of poor-quality pasture hay. With each successive increase in the supplement intake up to 446 g DM day^{-1}, both the overall and especially the incremental rates of substitution increased markedly. The last increase in supplement intake resulted in only a small decline in roughage intake, since this was already very low (Table 6.2). In contrast, Langlands (1969) fed increasing quantities of wheat to grazing sheep and found that the rate of substitution did not alter with successive increments of supplement.

5. For a given amount of pasture and supplement, the degree of substitution can also alter, depending on the physiological state of the animal. In general, animals with a greater demand for nutrients, such as rapidly

Table 6.2. Intakes of low-quality hay, supplement, metabolizable energy (ME) and nitrogen (N) of lambs in yards, together with estimated rates of substitution and liveweight gain (adapted from tabulated data in Freer *et al.*, 1988).

	Weight of air-dry supplement offered (g day^{-1})				
	0[a]	200	400	600	*Ad libitum*
Intake					
Supplement (g day^{-1})	75	176	313	446	1076
Hay (g day^{-1})	386	366	271	114	39
Total (g day^{-1})	461	542	584	560	1115
ME (MJ day^{-1})	3.50	4.48	5.32	5.69	12.11
N (g day^{-1})	4.2	7.1	10.8	14.0	32.5
Substitution (%, total)[b]	–	19.8	48.3	73.3	34.6
Substitution (%, incremental)	–	19.8	69.3	118.0	11.9
Weight change (g day^{-1})	–25	–17	39	54	142

[a]Animals on this treatment received 100 g day^{-1} supplement after second week.
[b]Total substitution calculated relative to lowest level of supplement offered. Incremental substitution calculated relative to previous level of supplement offered.
Hay ME content 6.9 MJ kg^{-1} DM and N content 5 g kg^{-1} DM. Supplement was 2 : 1 oat-grain (13 g N kg^{-1} DM) : sunflower meal (65 g N kg^{-1} DM) with ME content of 11 MJ kg^{-1} DM.

growing weaners and lactating ewes, will show a lower degree of substitution than, say, wethers or ewes in early pregnancy. The results shown in Fig. 6.2, calculated from Dove *et al.* (2000), show the level of substitution that resulted when ewes grazing green pastures based on *Phalaris aquatica* were offered 400 g OM day^{-1} of a pelleted supplement (1 : 1 milled oat-grain : sunflower meal). At both high (30.8 ewes ha^{-1}) and medium (17.1 ewes ha^{-1}) grazing pressures, there was a marked decline in substitution rate between late pregnancy, early lactation and mid-lactation. This decline occurred despite the fact that both the amount and the quality of the pasture improved over this period, which would be expected to result in increased, rather than decreased, substitution (see above).

6. The method and particularly the frequency of feeding may influence the rate of substitution, though this may only be observed with certain classes of sheep. For example, McCrabb *et al.* (1990) reported that, when lean ewes in late pregnancy were given lupin-grain supplements at rates of either 250 g day^{-1} or 875 g twice weekly, substitution was greater in the latter case.

Compared with concentrate supplements, it is much more difficult to obtain data about substitution rates between pasture and hay supplements. Again, this is related in part to the difficulty in obtaining field estimates of the intake of both. Birrell (1984) examined the interaction between hay intake and pasture availability in grazing sheep given hay every 2 days in self-feeders. For sheep grazing winter pastures in year 1, a sigmoidal relationship was established between hay intake and pasture availability (Fig. 6.3). Hay intake was highest when pasture availabilities were around 0.7 t DM ha^{-1} and then decreased as the amount of pasture on offer increased. Nevertheless, even at pasture availabilities above 5 t DM ha^{-1}, small amounts of hay were eaten (Fig. 6.3). Substitution rates between hay and

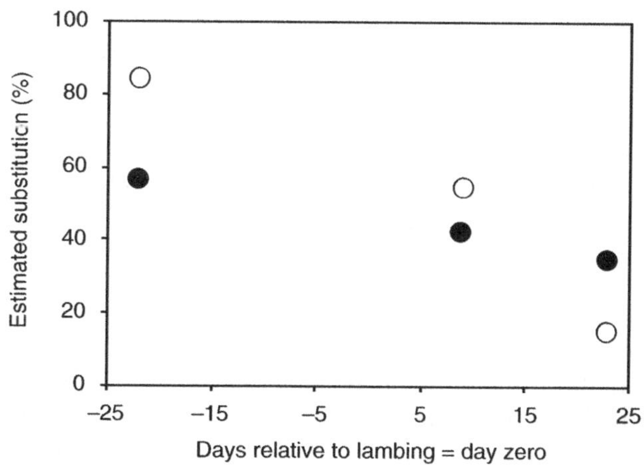

Fig. 6.2. Effect of stage of pregnancy/lactation on the estimated substitution rate between green pasture (based on *Phalaris aquatica*) and pelleted supplement (1 : 1 milled oat-grain : sunflower meal), at two grazing pressures (calculated from Dove *et al.*, 2000). ●, 31 ewes ha^{-1}; ○ 17 ewes ha^{-1}.

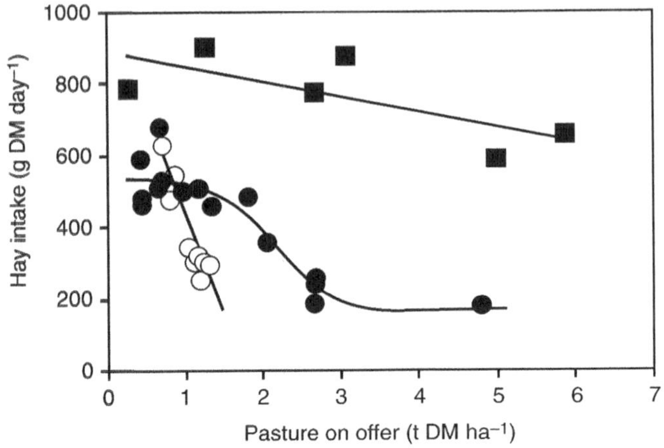

Fig. 6.3. Influence of the amount of pasture on offer on the intake of hay from self-feeders by grazing sheep (adapted from Birrell, 1984). ●, Winter, year 1; ○ winter, year 2; ■, summer, year 2.

pasture were not estimated in this study but in a subsequent experiment (winter, year 2), both hay intake and pasture intake were estimated and related to pasture availability. From these relationships, it can be calculated that the substitution rate between hay and pasture was 169%. This very high substitution rate reflects the fact that hay intake in the second experiment declined much more rapidly with increased pasture supply (Fig. 6.3), probably because the pasture on offer in the winter of year 2 was more digestible (70%) than the hay that was fed (61%). This interpretation is supported by other data showing the effect of increasing amounts of dead summer pasture on offer on the intake of hay (Fig. 6.3). In this case, the hay was much more digestible than the pasture and there was little decline in hay intake with increasing dry-pasture availability; it was not possible to calculate substitution rates from these latter data. In part, the unpredictable effects of hay supplementation on herbage intake and animal performance can be related to such interactions between the quality of the hay and the pasture itself. In general, there are unlikely to be economic benefits from supplementing sheep with hay that is of lower quality than the pasture itself, except when pasture availability is very low.

It must be stressed that the fact that there is substitution between herbage and supplement does not mean that there has been no response to the supplement, only that the response is less than might have been expected had supplement been consumed without an effect on herbage intake. This is clear in the data in Table 6.2; despite substantial substitution, the total intake of supplemented animals was increased. More importantly, because of the high quality of the supplement, the ME and N intakes of these lambs were increased even more markedly, such that liveweight gain was improved by 167 g day^{-1}, compared with lambs at the lowest level of supplementation.

Complementation

Assuming that there are no deficiencies of essential minerals or vitamins, the phenomenon of complementation is most likely to occur when sheep consuming poor-quality, low-N roughages are given supplements that increase the supply of N required for microbial fermentation of fibre in the rumen. Increased soluble-N supply to the rumen increases the rate of digestion of the roughage component of the diet, which in turn increases rumen outflow rate and thus intake. Two examples of complementation are shown in Fig. 6.4. In the first (Fig. 6.4a; see Freer *et al.*, 1988), lambs grazing mature pasture (OM digestibility 50–52%, N content 1.2%) were supplemented with increasing quantities of a supplement consisting (2 : 1) of oat-grain (1.3% N) : sunflower meal (6.5% N). Consumption of 160 g DM day^{-1} of this supplement increased pasture intake by 49% and total intake by 78%. A doubling of supplement intake resulted in further, though smaller, increases in both pasture and total intakes. Note that, as supplement intake was doubled from 324 to 640 g DM day^{-1}, the relationship between supplement and pasture intake became substitution rather than complementation, and at the rate of 110%.

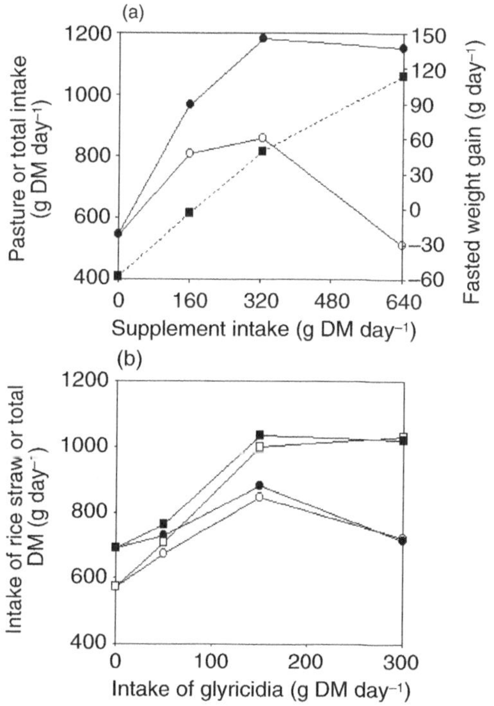

Fig. 6.4. Relationships between the intake of supplements providing rumen-degradable nitrogen and the intake of low-quality basal ration. (a) Data from lambs grazing mature pasture (experiment 2; Freer *et al.*, 1988). ○, Pasture intake; ●, total intake; ■, fasted weight gain (including wool growth). See text for details of nutrient content of pasture and the oat : sunflower meal supplement. (b) Data cited in Orskov (1999) for sheep offered rice straw plus supplements of gliricidia leaf. ○, Intake of rice straw, – urea; ●, intake of rice straw, + urea; □, total intake, – urea; ■, total intake, + urea.

This very high rate of substitution following a period of complementation has been observed in several other studies (e.g. Freer *et al.*, 1985; Doyle *et al.*, 1988). The 'switch' from complementation to substitution suggests that rumen requirements for soluble N had been met and that other constraints on intake were operating. This emphasizes the point that substitution and complementation must be regarded as parts of the same continuum, rather than as separate effects. Despite the fact that complementation gave way to substitution, total intake was not decreased (Fig. 6.4a) and ME intake was actually increased (Freer *et al.*, 1988). As a result, animal performance continued to improve with each successive increase in supplement intake.

In the second example (Fig. 6.4b; see Orskov, 1999), sheep consuming rice straw were supplemented with fresh leaves from the fodder legume gliricidia (*Gliricidia sepium*). As the level of supplementation increased from zero to 150 g DM day^{-1}, the intake of rice straw increased markedly, but then, with further supplementation, declined in the same manner as that observed by Freer *et al.* (1988). Despite this, total intake was maintained even at the highest level of supplementation. Some of the effect of gliricidia supplementation on rice straw intake was related to the provision of rumen-soluble N, since the inclusion of 2% urea (a source of rumen-soluble N) in the rice straw resulted in an increase in intake of about 20%, which was similar to the response observed with 50 g DM day^{-1} of gliricidia. However, the fact that there was also an intake response to gliricidia in sheep given the rice straw with urea suggests either that 2% urea was not sufficient to provide the soluble-N needs of the rumen or that intake was stimulated by other nutrients provided by the gliricidia.

Types of Supplementary Feed and their Nutritive Value

A wide range of supplements is fed to sheep within the grazing systems of the world and, to a large extent, any classification of these can only be in general terms. However, in production systems based on sown pastures in temperate areas, it is convenient to classify supplements into the general categories in Table 6.3.

Energy/high-carbohydrate supplements

Cereal grains, such as barley, wheat, oats, sorghum and maize, typify the 'energy' or 'high-carbohydrate' supplements. These contain large amounts of readily digestible carbohydrate, primarily as starch. It follows that an understanding of the differences in starch content and degradability between grains and the factors that influence these will lead to better understanding of the differences in nutritive value of different grains for different classes of livestock. However, recent research has also indicated that more attention needs to be paid to the non-starch polysaccharide, fibre and protein con-

Table 6.3. General classification of supplementary feeds for use in sheep grazing systems, with their advantages and disadvantages.

	Example	Advantages	Disadvantages
'Energy' or high-carbohydrate supplements	Cereal grains, crop by-products (e.g. bran, molasses)	Highly digestible, easy to store feed Relatively cheap ME source Can be produced on farm	Must be introduced gradually to avoid rumen problems May result in high levels of substitution if fed with poor-quality roughage
'Protein' or N supplements	Grain legumes, pulses, oilseeds and oilseed meals Non-protein N sources such as urea	Grain legumes, pulses, oilseed meals palatable, easily handled or mixed with cereals Pose few rumen problems	Urea potentially toxic Oilseed meals expensive source of ME; relatively cheap per kg CP
Conserved forage	Hay, silage	Most farmers have capacity to produce, especially hay Cheap per kg DM	Difficult to produce high-quality product Bulky to store, feed out May end up expensive per MJ ME Possible high substitution with hay, palatability problems with silage
Forage crops	Forage brassicas (rape, kale) and root crops (turnips, swedes, chou moellier); chicory Forage oats, winter wheats Forage maize, sorghums, Japanese millet	Produce large quantities of highly digestible forage Forage brassicas and root crops can be held in paddock for future use Feed grain from winter cereal can pay for crop costs	'Cropping penalty' (increase in grazing pressure during crop growth stage) Low DM content can limit intake Secondary compounds (brassicas) Growth rates sometimes disappointing

tents of cereal grains, as they influence the processes of digestion (see review by van Barneveld, 1999). The extent to which these effects can be manipulated by grain processing (e.g. cracking, steam-flaking, pelleting) have recently been reviewed by Rowe *et al.* (1999).

In future evaluations of the nutritive value of feed grains for ruminants, van Barneveld (1999) suggested that more attention needed to be paid to the following points.

1. The rate and extent of starch fermentation, between and within feed grain species and in different compartments of the gut.
2. The contribution of fibre to the nutritive value of feed grains, and especially clarification of the contribution of cellulose and hemicellulose components. For example, it is apparent that there are major differences in the contribution of fibre to the energy value of oat, wheat, barley and triticale grains (see van Barneveld, 1999).
3. Protein solubility in the rumen, its variability across species, cultivar and growing conditions and the extent to which protein solubility interacts with the rate of release and fermentation of starch.
4. The lipid content of feed grains as a contributor to their total ME contribution and as a possible negative influence on efficient fibre digestion (see Annison *et al.*, Chapter 5, this volume).
5. Fermentation patterns of non-starch polysaccharides in both cereal grains (e.g. the β-glucans of barley) and legume grains (see below).

While it is clear that grain processing can alter or negate some of the differences between grains in the above characteristics, it is also clear that the nutritive value of feed grains would be better predicted with more information on the above points.

Energy supplements, such as the cereal grains, have the added advantages of being readily produced and stored on farm and being easily fed out to sheep. This means that they are relatively cheap supplements, especially when evaluated in terms of cost per MJ ME, which is the appropriate criterion to use. In contrast, their relatively low and variable protein contents (especially in oat grain) mean they are likely to be expensive supplements when costed per kg of crude protein (CP), and they are thus both inefficient and expensive protein supplements. Perhaps the major difficulty encountered in using the high-starch cereal grains is the need for animals to be introduced to them gradually, in order to avoid problems with excessive lactic acid production in the rumen, as discussed by Mackie *et al.* (Chapter 4, this volume).

'Protein' supplements

'Protein' supplements are fed either to increase the supply of RDP in the rumen and thereby improve the efficiency of fibre digestion (e.g. protein supplements for sheep grazing low-quality roughages) or to effect an increase in the amount of MP leaving the rumen for digestion in and absorption from the small intestine. Increased MP supply can itself result from either increased microbial protein production in the rumen or an increase in the rumen outflow of UDP or, more commonly, from a combination of these.

The most widely used of the non-protein N supplements is urea, which is rapidly degraded to ammonia in the rumen. Provided there is a source of readily available carbohydrate (e.g. molasses), the ammonia can then be incorporated into the protein of rumen microbes. The main issues in relation to urea supplementation of sheep are discussed by O'Reagain and McMeniman (Chapter 12, this volume). Positive responses to urea supplements are more erratic in grazing sheep than in cattle, partly because the greater grazing selectivity of the former can result in their consuming a higher-quality diet, containing sufficient RDP to support rumen fermentation. Another feature of urea supplementation is large between-sheep variability in intake from the block or lick. This has two consequences. First, some animals might consume enough of the mix to receive a toxic dose of urea. Secondly, large variability in intake results in only some animals responding, so that the mean response is low and the cost of supplementation may be higher than might have been the case with a true protein supplement (e.g. lupins; see Rowe and Ferguson, 1986).

The true protein supplements include plant protein sources, such as grain legumes (e.g. lupins, vetches), pulses (e.g. peas, faba beans), oilseeds and oilseed meals (e.g. whole cottonseeds, cottonseed meal, soybean meal, sunflower meal), plus animal protein sources, such as fish meal. It is likely that the importance of plant protein sources will increase, with increasing worldwide concern about transfer of disease into human populations through the feeding of animal proteins to animals. This is already banned in several sheep-producing countries.

Plant protein supplements, such as those listed in Table 6.3, differ in their protein, starch, non-starch polysaccharide and lipid contents, depending on species and degree of processing (see van Barneveld, 1999), but all have much higher protein contents than the cereal grains (30–40% CP, cf. 7–14% CP in cereal grains). The rumen degradability of the protein varies with the extent of processing, particularly degree of grinding and of heat treatment. Fish meal usually has a higher protein content (60–70% CP) than the plant protein supplements and considerably lower protein degradability in the rumen. The lipid and protein contents of the oilseed meals depend on whether oil has been removed by mechanical expellers or by solvent extraction and on the extent to which the seeds have been dehulled.

All of these protein sources thus provide ME, RDP and UDP; the extent of animal response will depend on the animal's requirement for these and their interaction with nutrients provided by the rest of the intake. These supplements are usually more expensive than cereal grains but may be cheaper per kg CP. If their protein content is judged to be too high for the purpose, they are readily mixed and fed together with cereal grains, which reduces costs. The storage carbohydrate of the plant protein supplements is either starch at a lower concentration than in cereal grains (e.g. peas) or a non-starch material, such as the β(1–4)-galactan of lupins. This results in a different pattern of storage carbohydrate digestion from that in cereal grains (see van Barneveld, 1999) and means that these supplements, especially the legume grains, can be fed to sheep with much less likelihood of the major disturbances to rumen function that can occur with the over-rapid introduction of cereal grains.

Conserved forages

There is an extensive literature on the production and feeding of hay and silage, especially the former, in sheep production systems. As a generalization, it is very difficult to make a hay or silage that has a nutritive value equivalent to the pasture from which it is made. This means that, while conserved fodder may not be regarded as expensive per tonne of DM, the cost per MJ of ME or per kg of CP may be much higher and may compare unfavourably with the energy or protein supplements. In addition, substitution effects with hay can sometimes be very large, depending on the relative digestibilities of the hay and pasture (see Fig. 6.3). The use of silage in the various sheep-production systems of the world is highly variable. For example, it is often used in feeding systems in the UK, but is relatively unimportant in grazing systems in Australia.

Forage crops

These are not strictly 'supplements', because they are not fed to animals that are grazing some other source of fodder. Rather, the forage crops are the principal source of fodder. However, they will be discussed here as supplements, since their role is to provide a fodder resource at a time when pasture supplies would be expected to be reduced (e.g. a winter or a summer 'feed gap'). They thus obviate the need to buy and feed other supplements, though fodder crops themselves may need supplementation (see below). The general place of forage crops in grazing systems and early research on their role as supplements have been discussed by Wheeler (1981) and by Nicol and Barry (1986).

Forage crops are sown annually for use in a specific season and fall into several categories: cereal crops grazed in their vegetative stage; forage brassicas, root crops or special-purpose species, such as chicory (*Cichorium intybus*); and summer-growing species, such as maize, sorghum and its hybrids, and Japanese millet.

Cereal crops can be used in sheep-grazing systems as a source of forage. In Australian grazing systems, for example, forage oats are used as a feed bank for winter grazing or perhaps for hay production, with the possibility of grain production being of lesser importance. More recently, with the successful breeding of winter wheats suitable for southern Australia, there has been considerable interest in using these as a dual-purpose crop

– that is, as a source of both grazing and feed grain. Theoretically, the grain crop that is ultimately harvested pays for the costs associated with the crop, so that the grazing value of the crop can be regarded as pure profit.

Forage brassicas and related root crops are used extensively in European and New Zealand sheep-grazing systems, but to a lesser extent in Australia. They are high-yielding crops, producing material of high digestibility (75–90%) (see Armstrong *et al.*, 1993) but low DM content (10–20%), which are grown and held for later use by animals with a high demand for nutrients (e.g. finishing lambs). They offer the added advantage that fodder quality does not alter significantly over a period of months, which confers flexibility in their management. A more detailed description of the role of brassica forage and root crops is given by Nicol and Barry (1986).

Forage crops for use in spring–summer include forage maize, sorghum and millet. These grass species exhibit the C4 pathway of photosynthesis, which can produce large quantities of high-quality herbage. Given the structure of the crop they produce, they may be more suited to grazing by cattle than by sheep. Interest in chicory is more recent and the species has potential as a spring–summer fodder crop for sheep (e.g. Hume *et al.*, 1995).

All forage crops that are sown specifically for grazing involve a 'cropping penalty', in that setting aside part of the farm to grow the fodder crop increases the grazing pressure on the rest of the property, for a period which may be as long as 4–6 months for winter cereals or forage brassicas. The extent of any cropping penalty must therefore be a component of any evaluation of the role of forage crops, and the improved performance of sheep while grazing the crop must also offset the reduced production that arises from increased grazing pressure prior to grazing the forage crop. The extent of any cropping penalty will be closely related to the stocking rate and the proportion of the farm that is sown to forage crop. If the latter is very small, then the penalty will be small, but so will the potential benefit.

A frequent observation with forage brassicas is that liveweight gains are less than might have been expected from pasture of the same quality. This can be related to effects on intake, to possible nutrient deficiencies and to the effects of secondary compounds in the plant tissues, especially leaf laminae.

The intake of brassica forage crops can be reduced both by their high water content and by their content of glucosinolates, which affect both preference (Sarwar *et al.*, 1997) and total intake (e.g. Armstrong *et al.*, 1993). The glucosinolates, via their conversion to isothiocyanates during chewing, can disrupt thyroid function and cause both clinical (goitre) and subclinical symptoms that reduce growth rate. Forage brassicas also contain S-methylcysteine sulphoxide (SMCO). This is converted in the rumen to the secondary toxin dimethyl disulphide, which is responsible for the haemolytic anaemia that can develop in animals grazing forage brassicas, especially kale. The adverse effects on animals of secondary compounds in forage brassicas are discussed in more detail by Prache (1994). Forage brassicas can also disturb mineral metabolism, especially copper and selenium metabolism (Nicol and Barry, 1986; Prache, 1994). These can be addressed by appropriate supplementation.

The rumen degradability of CP in forage brassicas is very high (Dove and McCormack, 1986) and, at the intakes likely to prevail in animals grazing this forage, could result in a deficiency of MP and a need for further protein supplementation. For example, Vipond *et al.* (1982) found that a supplement of only 44 g day^{-1} of soybean meal increased swede intake by 14% and significantly improved the liveweight gains of both housed lactating ewes and their lambs. Similarly, when lambs grazing forage rape were offered small supplements (50 g day^{-1}) of formaldehyde-treated soybean meal, a source of UDP, liveweight gain and protein gain in grazing lambs were increased, without any increase in carcass fatness (Table 6.4). The effect was especially evident in lambs grazing 'stemmy' rape, which itself had a lower protein content. Taken together, these studies suggest that, on occasion, forage brassicas will not supply sufficient protein for the desired animal performance.

Energy and protein supplements revisited

It will be clear from the above discussion that the distinction between 'energy' and 'protein' supplements is only a general distinction and one of convenience. Ultimately, both types of supplement have the capacity to alter ME supply to the animal, the efficiency of utilization of ME (e.g. Dixon and Egan, 2000), the amount of microbial protein synthesized and the amount of dietary protein that escapes rumen degradation. In addition, once nutrients are absorbed from the gastrointestinal tract, there can be a further nutrient flux, principally energy, in the form of mobilized reserves of body fat. A good example of such interactions between grazed herbage, supplement and body-fat reserves is shown in Table 6.5, constructed from the data of Dove *et al.* (1985).

In unsupplemented, twin-suckling ewes, the pasture supported a milk yield of about 2 kg day^{-1}. Ewes maintained weight over 80 days of lactation, due mainly to increased pasture supply in later lactation. The provision of

Table 6.4. Influence of type of forage rape crop ('leafy', 'stemmy') and supplementary feeding on weight gains and carcass characteristics of weaned lambs (adapted from unpublished data of J.A. Milne and H. Dove).

	Leafy crop supplement			Stemmy crop supplement		
	Nil	RB	RB/FSBM	Nil	RB	RB/FSBM
Weight gain (g day^{-1})	167	157	198	118	116	141
Carcass protein gain (g day^{-1})	21	21	23	11	11	17
Carcass fat (%)	23.0	23.5	22.6	22.2	23.3	22.0

'Leafy' and 'stemmy' crops obtained using 28 kg Scottish Blackface lambs in a leader–follower grazing system. Herbage availabilities were 4–5 t DM ha^{-1} (leafy) and 1–2 t DM ha^{-1} (stemmy).
RB, rolled barley offered at the rate of 275 g DM day^{-1} per lamb; RB/FSBM, rolled barley at the same rate plus 50 g DM day^{-1} per lamb of formaldehyde-treated soybean meal.

Table 6.5. Influence of 'energy' and 'protein' supplements on digesta flow, milk yield and liveweight change of grazing ewes, and the weight gains of their lambs (adapted from data in Dove *et al.*, 1985).

	Supplement[a]		
	Nil	'Energy'	'Protein'
Rumen ammonia (mM)	24.1	16.4	20.1
DM flow (g day^{-1})[b]	1065	1288	1340
CP flow[c]	276 (0.934)	344 (0.851)	431 (0.772)
Milk yield (g day^{-1})	2048	2133	2846
Lamb weight gain (g day^{-1})	254	308	331
Ewe weight change (kg)[d]	0	5.1	−0.9

[a]Energy supplement 600 g day^{-1} (air-dry) of molassed sugarbeet pulp (CP 9%). Protein supplement 600 g day^{-1} (air-dry) of a mixture (1 : 1) of molassed sugarbeet pulp and formaldehyde-treated soybean meal. Ewes grazed perennial ryegrass pasture of 750–850 kg DM ha^{-1} and digestibility > 85%.
[b]All flows measured at abomasum and expressed in g day^{-1}. Values are means of measurements in weeks 3, 5 and 7 of lactation.
[c]Values in parentheses are the proportion of CP flow that is of microbial origin.
[d]Weight change to day 80 of lactation.

the 'energy' and the 'protein' supplements increased digesta flow at the abomasum by about 21 and 26%, respectively. Given the extent of digestion of the supplements in the rumen, both these values imply that substitution between supplement and herbage was low. The 'protein' supplement resulted in a large increase in CP flow in digesta (56%), of which significantly less was of microbial origin, as might be expected from a supplement that had been treated to resist rumen degradation. However, the 'energy' supplement also resulted in increased digesta CP flow, which may be related in part to increased 'capture' of rumen ammonia and conversion into microbial protein. Both supplements improved milk yield and lamb liveweight gains. This was especially so with the 'protein' supplement, on which ewes lost weight slightly over the lactation. In contrast, ewes given the energy supplement gained substantially. While some of these observations are consistent with the description of the supplements as 'energy' or 'protein' supplements, note that the 'energy' supplement influenced N transactions in the rumen and the 'protein' supplement influenced the mobilization of body energy reserves.

Supplementary Feeding: Some Practical Considerations

In grazing systems, the economics of supplementary feeding are influenced not only by the nutritional principles discussed in this chapter, but by practical considerations, including the rate at which animals become accustomed to the supplement, the variability of supplement intake within the group of animals and how frequently the supplement needs to be fed.

There are occasions on which it is appropriate to introduce animals to supplements very gradually (e.g. wheat feeding), but, in general, the profitability of supplementary feeding will be compromised if animals take a lengthy period to become accustomed to the supplement. The rate at which lambs or young sheep become used to a supplement can be greatly reduced by earlier exposure to the supplement, especially in the presence of older sheep (Green *et al.*, 1984; Mulholland, 1986). Green *et al.* (1984) gave unweaned Merino lambs access to supplement, in the presence or absence of their mothers. The lambs were weaned at 10 weeks of age and then tested for acceptance of the supplement at 3, 6, 12, 24 and 34 months of age, as described in Fig. 6.5. Sheep initially exposed to wheat with their mothers always ate much more than either control (unexposed) sheep or those exposed to wheat without their mothers (Fig. 6.5a). The latter group ate significantly more than control animals on only one occasion (12 months). Lambs previously exposed to supplement with their mothers not only ate more (Fig. 6.5a), but on their first day of re-exposure ate 40% of their ultimate intake (averaged across all testing ages) (Fig. 6.5b). In contrast, after 5 consecutive days of exposure, control lambs and those previously exposed without their mothers were only consuming 20% of the amount eaten by

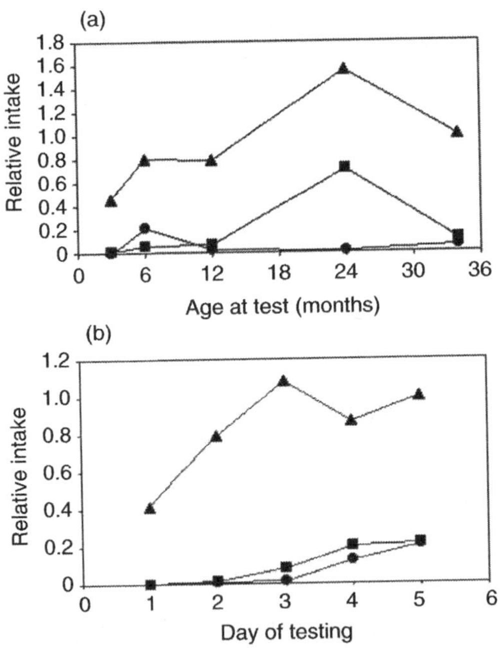

Fig. 6.5. Effect of prior exposure to supplements on their later acceptability to Merino lambs (Green *et al.*, 1984). ▲, Lambs exposed before weaning, in the presence of their mothers; ■, lambs exposed before weaning, in the absence of their mothers; ●, control lambs, no prior experience of the supplement. (a) Intakes, relative to the amount consumed by ▲ when tested at 34 months of age. (b) Intakes, relative to the amount consumed by ▲ on the fifth day of testing (mean across all ages of testing).

those exposed with their mothers. In newly weaned crossbred lambs with no prior experience of lupin grain, Mulholland (1986) reported that the presence of 5% of 'trainer ewes' (ewes previously exposed to lupins) was sufficient to ensure that lambs rapidly accepted the supplement under grazing conditions. These results strongly suggest that there would be economic value in exposing young sheep to supplements in the presence of experienced older animals, as a means of ensuring later rapid acceptance of the supplement.

In sheep that have not been exposed to supplements, there can be substantial variability in supplement intake between animals. Low supplement intakes in some sheep ('shy feeders') then result in a lower mean response and a more variable response to the supplement. The impact of shy feeders on the response to the supplement can be reduced by the training described above and also by less frequent feeding of supplements (e.g. every third day rather than daily) or by offering supplements in self-feeders. There is usually little penalty incurred in supplement response by feeding supplements less frequently than daily (though see McCrabb *et al.*, 1990), and there may be some advantage, especially for wool growth and particularly with cereal grains. For example, Fredericks *et al.* (1986) demonstrated a small extra response in the liveweight gain of Merino weaners when supplemented at the equivalent of 150 g day^{-1} every third day rather than daily. Supplements of oat or triticale grain that did not significantly increase wool growth when fed daily increased it by 25% when fed every third day. Responses to supplements of lupins, sunflower meal or formaldehyde-treated sunflower meal were greater than to the cereal grains, but were unaffected by feeding frequency.

Conclusion

Supplementary feeding is a deceptively simple concept but, in practice, requires the assessment of information concerning the current state of the animals and their body reserves, the amount and nutritive value of the herbage on offer and the nutritive value and amount of the supplement that is to be fed. As the discussion in this chapter has indicated, there are usually marked interactions, sometimes positive, sometimes negative, between supplement and herbage intakes. This means that the ultimate mix of nutrients absorbed from the gut of the animal is not easy to predict. Absorbed nutrients also interact with energy from the body reserves of the animal.

The sheep producer is also faced with questions concerning the supplement and labour costs of supplementary feeding (cost kg^{-1} DM vs. cost MJ^{-1} ME vs. cost g^{-1} CP; daily vs. infrequent feeding) and must also consider the target market. For example, in finishing lambs, should the aim be rapid weight gain to dispose of animals early, or slower weight gain to target a later, higher-priced market? Similarly, if supplementation for wool growth increases wool-fibre diameter, how does the price penalty of increased diameter compare with the extra income from more wool and the possible price premium of increased wool strength?

Given the complexity of the decisions involved in supplementary feeding, it is perhaps not surprising that responses to supplements can be variable in either physical or financial terms. One approach to assisting the decision making involved has been to incorporate current knowledge about supplementary feeding into computer-based 'decision support tools' (e.g. Freer *et al.*, 1997). Such tools can then be used by farmers or their advisers to simplify the process of establishing a supplementary feeding programme. The use of such tools for supplementary feeding decisions and for addressing wider questions of the nutritional management of sheep is the subject of the final chapter of this volume (Freer, Chapter 16).

References

Allden, W.G. (1981) Energy and protein supplements for grazing livestock. In: Morley, F.H.W. (ed.) *World Animal Science B1 Grazing Animals*. Elsevier, Amsterdam, pp. 289–307.

Armstrong, R.H., Beattie, M.M. and Robertson, E. (1993) Intake and digestibility of components of forage rape (*Brassica napus*) by sheep. *Grass and Forage Science* 48, 410–415.

Birrell, H.A. (1984) Effects of pasture availability and liveweight on the feeding of grass hay to grazing sheep. *Australian Journal of Experimental Agriculture and Animal Husbandry* 24, 26–33.

Degen, A.A., Benjamin, R.W., Mishorr, T., Kam, M., Makkar, H.P.S. and Schwartz, H.J. (2000) *Acacia saligna* as a supplementary feed for grazing desert sheep and goats. *Journal of Agricultural Science, Cambridge* 135, 77–84.

Dixon, R.M. and Egan, A.R. (2000) Response of lambs fed low quality roughage to supplements based on urea, cereal grain, or protein meals. *Australian Journal of Agricultural Research* 51, 811–821.

Dixon, R.M. and Stockdale, C.R. (1999) Associative effects between forages and grains: consequences for feed utilisation. *Australian Journal of Agricultural Research* 50, 757–773.

Dove, H. and Coombe, J.B. (1992) A comparison of methods for estimating supplement intake and diet digestibility in sheep. *Animal Production in Australia* 19, 239–241.

Dove, H. and McCormack, H.A. (1986) Estimation of the ruminal degradation of forage rape after incubation in nylon bags in the rumen of sheep. *Grass and Forage Science* 41, 129–136.

Dove, H., Milne, J.A., Lamb, C.S., McCormack, H.A. and Spence, A.M. (1985) The effect of supplementation on non-ammonia nitrogen flows at the abomasum of lactating grazing ewes. *Proceedings of the Nutrition Society* 44, 63A.

Dove, H., Freer, M. and Foot, J.Z. (2000) The nutrition of grazing ewes during pregnancy and lactation: a comparison of alkane-based and chromium/*in vitro*-based estimates of herbage intake. *Australian Journal of Agricultural Research* 51, 765–777.

Doyle, P.T. (1987) Supplements other than forages. In: Hacker, J.B. and Ternouth, J.H. (eds) *The Nutrition of Herbivores*. Academic Press, Sydney, pp. 429–464.

Doyle, P.T., Dove, H., Freer, M., Hart, F.J., Dixon, R.M. and Egan, A.R. (1988) Effects of a concentrate supplement on the intake and digestion of a low-quality forage by lambs. *Journal of Agricultural Science, Cambridge* 111, 503–511.

Fredericks, F., Dixon, R.M., Holmes, J.H.G. and Egan, A.R. (1986) Effect of daily or infrequent supplementation of weaner sheep on liveweight change and wool growth. *Animal Production in Australia* 16, 207–210.

Freer, M., Dove, H., Axelsen, A., Donnelly, J.R. and McKinney, G.T. (1985) Responses to supplements by weaned lambs grazing mature pasture or eating hay in yards. *Australian Journal of Experimental Agriculture* 25, 289–297.

Freer, M., Dove, H., Axelsen, A. and Donnelly, J.R. (1988) Responses to supplements by weaned lambs when grazing mature pasture or eating hay cut from the same pasture. *Journal of Agricultural Science, Cambridge* 110, 661–667.

Freer, M., Moore, A.D. and Donnelly, J.R. (1997) GRAZPLAN: decision support systems for Australian grazing enterprises. II. The animal biology model for feed intake, production and reproduction and the GrazFeed DSS. *Agricultural Systems* 54, 77–126.

Green, G.C., Elwin, R.L., Mottershead, B.E., Keogh, R.G. and Lynch, J.J. (1984) Long term effects of early experience to supplementary feeding in sheep. *Animal Production in Australia* 15, 373–375.

Hafi, A. and Rodriguez, A. (2000) *Projection of Regional Feed Demand and Supply in Australia*. Australian Bureau of Agricultural and Resource Economics and Grains Research and Development Corporation, Canberra, 62 pp.

Hume, D.E., Lyons, T.B. and Hay, R.J.M. (1995) Evaluation of 'Grasslands Puna' chicory (*Cichorium intybus* L.) in various grass mixtures under sheep grazing. *New Zealand Journal of Agricultural Research* 38, 317–328.

Kahn, L.P. (1994) The use of lithium chloride for estimating supplement intake in grazing sheep: estimates of heritability and repeatability. *Australian Journal of Agricultural Research* 45, 1731–1739.

Langlands, J.P. (1969) The feed intake of sheep supplemented with varying quantities of wheat while grazing pastures differing in herbage availability. *Australian Journal of Agricultural Research* 20, 919–924.

Mayes, R.W. and Dove, H. (2000) Measurement of dietary nutrient intake in free-ranging mammalian herbivores. *Nutrition Research Reviews* 13, 107–138.

McCrabb, G.J., Egan, A.R. and Hosking, B.J. (1990) The relationship between feed intake and the method of supplementation, body composition and stage of pregnancy/lactation. *Animal Production in Australia* 18, 520.

Milne, J.A., Maxwell, T.J. and Souter, W. (1981) Effect of supplementary feeding and herbage mass on the intake and performance of grazing ewes in early lactation. *Animal Production* 32, 185–195.

Mulholland, J.G. (1986) Introducing supplements to newly weaned lambs. *Animal Production in Australia* 16, 287–290.

Nicol, A.M. and Barry, T.N. (1986) The feeding of forage crops. In: Drew, K.R. and Fennessy, P.F. (eds) *Supplementary Feeding*. New Zealand Society of Animal Production Occasional Publication No. 7, Mosgiel, New Zealand, pp. 69–106.

Orskov, E.R. (1999) Supplement strategies for ruminants and management of feeding to maximize utilization of roughages. *Preventive Veterinary Medicine* 38, 179–185.

Prache, S. (1994) Haemolytic anaemia in ruminants fed forage brassicas: a review. *Veterinary Research* 25, 497–520.

Rowe, J.B. and Ferguson, J. (1986) Lupin grain as a supplement to sheep grazing cereal stubble. *Animal Production in Australia* 16, 343–346.

Rowe, J.B., Choct, M. and Pethick, D.W. (1999) Processing cereal grains for animal feeding. *Australian Journal of Agricultural Research* 50, 721–736.

Sarwar, M., Kirkegaard, J., Gowers, S. and Garrett, B.C. (1997) Glucosinolate content and animal acceptability of forage brassicas. *Cruciferae Newsletter* 19, 13–14.

van Barneveld, S.L. (1999) Chemical and physical characteristics of grains related to variability in energy and amino acid availability in ruminants: a review. *Australian Journal of Agricultural Research* 50, 651–666.

Vipond, J.E., Hunter, E.A. and King, M.E. (1982) Effects of cereal and protein supplements to swedes (*Brassica napus*) on intake and performance of pregnant and lactating ewes kept indoors. *Animal Production* 34, 131–137.

Wheeler, J.L. (1981) Complementing grassland with forage crops. In: Morley, F.H.W. (ed.) *World Animal Science B1 Grazing Animals*. Elsevier, Amsterdam, pp. 239–260.

7 Nutrition for Maintenance

J.L. Corbett[1] and A.J. Ball[2]

[1]*Animal Science, University of New England, Armidale, New South Wales 2351, Australia;* [2]*Meat and Livestock Australia, c/o Animal Science, University of New England, Armidale, New South Wales 2351, Australia*

The state of maintenance is often thought of as the preservation of constant live weight by animals. In practice, feeding sheep for this condition is sensible only for those that are mature, such as adult wethers (castrates) kept for wool production, that are non-breeding or in early pregnancy, or in the special circumstances of feed scarcity, such as in drought. At the maintenance level of feeding, rigorously defined, the basal requirements of the animal for the following are met:

1. Maintenance of homothermy and the normal continuance of vital processes within the body.
2. Replacement of obligatory losses in faeces and urine and from the skin.
3. Essential physical activities.

Thus the net gain or loss of energy and nutrients from the tissues of the animal as a whole is zero.

There is no single, universal index of maintenance. Constant live weight does not imply zero net change in the energy of the body tissues, nor does the latter mean that there is a constant content of protein, fat or any other constituent in the body. While any of these conditions and growth are mutually exclusive, in practice a part of the diet of an animal fed for the production of meat and wool or for reproduction is seen as being required to meet the demands for energy and nutrients of 'maintenance'. These demands are the overhead costs of the production, the costs of the supporting metabolism.

Effective nutritional management of animals requires definition of those costs, whether to identify how much of a known feed intake is required to meet them and thus assess if the remainder of the intake will provide for the desired production, or to formulate a ration that will provide for maintenance plus the production. In practical feeding, the primary concern is the energy cost of maintenance.

Energy

In 1839 Sarrus and Rameaux, in France, proposed that there was a relationship between the metabolic rate of animals (*H*) (heat production per unit time) and their surface area. Bodies of similar dimensions have surface areas (*S*) proportional to the squares of their linear dimensions and so to the two-thirds power of their volumes. In order to establish a relationship between *H* and *S*, various formulae have been proposed for the estimation of *S* from live weight (*W*) to the power 0.66 (or thereabouts, because animals are not spheres); these are unreliable because measurement of *S* is highly uncertain, and the relationship with *H* has no sound theoretical base (Kleiber, 1961).

An alternative approach is to use regression analysis to relate metabolic rate and live weight. A regression equation of the form

$$\ln H = b_0 + b_1(\ln W)$$

yields a value, b_1, for the exponent of *W* that best relates the two variables. For resting mature animals of many species differing widely in *W*, Kleiber (1961) estimated b_1 as 0.75 (i.e. $W^{0.75}$), which is now taken to represent 'metabolic body size' (MW), superseding the $W^{0.73}$ proposed by Brody (1935).

Measurement

Metabolizable energy (ME) (see Table 7.1; Fig. 1.1 in Coleman and Henry, Chapter 1, this volume) is used by the body tissues with an efficiency (*k*) of less than 1.0, resulting in the production of heat (*H*). The energy balance (EB) of the animal, its net energy (NE) gain, is then given by:

$$\text{EB} = (\text{ME} - H)$$

At maintenance, EB is zero and so the maintenance intake (ME_m) equals *H*, the energy loss by the animal as heat.

With intakes below maintenance, the efficiency with which ME is used to spare body tissues from catabolism (k_m) is the change in EB from more negative to less negative that is promoted by the intake of a given amount of ME (i.e. ΔEB/ΔME) (see Fig. 7.1). Similarly, above the ME_m, with animals growing, lactating, etc., the efficiencies with which ME is used for growth and fattening or for the production of milk are identified as k_g and k_l respectively; their values, like those for k_m, vary directly with the feed ME (metabolizable energy of dry matter (M/D), MJ kg^{-1} dry matter (DM)) (see Table 1.1 in Coleman and Henry, Chapter 1, this volume).

The US National Research Council (NRC) matches the requirements of livestock for maintenance, growth and lactation, expressed as net energy (NE = ME − *H*), with feed NE values, rather than ME as in the British (ARC, 1980) and Australian (SCA, 1990) systems. Their determination (NE_m, NE_g, NE_l, respectively) requires measurement of EB at two or more levels of feed intake: feed NE value per unit intake = ΔEB = ΔME − Δ*H*.

The three main methods for the measurement of animal requirements for maintenance, expressed as ME_m and/or NE_m, are feeding trials, estimation of ΔEB by the comparative slaughter (CS) technique and calorimetry.

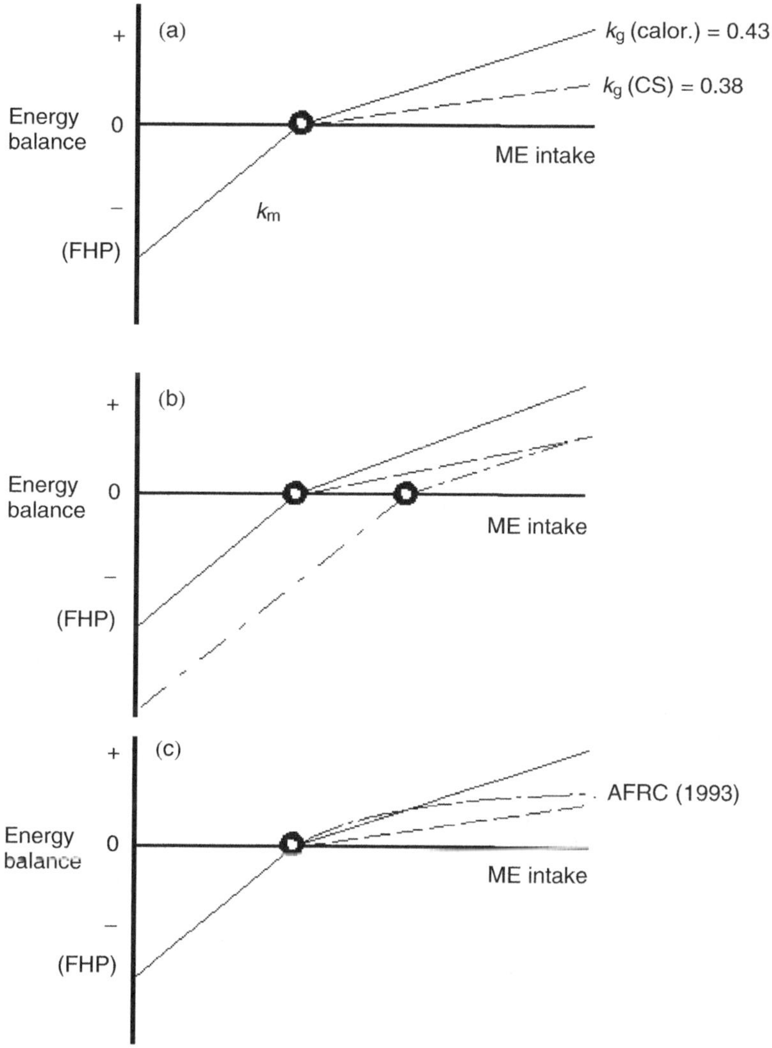

Fig. 7.1. Effect of method of measurement on the estimate of the efficiency of use of metabolizable energy (ME) for growth and fattening (k_g): (a) k_g determined by calorimetry (k_g calor.) and by comparative slaughter (k_g CS) for a feed with 10 MJ ME kg^{-1} DM and a value of 0.7 for the efficiency of use of ME for maintenance (k_m); (b) the same k_g in calorimetric and CS (broken line) situations, the difference in (a), taken to be methodological in origin, implies an increase in the maintenance metabolism in animals fed for production that is detectable (see text) in measurements of ME for maintenance and of fasting heat production (FHP); (c) k_g (calor.) adjusted for level of feeding (AFRC, 1993) on the assumption that ME_m is invariant.

Feeding trials

Feeding trials to assess maintenance needs are usually made in practical or near-practical conditions; their simplest form is exemplified by the studies made to establish the minimum amounts of feeds required to maintain non-breeding sheep during drought (CSIRO, 1958). Estimates can be obtained from the regression of live weight (W), change in live weight (ΔW) and milk production (M), if any, on intake (I) of digestible organic matter (DOM) or a related measure:

$$\text{DOMI} = bW^{0.75} + cM + d\,\Delta W$$

The values of the coefficients c and d are taken to be, respectively, the quantities of DOM used for the milk production and change in W, and coefficient b (DOMI per unit MW) is taken to indicate the maintenance cost. While such relationships can be used to obtain estimates of ME_m, they frequently involve correlated errors (e.g. inaccurate measurements of W will cause incorrect ΔW), so that the regression coefficients, though mathematically valid, do not provide reliable estimates.

Comparative slaughter

In the CS technique, representative animals from a group are slaughtered at the beginning of an experiment and the composition of their whole empty bodies, including blood but excluding gut contents, is determined. The initial composition of the remaining animals is estimated with regression equations derived from the slaughter results that relate carcass weight and total body energy, protein, fat, etc., to, usually, fasted W. At the end of a feeding period, usually of 3 months or more, the animals or a representative sample are slaughtered. Body composition is determined and the values are compared with the corresponding initial estimates to obtain values for their gains of energy, etc.

In some studies changes with time in the composition of the bodies of live animals have been estimated from serial measurements of their water content by marker dilution techniques. An injected dose of water labelled with deuterium (D_2O) or tritium (TOH) becomes distributed throughout the body water; the concentration of the marker in a sample, often obtained from blood, relative to the amount administered yields an estimate of D_2O or TOH space (l). Because there is virtually no water in body fat, the space in a fat animal is a smaller proportion of fasted W than in one which is less fat. This relationship enables establishment of equations for the prediction from the space of the quantities of fat and protein in the body and body gross energy. Other, more recent, techniques to estimate composition *in vivo* include computerized tomography (Perry *et al.*, 1998).

With determined ME intakes and body energy gains (EB), a relationship can be established of the form:

$$\text{EB} = a + b\text{ME}$$

Maintenance requirement can then be estimated as $ME_m = a/b$; the coefficient b is an estimate of k_g.

Calorimetry

The standard procedure for measuring the fasting metabolism (FM) (Table 7.1) of ruminants (a direct measure of NE_m) requires that feed but not water be withheld for 4 days. Heat production is usually measured during the third and fourth days of fast and this 'fasting heat production' (FHP) plus the gross energy of the urine excreted is the FM. Animals should be trained and well accustomed to the calorimeter so that, though they will not be at rest, as required for the determination of basal metabolic rate in human subjects (BMR), they are reasonably at ease. They must be kept in a thermoneutral environment. During the measurement the respiratory quotient (CO_2 produced/O_2 consumed) should have decreased to about 0.7 and a sheep should be producing no more than about 0.5 l day^{-1} of methane. Strictly speaking, a postabsorptive state is required for the determination of BMR, but this cannot be achieved with ruminants and low methane production indicates that the nearest practical approach to this condition has been achieved. The value of FHP varies directly with the level of feeding before fast (see below); to obtain results repeatable over time, feeding for the 3 weeks immediately before measurement has been standardized at approximately the maintenance level.

For practical use, the FM values have to be adjusted for the difference between the fasted weight (FW) of an animal and its live weight when it is fed. The relationship for sheep assumed by the Agricultural Research Council (ARC, 1980) that $FW^{0.75} = (W/1.08)^{0.75}$ is commonly used.

Table 7.1. Energy requirements: definitions of terms.

Term		Definition
Metabolizable energy of feed	$ME = GE - (FE, UE, CH_4E)$	Gross energy (heat of combustion) of feed consumed minus energy in the faeces (FE), urine (UE) and methane (CH_4E)
Energy balance	$EB = ME - H$	ME intake by the animal minus its heat production (*H*)
Maintenance	$EB = 0$ thus $ME = H$	Net gain or loss of energy by the animal is zero
Basal metabolic rate	BMR	Heat production by a fasting animal in a postabsorptive state in a thermoneutral environment and at rest
Fasting heat production	FHP	BMR plus energy for minimal activity
Fasting metabolism	FM	FHP plus the GE of urine excreted
Net energy for maintenance	NE_m	FM plus the energy costs of physical activities, including grazing, maintenance of homothermy and (SCA, 1990) energy costs related to level of feeding
Net efficiency of use of ME for maintenance	$NE_m/ME_m = k_m$	$NE_m = ME_m \times k_m$
ME for maintenance	ME_m	NE_m plus heat losses in metabolism $= ME_m \times (1 - k_m)$

When ME intakes and H are measured in grazing sheep (e.g. Young and Corbett, 1972) and analysed in the form:

$$H = p + q\text{ME}$$

then, since $H = \text{ME}_m$ at zero EB, ME_m can be calculated from the above equation as $p/(1 - q)$.

Components of the requirement

An index of the energy costs of a number of essential physiological activities is provided by measurements of the associated oxygen consumption, made by *in vitro* and *in vivo* techniques that are described by Seal and Reynolds (1993). Incubation of a small sample of tissue from, say, the liver can yield a value for oxygen consumption g^{-1} of tissue and, by extrapolation, by the whole organ. *In vivo* values for oxygen removal by a whole organ can be obtained from measurements of the rate of blood flow across the organ and the arteriovenous difference in oxygen concentration.

Two major contributors to oxygen consumption are the transfer by the gastrointestinal tract of nutrients from the lumen of the gut into the bloodstream and the moderation of these nutrients by the liver for use by other tissues. These two anatomical entities are together termed the splanchnic bed and represent some 0.10–0.13 of W, but their oxygen consumption in sum amounts to about half of whole body oxygen consumption (Webster, 1989; Seal and Reynolds, 1993). Skin, kidneys and nervous tissue are responsible for about one-third of the consumption and muscle, including the heart muscle, for the remainder.

Maintenance heat production, H_m (= ME_m), can also be analysed in terms of metabolic processes. There is substantial oxygen consumption in ion pumping by the active transport system Na^+K^+-ATPase, in an amount estimated from *in vivo* studies (Huntington and McBride, 1988) to be 0.36 of H_m. The remaining oxygen consumption was the result of protein synthesis (0.25), protein degradation (0.10), substrate cycling (0.12) and urea synthesis (0.17). These processes in the gut plus liver were estimated to account for 0.72 of H_m and in the rest of the body for 0.28.

Adipose tissue is by no means inert but differences in H_m between and within breeds of sheep are reduced when expressed in relation to lean body mass rather than W (e.g. Ball *et al.*, 1998).

Variation in requirement

Genotype

There is much evidence of variation in FHP between and within breeds of cattle but not for sheep, perhaps because there is not the range in genotypes represented in cattle by the extreme dairy and beef types that have resulted from selective breeding. Blaxter (1962) found no difference between the values for ewes and wethers (MJ day^{-1} per 50 kg *W*) obtained for Scottish Blackface, Cheviot and Down crosses and those reported from the USA for Durham and Hampshire and for Merinos from Australia. Freetly *et al.* (1995) found that, at a common *W*, Texel ewes had a lower FHP than Suffolk ewes, but not when the values were related to $W^{0.75}$ or when the ewes were compared at common proportions of their mature weights.

The Merino is distinguished from other breeds by having a much higher rate of wool growth and the energy cost of that growth, which continues even in sheep that are severely undernourished, is an often unacknowledged contributor to FHP. The daily additional energy cost of the extra few grams of wool grown by a Merino would, however, be towards the limits of measurement by calorimetry, though it might be detected in determinations of ME_m by longer-term feeding trials that used many animals.

There is undoubtedly variation between individuals to be exploited for increasing efficiency of conversion of feed to gain. Blaxter (1962) found that there were large differences in FM between individual sheep and that these differences persisted through repeated measurements made over several years. A study by Graham (1968) indicated that a low FM might not be advantageous for wool production because Merino rams bred for high wool production had a higher FM per unit MW and per kg fat-free *W* than rams with a production 40–50% lower.

Age and physiological state

A single value for *H* per unit MW derived from measurements at various ages underpredicts the maintenance requirement of young sheep and overpredicts for adults, and there is evidence that for growing animals, an exponent of 0.45–0.60 is more appropriate (Graham *et al.*, 1974; Freetly *et al.*, 1995). Published data suggest a fall of 3–8% per year in FHP (Blaxter, 1962; Graham *et al.*, 1974).

Activity of Na^+K^+-ATPase in both liver and skeletal muscle decreases with age and increases during lactation (Kelly and McBride, 1990). During pregnancy and lactation there are increases in the size of the visceral organs and in the blood flow through and the oxygen uptake by the liver and portal-drained viscera (PDV) (e.g. Freetly and Ferrell, 1997). Cristian *et al.* (1980) reported that, compared with early pregnancy, the ME_m per unit MW for ewes just before parturition was greater by 46% and, during the first 2 months of lactation, was greater by 17%. Estimates by Corbett *et al.* (1980) indicated no significant differences in ME_m between grazing Merino ewes 54 and 100 days pregnant and those non-pregnant, but a significant increase of 14% at 130 days. In a later experiment with unshorn Border Leicester ewes at a similar stage of gestation (Corbett *et al.*, 1982), the increase was 18%, but was 40% for pregnant ewes that had been shorn and were in ambient temperatures below their lower critical temperature. During the sixth week of subsequent lactation, ME_m was 33% greater than that of non-lactating ewes.

Several studies support the calorimetric measurements of Graham (1968), which show that, while ewes and castrates have similar ME_m, the requirement for rams can be taken to be 15% greater. This is due in part to their relatively greater lean body mass as a proportion of *W*, but Ball *et al.* (1998) found that a 5% higher ME_m could not be accounted for by differences in body composition.

Season of year

Studies with grazing sheep (Corbett *et al.*, 1980, 1982) indicated that ME_m was greater in spring than during the preceding winter. This result was confounded with the effects of the greater pasture intakes in spring in both years and with increasing day length. Sheep show an annual cycle of feed intake, a direct relationship with day length probably reflecting corresponding variation in hormone secretion by the pineal gland (Forbes, 1982).

With sheep fed year-long at a near-maintenance level, Walker *et al.* (1991) found a seasonal pattern in their heat production under natural light/dark; the periods of peak and trough values coincided with maximum and minimum day lengths, respectively. With an artificial light regimen the reverse of the natural seasonal cycle, there was an almost corresponding shift in the heat-production pattern. The variation about the mean value for *H* was similar to the ±14% amplitude in the annual periodicity apparent from measurements made over several years by Blaxter and Boyne (1982) of the FHP of sheep consistently given a maintenance ration. It is not clear whether such variation in FHP is the cause or the result of the seasonal variation of similar amplitude in the body composition of sheep reported by Ball *et al.* (1996).

Disease and parasitism

It can be expected that there will be energy costs for the animal from bacterial and viral infections and from ectoparasitism (e.g. lice, maggots from 'fly strike'), but these will occur for little longer than the period of the recovery promoted by appropriate treatments. Endoparasitism is, however, a ubiquitous and chronic condition in sheep, and one major cause for reduced production by sheep with gastrointestinal helminthiasis is a reduction in feed intake, which can reach 50% even in subclinical cases (Sykes, 2000; see also Coop and Sykes, Chapter 14, this volume). Efficiency of feed conversion (e.g. intake : ΔW) also deteriorates but in the first instance this is due to a reduction in the digestibility and hence in the M/D of the feed. Calorimetric studies (MacRae, 1993) on the efficiency of use of the reduced quantity of ME gained from the feed showed that this was indistinguishable from the efficiency value measured with pair-fed sheep that had been reared in a controlled environment to be parasite-free (PF). Though energy balances in the sheep with parasites were similar to those in the sheep without, live weights of the former group remained virtually unchanged over a 10-week period of the experiment, while the PF sheep gained 5–10 kg during the same period. This difference indicates a substantially greater energy cost for maintenance in the parasitized sheep, their maintenance involving two identifiable energy-costly processes: the cost of repair of the gastrointestinal tissue damage caused by the helminths and the cost of mounting an immune response and so limiting or preventing further tissue damage (Sykes, 2000).

Level of feeding

The relationship ΔEB/ΔME is curvilinear, the proportion of feed energy retained by the animal decreasing with increasing intake, but by convention it is represented by two straight lines (Fig. 7.1a). The slopes of the lines below and above maintenance intake are estimates of the efficiencies of use of ME for maintenance (k_m) and growth (k_g), respectively. In this example, 0.7 and 0.43 for k_m and k_g (calorimetry (calor.)), respectively, are predicted for a feed with M/D = 10 using the equations k_m = 0.02 M/D + 0.5 and k_g = 0.043 M/D, derived from ARC (1980) by the Standing Committee on Agriculture (SCA, 1990). At the same M/D, the NRC (1985) value for k_g (CS) derived by CS is 0.38; CS values are usually lower than those obtained by calorimetry (e.g. Thomson and Cammell, 1979).

Despite this difference, estimates of ME_m obtained by the two techniques are similar, because those obtained by CS reflect the performance of the group of animals that, as for determinations of FM, are fed at about the maintenance level. However, the fact that the performance of the CS animals at a higher level of feeding implies a lower k_g does not mean that the metabolic processes in their tissues are less efficient. Rather, it implies that the proportion of the ME intake being used by those animals to satisfy overhead energy costs is greater than the maintenance cost measured when EB is approximately zero; that is, there is an effect of level of feeding on the maintenance requirement. This is illustrated in Fig. 7.1b, with k_g (CS) parallel to k_g (calor.) on the basis that the efficiency of ME use does not differ between feedlot and calorimeter. This also implies that, if the FHP of the full-fed animals were to be determined without an intervening period of ME_m, then its value would be substantially greater (*x* intercept, Fig. 7.1b) than that which would have been obtained under the standardized conditions for measurement of FHP. There is extensive evidence that ME_m and FHP do increase with intake, and of the corollary that both are reduced by undernourishment (e.g. Lines and Peirce, 1931; CSIRO, 1958; Graham and Searle, 1979).

This variation reflects identifiable physiological responses. Ferrell *et al.* (1986) found that, with increasing level of feeding (*L*), along with increasing FHP, there were significant increases in the weights of liver, kidney, stomach and small and large intestines, both in absolute terms and as percentages of empty body weight. There is unequivocal evidence that thermogenesis by the organs varies directly with *L*, as indicated by the reports of positive relationships with portal and hepatic blood flows and oxygen uptake by liver and PDV (e.g. Ortigues and Durand, 1995) and with Na^+K^+-ATPase-dependent respiration in duodenal tissue (McBride and Milligan, 1985).

Graham (1982) suggested that the differences between calorimetric and CS measurements of energetic efficiency exist because the physiological responses to change in L occur rather slowly. With CS, animals are fed at a given L for, usually, 3 months or more. In contrast, calorimetric studies (Fig. 7.1a) usually comprise measurements of EB at a number of widely differing feeding levels and during fasts, and an animal is fed at one L for only 2–3 weeks before a change to another. At high L, therefore, the energy cost of the support metabolism is likely to be less enhanced and the proportion of dietary energy available for storage in tissue greater than in an animal long accustomed to that level. This view is substantiated by studies indicating that it may take 4 or more weeks for animals to adapt, in terms of the energy cost of support metabolism, to a new feeding regimen (e.g. Turner and Taylor, 1983).

Feeding management

Compensatory, or 'catch-up', growth occurs when animals that have been underfed for a considerable time are provided with abundant good-quality feed. Reasons for an ensuing rate of liveweight gain that is higher than by similar animals also given abundant feed but without earlier restriction (Ball *et al.*, 1997) include a feed intake (g kg W^{-1}) that for some time is greater than that of the unrestricted animals. It is also found that gross efficiency of feed conversion, both as ΔW kg per kg intake and ΔEB MJ per MJ feed NE, is increased during the compensation period; a preceding reduction in FM persisting as a lower maintenance cost results in a greater proportion of the diet being available for growth than under a steady feeding regimen.

When sheep at pasture have to be fed a supplement for their maintenance or survival, it saves labour and costs to provide their ration once or twice weekly rather than in smaller daily amounts; also, while dominant animals may eat most of a daily ration so that 'shy feeders' eat little or none, this is less likely when the ration for several days is provided at one time. A reduction in frequency of feeding does, however, result in some increase in ME_m (Perry *et al.*, 1998).

Practical definition

Though it is evident that, with increases in feed intake, the energy cost of the supporting metabolism also increases, most definitions of energy requirements regard maintenance as a fixed cost per unit MW. So expressed, the NRC (1985) predicts NE_m for sheep of all ages and sex type as 0.234 MJ. The ARC (1980) has six 'preferred values' for the FM in sheep, decreasing from 0.35 MJ for unweaned lambs to 0.21 MJ at age 2 years and more (all 15% greater for rams), though in practice the Agricultural and Food Research Council (AFRC, 1993) recommends only 0.23 MJ up to 2 years of age and 0.215 MJ for older sheep. The progressive reduction in energy gain per unit ME intake by growing animals is regarded as being due to a progressive decrease in efficiency (k_g) above a constant ME_m and the value for k_g is reduced as level of feeding increases (Fig. 7.1c); the NRC (1985) k_g values do not require this adjustment.

The Australian feeding system (SCA, 1990) explicitly allows for variation in ME_m with level of feeding, using a modification (Corbett *et al.*, 1987) of the equation of Graham *et al.* (1974) that took account of the feed intake (including the contribution from milk), ΔW and the age of sheep, so that, when ME intake is known or predicted, it became:

$$ME_m = (KSM\ 0.26W^{0.75}\exp(-0.03A))/k_m + 0.09MEI + ME_{graze} + E_{cold}$$

The calculation of ME_m in ration formulation allows for the ME used for production, not total ME intake, so that the coefficient 0.26 for $W^{0.75}$ in the above equation becomes 0.28:

$$ME_m = (KSM\ 0.28W^{0.75}\exp(-0.03A))/k_m + 0.1ME_p + ME_{graze} + E_{cold}$$

where:

K = 1.0 for sheep
S = 1.0 (females and castrates) or 1.15 (intact males)
M = a factor based on the proportion of dietary energy from milk; estimated as [1 + (0.26 – 0.015a)], where a is week of life; weaning at age 17 weeks is assumed, when M = 1.0
W = live weight (kg)
A = age (years) with a maximum value of 6.0, when the value of [exp(0.03A)] is 0.84
k_m = net efficiency of use of ME for maintenance (0.85 for milk diets; calculated as (0.02M/D + 0.5) for other diets (ARC, 1980))
MEI = total ME intake (MJ day^{-1})
ME_p = the ME (MJ) being used directly for production
ME_{graze} = additional energy costs incurred in grazing
E_{cold} = energy expenditure in cold stress

Values for FM predicted with the first term ($KSM\ 0.28W^{0.75}\exp(-0.03A)$) are similar, at corresponding ages, to the several 'preferred values' of the ARC (1980). The term has an additional, useful attribute. It allows the effective biomasses of widely varying types of animals to be compared on the objective, common, basis of their NE_m, instead of by uncertainly based livestock units. With *Bos taurus*, K = 1.4 and, for example, ten female or castrate sheep, each 35 kg W and 6 months old with NE_m = 4.73 MJ, are nearly equivalent to one bull of 600 kg W and 4 years old (NE_m = 48.8 MJ).

These equations define ME_m for animals accustomed to a given MEI. Oltjen and Sainz (2000) have recently proposed an additional term that can take account of 'nutritional history', such as a change from the MEI at t_0 to another MEI at t_1. The ME_m at t_0 is multiplied by the term $1 + b(MEI_{t1}/MEI_{t0}-1)[1-\exp(-t/\tau)]$. The proposed value for b is 0.117 and for τ is 48 days, which implies that nearly 7 weeks after a change in level of feeding the adjustment in an animal's metabolism is barely two-thirds (only 0.63) complete.

No feeding system allows for seasonal variation in ME_m. Augmentation of maternal metabolism during pregnancy is accounted for by the use of a gross, not net, efficiency value for the utilization of ME for conceptus energy gain (SCA, 1990).

Physical activity

The NRC (1985) makes no allowance for energy costs of grazing. The ARC (1980) allowances revised by the AFRC (1993) are based on assumed distances walked, time spent standing and number of position changes. The fixed NE values (MJ per unit MW) for housed sheep are 0.0054 (pregnant ewes), 0.0096 (lactating ewes) or 0.0067 (fattening lambs); the allowance for 'lowland ewes out of doors' is 0.0107 and for 'ewes on hill grazing' is 0.024. With these allowances the NE_m for housed sheep aged 1 or more years are some 10–15 kJ per unit MW lower than those of the SCA (1990).

The requirement as ME_m (= NE_m /k_m) already allows for the physical activities associated with eating for maintenance. Consequently, when the additional energy costs incurred by grazing animals, ME_{graze} (MJ per kg W per day), are to be assessed, it is not the total time they spend in eating (about 2.5 kJ (kg^{-1} W h^{-1}), the total distance they walk (2.6 kJ per horizontal km and 28 kJ per vertical km, both per kg W), etc. that are of concern; it is the extra time, extra distance, etc., which will vary with grazing conditions, that have to be allowed for, as in the equation from SCA (1990):

$$ME_{graze} = \{0.05[DMI(0.9 - D)] + [0.05T/(GF + 3)]\}/k_m$$

where:

DMI = dry-matter intake (kg day^{-1})
D = digestibility of the dry matter
T = a value varying with terrain from 1.0 for level ground to 2.0 for steep, hilly ground
GF = the quantity of green forage available (t DM ha^{-1})

The first term predicts the additional cost of grazing the DMI rather than eating it from a trough. The second term predicts the additional costs of the walking and related physical activities associated with grazing over distances of up to about 7 km day^{-1} on the given terrain (T). These costs decrease as GF increases, because of the decreasing need to search for feed. When there is very little GF in a larger mass of dry forage (e.g. < 0.1 t DM ha^{-1}), animals are likely to abandon attempts at selection of the green material; in these circumstances, GF is replaced by the value for the total forage DM (t ha^{-1}). No account need be taken of rumination, because it can be assumed that, for any given amount and quality of feed, the time and energy spent on this activity will be the same whether the feed is eaten from a trough or is grazed from pasture. The equation is also applicable to cattle; the coefficient 0.05 in the first term becomes 0.006, implying that the relative pasture intake rates (kg DM per head) by sheep and cattle are 1 : 8, respectively.

Predicted ME_{graze} is consistent with the results of calorimetric measurements of the energy expenditures of freely grazing animals (e.g. Young and Corbett, 1972; Corbett *et al.*, 1980, 1982), which showed that, in the absence of cold stress, the value of ME_m at pasture would not be more than 40–50% greater than the ME_m for a similar housed animal, even in the most severe grazing conditions. With abundant and highly digestible pasturage, the difference might be as little as 10% (Langlands *et al.*, 1963).

Temperature

There is a range in ambient temperature (T_a), the 'zone of thermoneutrality', within which a sheep loses heat by evaporation, conduction, convection and radiation at a rate consistent with maintaining body temperature at about 39°C. The lower end of that variable range is the lower critical temperature (LCT), below which its heat production from metabolism in its tissues and from fermentation in its rumen is less than the rate of loss. Unless additional feed is provided, the sheep must then generate additional heat, which can to a limited extent be by shivering (i.e. muscular work) but is mainly from the catabolism of body fat; any contribution from protein breakdown is small. Additional ME is taken to be used with an efficiency of 1.0 for the alleviation of cold stress.

There is an inevitable evaporative heat loss via the lungs, expired gas being saturated with water vapour, and this loss decreases with T_a to a minimum at about the LCT. The rate of heat loss from the body other than via the lungs depends on the sheep's thermal insulation provided, first, by the cutaneous tissues (I_t), secondly, by its fleece (I_f) and, thirdly, by the boundary layer of air at the fleece surface (I_a). Some of the heat conducted through the cutaneous tissues is lost by evaporation at the skin surface and the remainder by conduction and convection through the fleece to its surface, where it is dissipated by conduction and radiation.

The equations and the numerical values for the several variables required for the calculation of LCT are given in SCA (1990), from which are taken the values in Table 7.2 for a 5 kg lamb and a 50 kg adult sheep. Wind reduces I_a, and when rain wets the fleece it reduces I_f, increasing its thermal conductivity and the rate of heat loss by the animal. Clearly, young lambs are very susceptible to cold stress (Table 7.2), as are newly shorn adult sheep, which respond with a persistent increase in heat production (Farrell and Corbett, 1970); both should be provided with shelter in adverse weather. An ME intake of less than maintenance results in an increase in LCT – that is, cold stress will occur at a higher ambient temperature, because of reduced heat production by the animal; if undernourishment is prolonged, then skin thickness and thus I_t can be reduced. Conversely, LCT becomes lower as ME intake increases.

When the other limit of the thermoneutral zone, the upper critical temperature, is exceeded, the animal cannot lose heat by conduction, convection or radiation. Cutaneous and respiratory (panting) evaporative heat loss increase to the extent allowed by the relative humidity (RH) of the air (nil if

Table 7.2. Lower critical temperatures of lambs and adult sheep with metabolizable energy intakes sufficient for maintenance in thermoneutral conditions. The values (°C) are for rainfalls of nil and 30 mm day^{-1} in calm and with 30 km h^{-1} wind at animal height (assumed to be 0.4 of velocity measured 10 m above ground, as at meteorological stations).

	Fleece depth (mm)	Calm		Wind 30 km h^{-1}	
		Dry	30 mm	Dry	30 mm
Lamb, 5 kg	6	21	24	28	29
	14	18	22	26	28
Adult, 50 kg	5	19	22	27	28
	20	10	16	23	25
	50	–5	1	18	20

RH = 100). Long-term hyperthermia is fatal, but over the short term some heat can be stored in the body, during a hot daytime, and later dissipated. An increased body temperature increases metabolic rate and therefore energy expenditure. The NRC (1996) suggests that the type and intensity of panting are an index of the increase in maintenance requirement consequent on hyperthermia, proposing an increase of 7% when there is rapid shallow breathing and 11–25% when there is deep open-mouth panting.

Protein

The immediate need is an intake of degradable protein or non-protein nitrogen sufficient to maintain active microbial fermentation in the rumen. The minimum dietary nitrogen (N) concentration required is approximately 10 g kg^{-1} DM, about 62.5 g kg^{-1} crude protein (CP); lower concentrations will increasingly impair microbial breakdown of ruminal digesta and retard its onward passage, so that feed intake will be severely reduced.

Endogenous losses

The protein requirement for maintenance is the amount that will make good the endogenous losses in urine and faeces and from the skin. Methods for determination are similar to those used for the measurement of maintenance energy. The minimum dietary N supply that results in N equilibrium can be established from feeding trials; endoparasitism, even subclinical infections, will inflate the result (Sykes, 2000). With a second method, analogous to the measurement of FHP, the N loss by the animal when fed an N-free diet is measured and, as with FHP, the results are affected by prior nutrition.

Animals on N-free diets continue to lose N in urine (U), mostly as urea resulting from catabolism of amino acids during protein turnover. Brody (1945) noted that, across many species, the loss was about 0.5 g N MJ^{-1} BMR, but it is substantially less in ruminants, because of their ability to recycle urea to the digestive tract. The ARC (1980) estimated (U × 6.25) (g day^{-1}) as ($0.147W + 3.375$).

A loss of N in faeces, termed metabolic faecal nitrogen (MFN), may be estimated from (faecal N = a + b(N consumed)), where a is MFN; its amount increases with increasing feed intake and is generally found to be about 5 g kg^{-1} DMI. The majority of the MFN is microbial debris, much of it from fermentation in the hind-gut, where microbial growth will be substantially dependent on urea entering through the gut wall, because there will be little available N in the digesta flow; the urea supply will be a cost to the protein economy of the animal. Endogenous N is present in the form of enzyme and sloughed cell residues. Hogan and Weston (1968) estimated, from the relationship between N in digesta flowing from the abomasum of sheep and in their faeces, that MFN from the intestines was 1.8 g kg^{-1} organic-matter flow. This value, much less than that for the entire digestive tract, would include a contribution from microbial debris from the hind-gut. Storm *et al.* (1983) maintained sheep by N-free intragastric infusions, so that there was no microbial contribution, and reported that the endogenous loss of N in faeces was 0.037 g per unit MW; with a maintenance DMI of 40 g per unit MW, the loss would be 0.9 g kg^{-1} DMI. The SCA (1990) estimate of the faecal endogenous loss (F) in normally fed sheep is 2.43 g kg^{-1} DMI (or, as CP, 15.2 g kg^{-1} DMI), the difference from Storm *et al.* (1983), 1.53 g kg^{-1} DMI, representing the microbial component.

Sustenance of ruminants solely by intragastric infusion of nutrients (Ørskov *et al.*, 1979) resolved the problem that, with N-free diets, the fermentation of feed and therefore feed intake are at risk, so that measurements of U are difficult and uncertain. With N-free infusates, a 'basal endogenous nitrogen' (BEN) loss was 0.35 g per unit MW; it was wholly in U, there being no voiding of faeces, and it was stated by the ARC (1984) to be applicable 'at a maintenance level of metabolizable energy intake'. It is applied by the AFRC (1993) at all L and is taken to encompass any endogenous N loss in faeces by normally fed animals; by implication, any increase in a faecal loss with increasing L is matched by a corresponding reduction in the urinary endogenous loss. The value for BEN is approximately the sum of endogenous losses estimated as U and MFN (ARC, 1984).

Dermal loss

With cattle, dermal loss (D) is as scurf and brushings (shed hair). Dermal loss by sheep is determined by the rate of wool growth, which continues even during severe underfeeding.

Practical definition

The maintenance need, expressed as [6.25(F + U + D)] or as [6.25(BEN + D)] in the AFRC (1993) system, is the amount of true protein that has to be digested in and absorbed from the small intestine. In practical feeding, it is the metabolizable protein (MP) to be supplied from the feed – that is, the amounts of truly digestible microbial true protein plus undegraded dietary protein. With true digestibility = 0.85, the efficiency with which MP is used to meet the requirement for BEN, k_{nb}, is taken to be 1.0 by the AFRC (1993); in its system, the efficiency value for D as scurf and hair, k_{nd}, is also taken to be 1.0, but with sheep its value for wool growth, k_{nw} = 0.26, would be appropriate. With the requirement as the sum of F, U and D, the k_{nm} = 0.8 of ARC (1984) allows for possible inefficiencies. The MP requirement for D, the wool growth, is discussed by Hynd and Masters (Chapter 8, this volume).

There would be major difficulties in expressing N requirements for maintenance in terms of individual amino acids and the proportions of the acids in MP and most body proteins are broadly similar. The exception is wool protein, which has a content of sulphur amino acids three to four times that in, for example, muscle and meat proteins. Liu and Masters (2000) have estimated that the requirement for absorbed methionine of the Merino sheep at maintenance is, depending on W, 0.45–0.75 g day^{-1} and for absorbed cysteine is 0.52–0.63 g day^{-1}.

Minerals and Vitamins

The net amount of a mineral required by the sheep for maintenance is the sum of the quantities lost from the body as endogenous excretions in urine and faeces and from the skin as suint (principally Na and K). Their conversion to dietary requirements presents a number of difficulties (for discussion, see SCA, 1990). These include variation in the absorbability of a mineral between feeds, with concentration in the feed, with animal need and from interactions with other minerals (e.g. Cu with Mo and S) (see Lee *et al.*, Chapter 13, this volume). Some feed components affect requirements; for example, those for I and S are affected by, respectively, goitrogenic and cyanogenic substances. The requirements listed in Table 7.3, given for convenience as dietary concentrations, should thus be taken only as a guide.

The requirement for S is determined primarily by its essentiality for protein synthesis and growth by the ruminal microbiota. Consequently the requirement is better expressed by reference to the N supplied by the diet rather than as a concentration; for sheep an S : N ratio of 0.08 – that is, 12.5 g N : 1 g S – has been recommended (SCA, 1990). Deficiencies of K and Cl are unlikely, and there has been no clear demonstration of a primary P deficiency in grazing sheep. Ca will be deficient when sheep are given cereal grains for their survival, for example, on drought-affected bare pastures; finely ground limestone to provide Ca should be added to grain at the rate of 15 g kg^{-1}.

Table 7.3. Guide to desirable concentrations of minerals in feed dry matter (DM) (from SCA, 1990).

Major minerals (g kg^{-1} DM)		Trace minerals (mg kg^{-1} DM)	
Calcium	1.5	Cobalt	0.11
Phosphorus	1.3	Copper	5
Chlorine	1.0	Iodine	0.5
Magnesium	1.2	Iron	40
Potassium	5	Manganese	15
Sodium	0.7	Selenium	0.05
Sulphur	2.0	Zinc	20

Compared with other nutrients, animals can be maintained for much longer periods on daily intakes of many of the minerals that are less than requirements. This is because they are sustained by the mobilization of the minerals held mainly in bone and liver, though these stores would eventually have to be replenished.

Only on rare occasions in the maintenance of sheep must attention be paid to their vitamin requirements (discussed by Lee *et al.*, Chapter 13, this volume). Vitamin D might be of concern in sheep with prolonged housing or, if outdoors, if the elevation of the sun were less than 35° for long periods. In both circumstances, because of low solar ultraviolet radiation, there would be very little synthesis in the animal body of D_2 (ergocalciferol) from ergosterol and of D_3 (cholecalciferol) from 7-dehydrocholesterol. If the diets included fresh or dried forages, it is likely that the requirement of around 0.2 μg kg^{-1} W would be met. Grazing sheep generally do not require supplementary vitamin A; even when drought rations of cereal grains are given, hepatic stores are sufficient for a period that, with grown sheep, can be as long as a year.

Water

During starvation, an animal can lose almost all of the fat and about half of the protein in its body and yet still survive, but the loss of one-tenth of its body water is probably fatal. Water has four main functions in the body: (i) elimination of waste products from digestion and metabolism; (ii) regulation of blood osmotic pressure; (iii) production of secretions (e.g. saliva and other digestive fluids); and (iv) thermoregulation, involving evaporative losses from the lungs and skin surface.

Water is gained by drinking, as water in feed and on feed as dew and rainfall, and as 'metabolic' water formed during oxidation of dietary nutrients and catabolism of body tissues. Lynch *et al.* (1972) reported that, when grazing ewes in a temperate climate were deprived of drinking-water for 12 months, they survived and even bore lambs. In practice, deprivation would be folly. Within the thermoneutral zone, the sensible heat losses by the animal are less than the evaporative losses and for each MJ lost by that means the animal loses from its body about 0.42 l of water. The water loss increases greatly at temperatures above the higher critical value – for example, a three- to fourfold increase with a change from 15 to 35–40°C.

Minimum water requirements can be calculated by summation of evaporative losses and minimal losses in excreta, but, unlike other nutrients, recommended values for requirements are generally based on observations of voluntary intakes, which show that total water intake (drunk and in feed) is positively related to DM intake. The SCA (1990) recommended total water intakes (l per kg DMI) for weaned sheep, not pregnant or lactating, of 2.0 at ≤ 15°C, 2.5 at 20°C, 3.5 at 25°C, 5.0 at 30°C and 7.0 at 35°C. These allowances are for drinking-water containing not more than 2000 mg total soluble salts (TSS) l^{-1} and for feed containing not more than 100 g ash (other than soil ash) kg^{-1} DM. For each 1000 mg TSS in excess, allowances should be increased by 3% and, for each 10 g ash in excess, by 5%.

Conclusion

Greater understanding of the maintenance metabolism from more knowledge of metabolism in tissues associated with normal body function and of those directly involved in growth, particularly associated variations in protein turnover, will facilitate identification of intrinsic differences in maintenance requirements between animals. There will be consequent improvements in models of energy utilization and opportunities for increasing productivity by selection of animals that are more efficient because of lower maintenance needs.

References

AFRC (1993) *Energy and Protein Requirements of Ruminants. An Advisory Manual Prepared by the AFRC Technical Committee on Responses to Nutrients.* CAB International, Wallingford, UK, 159 pp.

ARC (1980) *The Nutrient Requirements of Ruminant Livestock. Technical Review by an Agricultural Research Council Working Party.* Commonwealth Agricultural Bureaux, Farnham Royal, UK.

ARC (1984) *Report of the Protein Group of the Agricultural Research Council Working Party on the Nutrient Requirements of Ruminants.* Commonwealth Agricultural Bureaux, Farnham Royal, UK.

Ball, A.J., Thompson, J.M. and Pleasants, A.B. (1996) Seasonal changes in body composition of growing Merino sheep. *Livestock Production Science* 46, 173–180.

Ball, A.J., Oddy, V.H. and Thompson, J.M. (1997) Nutritional manipulation of body composition and efficiency in ruminants. In: Corbett, J.L., Choct, M., Nolan, J.V. and Rowe, J.B. (eds) *Recent Advances in Animal Nutrition in Australia, 1997.* Department of Animal Science, University of New England, Armidale, Australia, pp. 192–208.

Ball, A.J., Thompson, J.M., Alston, C.L., Blakely, A.R. and Hinch, G.N. (1998) Changes in maintenance energy requirements of mature sheep fed at different levels of feed intake at maintenance, during weight loss and realimentation. *Livestock Production Science* 53, 191–204.

Blaxter, K.L. (1962) The fasting metabolism of adult wether sheep. *British Journal of Nutrition* 16, 615–626.

Blaxter, K.L. and Boyne, A.W. (1982) Fasting and maintenance metabolism of sheep. *Journal of Agricultural Science, Cambridge* 99, 611–620.

Brody, S. (1935) The relation between feeding standards and basal metabolism. In: *Report of the Conference on Energy Metabolism, State College, Pennsylvania*. Committee on Animal Nutrition, National Research Council, Washington, DC, pp. 12–23.

Brody, S. (1945) *Bioenergetics and Growth*. Rheinhold Publishing, Baltimore, Maryland, 1023 pp.

Corbett, J.L., Furnival, E.P., Inskip, M.W., Pickering, F.S. and Plaza, J. (1980) Pasture intake and heat production of breeding ewes. In: Mount, L.E. (ed.) *Energy Metabolism*. Butterworths, London, pp. 319–323.

Corbett, J.L., Furnival, E.P. and Pickering, F.S. (1982) Energy expenditure at pasture of shorn and unshorn Border Leicester ewes during late pregnancy and lactation. In: Ekern, A. and Sundstøl, F. (eds) *Proceedings of the 9th EAAP Symposium on Energy Metabolism of Farm Animals*. Agricultural University of Norway, Ås, Norway, pp. 34–37.

Corbett, J.L., Freer, M. and Graham, N.McC. (1987) A generalized equation to predict the varying maintenance metabolism of sheep and cattle. In: Moe, P.W., Tyrrell, H.F. and Reynolds, P.J. (eds) *Proceedings of the 10th EAAP Symposium on Energy Metabolism of Farm Animals*. Rowman and Littlefield, New Jersey, pp. 62–65.

Cristian, A., Meneses, E.E., Burlacu, G. and Stavri, J. (1980) Efficiency of utilization of corn silage diets by pregnant and lactating sheep. In: Mount, L.E. (ed.) *Energy Metabolism*. Butterworths, London, pp. 363–365.

CSIRO (1958) *Drought Feeding of Sheep*. Leaflet Series no. 23, CSIRO, Melbourne, 32 pp.

Farrell, D.J. and Corbett, J.L. (1970) Fasting heat production of sheep at pasture before and after shearing. *Proceedings of the Australian Society of Animal Production* 8, 267–271.

Ferrell, H.C., Koong, L.J. and Nienaber, J.A. (1986) Effect of previous nutrition on body composition and maintenance energy costs of growing lambs. *British Journal of Nutrition* 56, 595–605.

Forbes, J.M. (1982) Effect of lighting pattern on growth, lactation and food intake of sheep, cattle and deer. *Livestock Production Science* 9, 361–374.

Freetly, H.C. and Ferrell, C.L. (1997) Changes in gut and liver glucose release and oxygen consumption during gestation and lactation in the ewe. In: McCracken, K., Unsworth, E.F. and Wylie, A.R.G. (eds) *Proceedings of the 14th EAAP Symposium on Energy Metabolism of Farm Animals*. CAB International, Wallingford, UK, pp. 35–38.

Freetly, H.C., Nienaber, J.A., Leymaster, K.A. and Jenkins, T.G. (1995) Relationships among heat production, body weight, and age in Suffolk and Texel ewes. *Journal of Animal Science* 73, 1030–1037.

Graham, N.McC. (1968) The metabolic rate of Merino rams bred for high or low wool production. *Australian Journal of Agricultural Research* 19, 821–824.

Graham, N.McC. (1982) Energy feeding standards: a methodological problem. In: Ekern, A. and Sundstøl, F. (eds) *Proceedings of the 9th EAAP Symposium on Energy Metabolism of Farm Animals*. Agricultural University of Norway, Ås, Norway, pp. 108–111.

Graham, N.McC. and Searle, T.W. (1979) Studies of weaned lambs before, during and after a period of weight loss 1. Energy and nitrogen utilization. *Australian Journal of Agricultural Research* 30, 513–523.

Graham, N.McC., Searle, T.W. and Griffiths, D.A. (1974) Basal metabolic rate in lambs and young sheep. *Australian Journal of Agricultural Research* 25, 957–971.

Hogan, J.P. and Weston, R.H. (1968) Digestion of protein in the intestines of the sheep. *Proceedings of the Australian Society of Animal Production* 7, 364–368.

Huntington, G.B. and McBride, B.W. (1988) Ruminant splanchnic tissues: energy costs of absorption and metabolism. In: Steffens, G.L. and Rumsay, T.S. (eds) *Biomechanisms Regulating Growth and Development.* Kluwer, Boston, Massachusetts, pp. 313–328.

Kelly, J.M. and McBride, B.W. (1990) The sodium pump and other mechanisms of thermogenesis in selected tissues. *Proceedings of the Nutrition Society* 49, 185–202.

Kleiber, M. (1961) *The Fire of Life*. John Wiley, New York, 454 pp.

Langlands, J.P., Corbett, J.L., McDonald, I. and Reid, G.W. (1963) Estimates of the energy required for maintenance by adult sheep 2. Grazing sheep. *Animal Production* 5, 11–16.

Lines, E.W. and Peirce, A.W. (1931) *The Basal (Standard) Metabolism of the Australian Merino Sheep*. Bulletin no. 55, Council for Scientific and Industrial Research, Melbourne.

Liu, S.M. and Masters, D.G. (2000) Quantitative analysis of methionine and cysteine requirements for wool production of sheep. *Animal Science* 71, 175–185.

Lynch, J.J., Brown, G.D., May, P.F. and Donnelly, J.B. (1972) The effect of withholding drinking water on wool growth and lamb production of grazing Merino sheep in a temperate climate. *Australian Journal of Agricultural Research* 23, 659–668.

MacRae, J.C. (1993) Metabolic consequences of internal parasitism. *Proceedings of the Nutrition Society* 52, 121–130.

McBride, B.W. and Milligan, L.P. (1985) Influence of feed intake and starvation on the magnitude of $Na^{+}K^{+}$-ATPase (*EC* 3.6.1.3)-dependent respiration in duodenal mucosa of sheep. *British Journal of Nutrition* 53, 605–614.

NRC (1985) *Nutrient Requirements of Sheep*, 6th edn. National Academy Press, Washington, DC, 99 pp.

NRC (1996) *Nutrient Requirements of Beef Cattle*, 7th edn. National Academy Press, Washington, DC, 242 pp.

Oltjen, J.W. and Sainz, R.D. (2000) Alternate forms for heat production in ruminant growth and composition models. In: Chwalibog, A. and Jakobsen, K. (eds) *Proceedings of the 15th EAAP Symposium on Energy Metabolism of Farm Animals, Snekkersten, Denmark.* Wageningen Pers, The Netherlands, pp. 39–42.

Ørskov, E.R., Grubb, D.A., Wenham, G. and Corrigall, W. (1979) The sustenance of growing and fattening ruminants by intragastric infusion of volatile fatty acid and protein. *British Journal of Nutrition* 41, 553–558.

Ortigues, I. and Durand, D. (1995) Adaptation of energy metabolism to undernutrition in ewes: contribution of portal-drained viscera, liver and hindquarters. *British Journal of Nutrition* 73, 209–222.

Perry, D., Ball, A.J., Thompson, J.M., Littlefield, P.L. and Howe, S. (1998) Body composition changes in response to different frequency of feeding of maintenance rations. *Animal Production in Australia* 22, 302.

SCA (1990) *Feeding Standards for Australian Livestock: Ruminants.* Standing Committee on Agriculture and CSIRO, Melbourne, 266 pp.

Seal, C.J. and Reynolds, C.K. (1993) Nutritional implications of gastrointestinal and liver metabolism in ruminants. *Nutrition Research Reviews* 6, 185–208.
Storm, E., Brown, D.S. and Ørskov, E.R. (1983) The nutritive value of rumen micro-organisms in ruminants. 3. The digestion of microbial amino and nucleic acids in, and losses of endogenous nitrogen from, the small intestine of sheep. *British Journal of Nutrition* 50, 479–485.
Sykes, A.R. (2000) Environmental effects on animal production: the nutritional demands of nematode parasite exposure in sheep. *Asian–Australasian Journal of Animal Sciences* 13 (Suppl. A), 343–350.
Thomson, D.J. and Cammell, S.B. (1979) The utilization of chopped and pelleted lucerne (*Medicago sativa*) by growing lambs. *British Journal of Nutrition* 41, 297–310.
Turner, H.G. and Taylor, St.C.S. (1983) Dynamic factors in models of energy utilization with particular reference to maintenance requirements of cattle. *World Review of Nutrition and Dietetics* 42, 135–190.
Walker, V.A., Young, B.A. and Walker, B. (1991) Does seasonal photoperiod directly influence energy metabolism? In: Wenk, C. and Boessinger, M. (eds) *Proceedings of the 12th EAAP Symposium on Energy Metabolism of Farm Animals.* Institut für Nutztierwissenschaften, Zurich, pp. 372–375.
Webster, A.J.F. (1989) Bioenergetics, bioengineering and growth. *Animal Production* 48, 249–269.
Young, B.A. and Corbett, J.L. (1972) Maintenance energy requirement of grazing sheep in relation to herbage availability. 1. Calorimetric estimates. *Australian Journal of Agricultural Research* 23, 57–76.

8 Nutrition and Wool Growth

P.I. Hynd[1] and D.G. Masters[2]

[1]*Department of Animal Science, Adelaide University, Roseworthy, South Australia, Australia;* [2]*CSIRO Livestock Industries, Wembley, Western Australia, Australia*

Introduction

The impact of nutrition on the wool growth of grazing sheep has long been appreciated, with periods of poor pasture growth or quality reflected in a reduction in total fleece growth per animal and per unit area of grazed land. As for all other forms of animal production, this relationship between nutrient intake and product output reflects changes in the supply of substrates – in this case, substrates essential for fibre synthesis in the wool follicle, the skin's fibre-producing 'factory'. This chapter examines the relative importance of amino acids, carbohydrates, minerals and vitamins for wool production and quality. The nutritional processes involved in fibre production within the follicle are outlined, along with the relationship between nutrient supply from the gastrointestinal tract and fibre growth rate, fibre diameter, fibre length, staple strength, clean fibre yield and wool colour.

The Process of Fibre Production in the Wool Follicle

Wool follicle initiation in the fetus

The wool follicle is an invagination (down-growth) of the epidermis formed during fetal life. The first (primary) follicles start forming 50–60 days after conception. By day 90–100, they are producing a fibre. There are two types of secondary follicle. The first are termed the 'original' secondary follicles and, like the primaries, they are produced from the overlying epidermis, but commencing from day 85–90 post-conception. The second type is known as the 'derived' or branched secondary follicles, because they are produced by budding of the already established original secondary follicles. Primary follicles are often larger in both diameter and length than original secondary follicles and therefore produce fibres that are longer and coarser. Similarly, original secondary follicles and fibres are usually larger than derived secondary follicles and fibres. Regardless of the type of follicle, the processes involved in fibre production described below are identical, even though the rate of processes may differ, depending on follicle size.

The cellular events in wool fibre synthesis

Figure 8.1 shows a photomicrograph of a longitudinal section of two follicles in the skin of a Merino sheep. One follicle is in the actively growing phase, known as anagen, and the other in the resting phase of the fibre cycle, known as telogen. A transverse section of a follicle and fibre is shown schematically in Fig. 8.2, along with a photomicrograph of a Merino wool follicle in anagen.

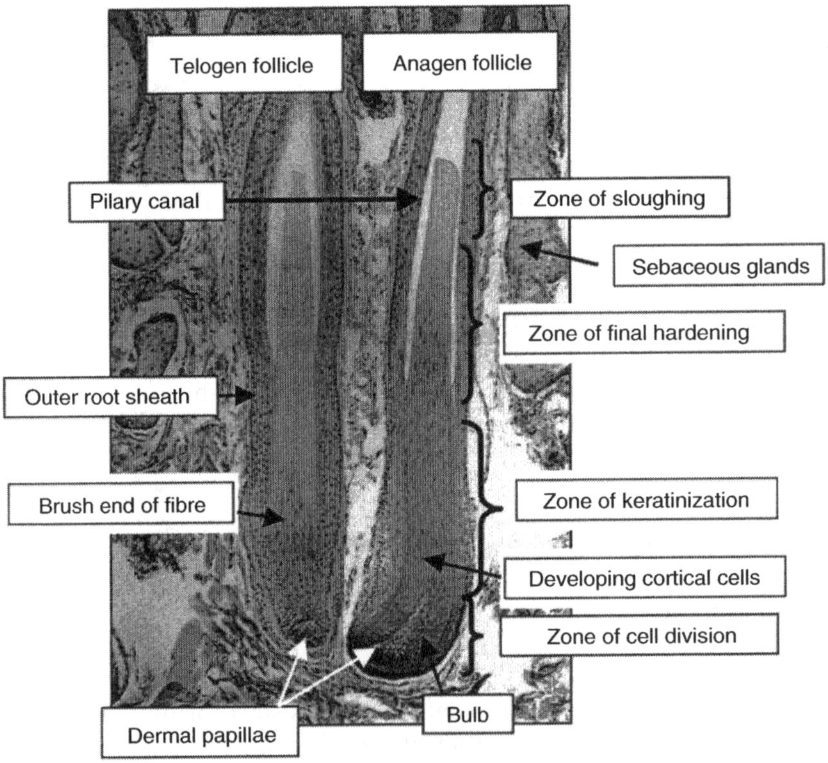

Fig. 8.1. Photomicrograph of sheep wool follicles from the face of a Merino sheep showing a follicle in the resting (telogen) phase of the fibre growth cycle (left-hand side) and the growing (anagen) phase of the fibre growth cycle (right-hand side). The telogen follicle is characterized by the presence of a fibre with a brush end, a dermal papilla that is condensed and circular in shape, and a shrunken and distorted outer root sheath and dermal sheath. (Photomicrograph courtesy of Dr Michelle Nancarrow.)

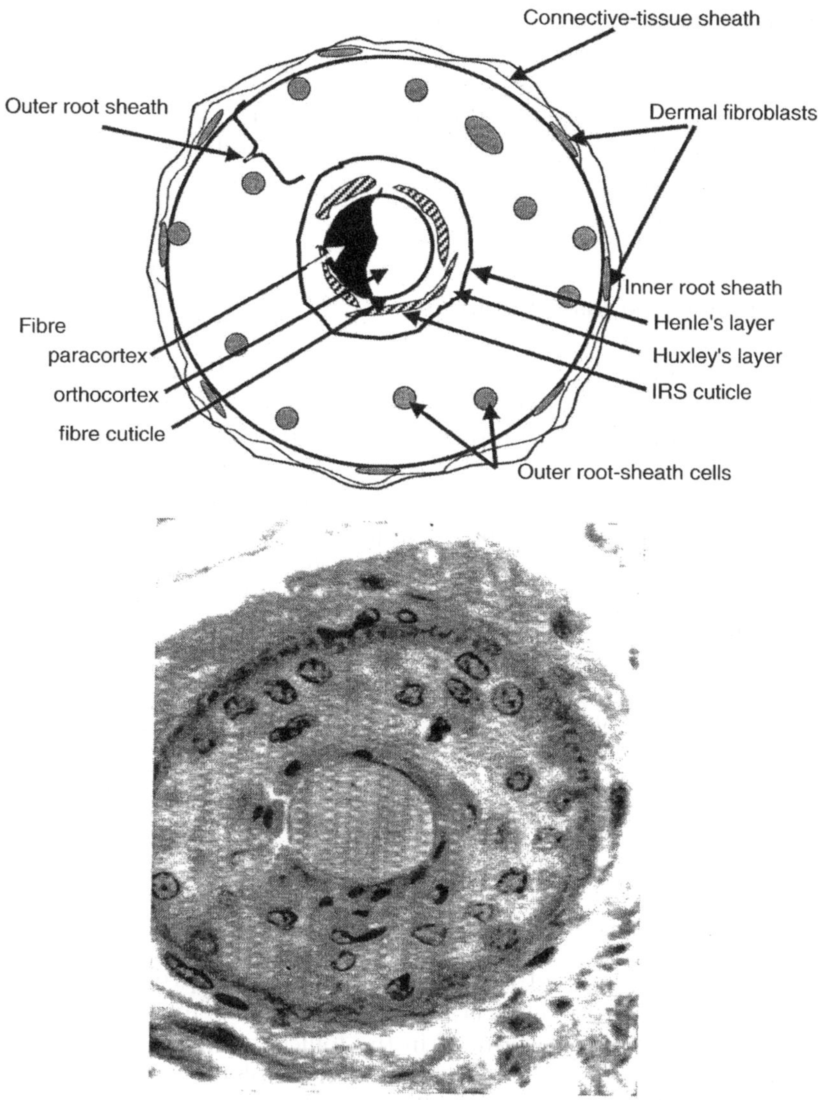

Fig. 8.2. Schematic diagram (top) and photomicrograph (bottom) of a transverse section of a wool follicle, showing the major regions of the follicle and fibre.

Fibre production commences with rapid division of the cells in the germinative region of the follicle bulb, defined as the area surrounding and extending to the tip of the dermal papilla (Fig. 8.1). The total volume of fibre produced depends partly on the total number of cells present in the follicle bulb and their turnover rate; together, these determine the total number of dividing cells per unit time. It also depends on the final volume of the cells after keratinization, the proportion of the dividing cells that enter the fibre versus the inner root sheath and the volume of the intercellular cement (Orwin, 1971). These processes are discussed briefly below.

Follicle bulb and papilla size

The diameter and length of the wool fibres are positively and closely related to the dimensions of the follicle bulb and the dermal papilla (diameter, volume and surface area) that produce them, regardless of whether the differences are generated by genetics or nutritional regimen (Hynd, 1994a, b).

Cell proliferation in the follicle bulb

Cell proliferation (reviewed by Chapman and Ward, 1979) occurs in the follicle bulb and in the outer root sheath along the entire length of the follicle. Recent evidence supports the notion that there is a population of follicle stem cells resident in the outer root sheath. These pluripotent cells give rise to daughter cells, which migrate downwards to eventually become the cells of the follicle bulb. It appears that all cells in the follicle bulb undergo mitosis, whereas the cells of the dermal papilla are mitotically inactive. There are between 500 and 1500 bulb cells, depending on nutrition and genotype. Between 16 and 44 of these cells undergo cell division each hour. The time taken to replace the entire bulb cell population (the turnover time) ranges from 19 to 44 h (Table 8.1), but it is unlikely that the extremes of wool growth rates have been investigated. The outer root sheath cells divide less frequently than the bulb cells. The greatest cell proliferation in the outer root sheath occurs in the thickened region adjacent to the region of keratinization of the fibre.

Cell migration

Cell migration in wool follicles is a well-ordered procedure, discussed in detail by Chapman *et al.* (1980). Cells destined to enter the inner root sheath and fibre are produced in the follicle bulb, while outer root-sheath cells replicate themselves along the length of the follicle (Fig. 8.1). The inner root-sheath precursor cells move out of the bulb ahead of the contemporaneously formed fibre cells (Chapman *et al.*, 1980). The inner root sheath is thought to play a role in the shaping of the newly formed fibre.

Gene expression and keratin synthesis

As cells migrate from the follicle bulb, they commence the process of differentiation, in which the expression of different genes produces different keratin and keratin-associated proteins. The keratin genes are activated in the cells destined to become the cuticle and cortex, and the trichohyalin gene is activated in the cells of the inner root sheath and medulla. It is thought that there may be more than 60 proteins produced in the fibre

Table 8.1. Effect of nutrition and genotype on follicle dimensions, cell volumes and cell kinetics.

Genotype		Nutrition	Bulb volume ($10^{-5} \times \mu m^3$)	Bulb cell volume (μm^3)	Bulb cell number	Mitoses (no. h^{-1})	Cortical cell volume (μm^3)	Cell turnover time (h)	Dividing bulb cells entering fibre (%)	References
Merino	MW	Low	2.26	426	543	16.9	764	32.1	15	1
	MW	Medium	3.33	404	814	30.8	1015	26.4	13	1
	MW[a]	High	3.00	511	588	30.3	1176	19.4	14	1
Romney		Winter	n.d.	n.d.	591	n.d.	n.d.	36.0	n.d.	2
Romney		Spring	n.d.	n.d.	709	n.d.	n.d.	19.0	n.d.	2
Merino	MW	Low	2.10	288	731	16.5	796	44.3	15	3
	MW	High	2.85	349	816	26.8	949	30.4	18	3
Merino	SW	Low	n.d.	n.d.	1005	26.8	918	37.5	32	4
	SW	High	n.d.	n.d.	1211	35.2	950	34.4	35	4
Corriedale[a]		Low	n.d.	n.d.	845	27	1031	31.3	30	4
Corriedale[a]		High	n.d.	n.d.	1479	44	1098	33.6	29	4
Merino	FW[a]	Low	n.d.	n.d.	493	20	841	24.7	26	4
	FW[a]	High	n.d.	n.d.	704	26	904	27.1	22	4
	FW	Medium	0.86	176	535	18.3	896	29.2	20	5
	SW	Medium	1.92	261	830	37.7	1061	22.0	35	5

[a]One animal only.

References: 1, Wilson and Short (1979); 2, Fraser (1965); 3, Short *et al.* (1965); 4, Hynd (1989); 5, Hocking Edwards and Hynd (1992).

MW, medium wool; SW, strong wool; FW, fine wool; n.d., not determined.

cells (Powell *et al.*, 1991). These proteins belong to two groups: the intermediate filament (IF) proteins and the intermediate filament-associated proteins (IFAP). The IF group comprises two families, IF type I and IF type II, with five genes in each encoding relatively low-sulphur (S) proteins. The IFAP group contains approximately 22 high-S genes, 16 ultra-high-S genes and 12 high-glycine/tyrosine genes. The production of a fibre is the result of a complex and well-coordinated expression of these keratin gene families, which have overlapping as well as discrete patterns of expression (Powell *et al.*, 1991). The large variation in the composition of the proteins encoded by the keratin genes provides a mechanism for nutrition to alter fibre composition through altered expression of the genes (see below).

The proportion of dividing bulb cells that produce fibre and inner root sheath

The proportion of the dividing bulb cells that enter the wool fibre is low. Of all the cells produced by cell division in the follicle bulb, only about 10–40% end up in the fibre cortex and cuticle (Short *et al.*, 1965). Presumably the other cells produce the three cell layers of the inner root sheath, which are ultimately resorbed or sloughed into the pilary canal of the follicle (Fig. 8.1).

The nutritional biochemistry of wool follicles

Given the high rate of cell division and protein synthesis in the wool follicle, one would expect a high sensitivity of the follicle processes and fibre growth to changes in the supply of energy, protein, lipids, vitamins and minerals. The relative influence of these nutrients on fibre growth will depend on the pathways operating in the follicle cells. These are discussed in this section.

Energy metabolism in the wool follicle

The development of serum-free culture of wool and hair follicles in minimal media (Philpott *et al.*, 1990) paved the way for detailed studies of metabolism in actively growing follicles. These studies have shown that follicles have developed some unusual features of energy metabolism, including anaerobic glycolysis, glycogen metabolism, an active pentose phosphate pathway and glutaminolysis.

Of all the fuels available to the follicle, it appears that the predominant substrates are glucose and glutamine (Kealey *et al.*, 1991). Acetate fails to maintain fibre growth *in vitro* and lipid catabolism is low. Of all the glucose utilized by the follicle, only about 10% is oxidized; the remaining 90% undergoes anaerobic glycolysis to produce lactate, even when oxygen is present.

This raises several questions that highlight the distinction between nutrition at the cellular level compared with the whole animal. First, why would follicles produce lactic acid via anaerobic pathways, yielding only 2 mol of ATP mol^{-1} of glucose utilized, when aerobic pathways yielding 36 mol of ATP mol^{-1} of glucose are available? Secondly, why is glutamine such an important fuel for follicles? Thirdly, what is the relevance of the pentose phosphate shunt to follicle function? Finally, what relevance has glycogen metabolism to follicle function?

The answer to the first question might relate to the necessity for the follicle to produce a fibre when blood flow and hence oxygen supply are reduced, a situation that arises in skin in response to low temperatures and noradrenaline release from the sympathetic nerves. While anaerobic glycolysis may appear inefficient from the point of view of the follicle, from a whole-animal viewpoint the return of the lactate to the liver for oxidation recovers the energy. From the follicle viewpoint, glucose is readily available from glycogen stored in the outer root sheath. Whether the follicle uses the aerobic or anaerobic pathways of carbohydrate metabolism is important, because it determines the total quantity of energy substrates required for wool growth. If the low-efficiency anaerobic pathway is used instead of the aerobic pathway, then 18 times more glucose would be required. This may explain why wool growth sometimes responds to energy substrates, while at other times it is entirely dependent on amino acid supply (see Fig. 8.3).

Glutamine oxidation in follicles is high and may yield as much energy as glucose metabolism. This would provide a large quantity of ammonia, which might buffer the pH changes induced by lactate production. The pentose phosphate pathway would supply a large amount of pentose required for DNA synthesis in the bulb cells and RNA synthesis in the migrating keratinocytes (Chapman and Ward, 1979). In addition, the large amounts of NADPH produced by this pathway would maintain the redox status of the cells.

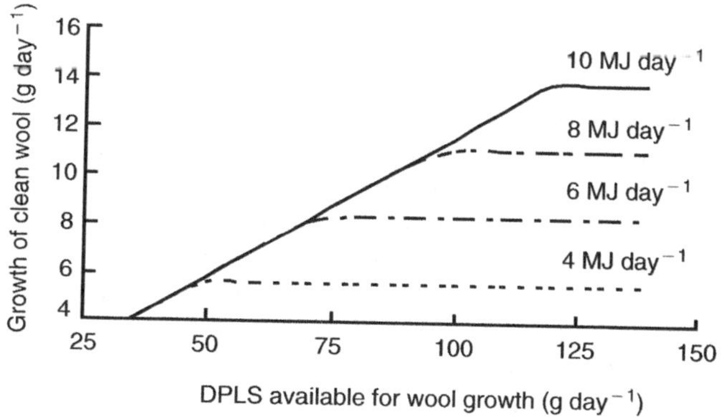

Fig. 8.3. Wool-growth response to digestible protein leaving the stomach (DPLS) at four levels of metabolizable energy intake (MEI): 4, 6, 8 and 10 MJ day^{-1}, assuming that the DPLS is used for wool growth with an efficiency of 11.6% (Hogan *et al.*, 1979) and that wool growth is determined by DPLS until DPLS/MEI exceeds 12 g MJ^{-1} (Kempton, 1979).

Protein metabolism in wool follicles

The effect of amino acids on the growth and composition of wool fibres is covered in detail by Reis (1979). Wool growth is limited by the supply of cysteine to the follicle in most classes of sheep. Wool contains about 10% cysteine compared with < 2% in other tissues of the body. This cysteine arises from several sources, including microbial cysteine entering the intestines, dietary cysteine that has escaped rumen degradation and cysteine that is produced from methionine by the trans-sulphuration pathway (Benevenga and Egan, 1983). When radiolabelled cysteine is introduced into the bloodstream, it rapidly enters the cells in the keratogenous zone (Downes *et al.*, 1962). Presumably the cysteine diffuses across the endothelium of the capillaries surrounding the follicle and traverses the extracellular space. The means by which cysteine then enters the cuticle and cortical cells, where it is required for keratin synthesis, is unclear. There are several cell layers through which the cysteine must travel (the dermal sheath, the outer root sheath, the inner root sheath and finally the cells that will form the cuticle and cortex). The amino acid may present itself to the fibre cells by moving between cells in these layers or it may travel through the cells by attaching to specific amino acid transport proteins. The former is unlikely, given the tight junctions between cells of the outer root sheath. Recently, complementary DNA (cDNA) encoding a neutral amino acid transport protein was isolated from follicles and shown to operate in precisely the same region as that in which the labelled cysteine enters the follicle (Nattrass, 2000).

It remains to be determined whether other amino acids involved in follicle function are transported by membrane-bound carrier proteins. However, lysine enters the cells of the lower follicle bulb, while leucine and alanine are uniformly taken up by cells in the outer root sheath, the follicle bulb and the keratinizing zone. The pattern of amino acid requirements of the bulb cells is presumably the same as that of most mammalian cells, in that the normal requirements for growth and metabolism would exist here. Lysine, for instance, would be required for the synthesis of histones required for DNA synthesis. However, once the cells migrate from the zone of cell division and commence keratin synthesis, the requirement for cysteine increases markedly relative to the other amino acids. Alterations to the balance of amino acids presented to the follicle are thus likely to alter the relative balance of cell division versus keratin synthesis. For instance, a supply of amino acids rich in cysteine but low in lysine might be expected to lead to a reduction in cell division in the bulb cells (Hynd, 1989). It might also lead to a disproportionately high supply of cysteine per migrating cell, resulting in larger cortical cells or cortical cells of different composition (see below).

The other S-containing amino acid, methionine, also increases wool growth over and above that expected by its increasing the supply of cysteine through trans-sulphuration. Methionine is a precursor for polyamine synthesis (Reis, 1979) and polyamines are important in fibre growth. Inhibition of ornithine decarboxylase, the rate-limiting enzyme for polyamine synthesis, results in a decrease in fibre length and an increase in fibre diameter in the absence of any change in feed intake (Hynd and Nancarrow, 1996). The composition of the fibres, the proportion of para-cortical cells in the fibre and the expression of a cysteine-rich family of keratin genes are also altered, suggesting that polyamines are involved in both cell division and gene expression. Methionine is also a precursor for *S*-adenosylmethionine, the major donor of methyl groups in the body. Methylation of cytosine may regulate gene activity and DNA repair. There are also many other key metabolites produced from methyl reactions involving methionine. A role for methionine in follicle metabolism, other than as a precursor of cysteine, is therefore highly likely.

Vitamins and wool growth

A deficiency of a vitamin may reduce or completely inhibit fibre growth, by reducing the feed intake of the animal and hence the supply of substrate to the follicle, by inhibiting the activity of enzymes involved in protein or energy metabolism, by reducing the production of nucleic acids required in the follicle for cell division and protein synthesis or by directly inhibiting keratinization (see review by Hynd, 2000).

Several of the vitamins play vital roles in protein synthesis, S-amino acid metabolism, nucleic acid synthesis or gene expression and keratinization. Thiamine (vitamin B_1) is a cofactor for the transketolase enzyme required for the pentose phosphate pathway. Pyridoxine (vitamin B_6) is required for amino acid metabolism in general and in the trans-sulphuration reaction in which methionine is converted to cysteine. Pyridoxine is also essential for polyamine synthesis and is involved in glycogen metabolism. Biotin may be involved in follicle function, because it is required for nucleic acid synthesis. Folic acid is essential for transferring one-carbon fragments from serine, glycine and histidine to other amino acids, purines and thymidine, thereby contributing to cell division and protein synthesis. Vitamin B_{12} is a cofactor in methionine synthetase, involved in methionine conservation and the provision of methyl groups for a range of molecules. Vitamin B_{12} is also essential for the activity of methylmalonyl coenzyme A (CoA) isomerase, a key enzyme in the production of glucose from propionate.

The only direct demonstration of a vitamin deficiency affecting wool growth occurred in preruminant lambs supplied with diets deficient in folic acid (Chapman and Black, 1981). The wool lacked crimp and in several cases fibre growth ceased completely, despite the fact that the animals were gaining weight. Provision of folic acid alleviated the condition, supporting the notion that this vitamin is essential for wool growth.

While microbial synthesis of the B-group vitamins in the rumen means that adult ruminants are unlikely to suffer deficiencies of these vitamins, perturbations to rumen function may reduce microbial supply. The presence of 'antivitamin' compounds in feeds (e.g. antithiaminase in bracken fern) may also induce a deficiency.

The fat-soluble vitamins A and D_3 probably have direct effects on follicle function, as both have specific receptors in various parts of the follicle.

Vitamin A affects keratin gene expression as well as cell division in the follicle bulb (Hynd, 2000). Vitamin E may play a role with selenium in maintaining the redox potential of the follicle cells, but there is no evidence of direct effects of vitamin E on fibre growth. Similarly, vitamin K has not been directly implicated in follicle function.

Minerals and wool growth

Minerals can influence wool growth by affecting feed intake (sodium, potassium, S, phosphorus, magnesium, cobalt and zinc), by altering rumen function and hence the supply of nutrients flowing from the rumen (S, sodium, potassium and cobalt) or by directly disrupting metabolism within the sheep (zinc, copper, selenium, iodine and cobalt). The wool matrix contains significant quantities of calcium, potassium, sodium, zinc, copper, manganese, iron and selenium (Lee and Grace, 1988), but only copper, zinc, iodine and possibly selenium alter follicle function and wool growth directly. Cobalt has no direct role, but, as part of the vitamin B_{12} molecule, may alter fibre growth.

COPPER. A deficiency of copper, either in the ration of sheep or induced by high levels of S and molybdenum in the diet, results in depigmentation of the wool of black sheep and the production of wool that lacks crimp and has low mechanical strength and a lustrous appearance. Depigmentation of black wool is due to low activity of the enzyme tyrosinase, which catalyses the hydroxylation of tyrosine to L-3,4-dihydroxyphenylalanine (dopa) and the subsequent oxidation of dopa to dopaquinone, the latter being essential for melanin synthesis (see review by Hynd, 2000). The production of weak and lustrous wool lacking crimp is a consequence of improper keratinization. Copper is thought to be essential for the oxidation of thiol groups to form the disulphide linkages required for keratin formation.

ZINC. Zinc deficiency in sheep results in a marked reduction in wool growth, over and above that associated with the reduced feed intake induced by the deficiency (White *et al.*, 1994). Some fibres are shed, and the fibres that are produced lack crimp and are lustrous and brittle. Cell division in the follicle bulb is marginally reduced by zinc deficiency, but the major effect appears to be on the keratinization of the fibre.

SELENIUM. Selenium deficiency reduces wool growth without a reduction in feed intake. While the exact mechanisms involved are not known, many of the selenoproteins have key metabolic roles as antioxidants and affect the redox status of cells. Uncontrolled peroxidation during severe selenium deficiency causes necrosis due to oxidative damage to cellular macromolecules. A lesser deficiency may result in a milder oxidative stress caused by increased concentrations of peroxides of hydrogen and lipids. Oxidative stress causes gene repression through modulation of transcription factors. Such changes may induce temporary growth arrest and lengthening of the cell cycle in the follicle (Morel and Barouki, 1999).

IODINE. Lack of iodine reduces the production of the thyroid hormones. These hormones interact with intracellular transcription factors to modulate gene expression (Taylor and Brameld, 1999). A deficiency of thyroid hormones causes abnormal follicle development in the fetus and, in adult sheep, reduces wool growth and quality (Hynd, 1994b). In extreme cases, the follicles of thyroid-deficient sheep cease fibre production completely (Hynd, 1994b).

Effects of Nutrition on Cellular Processes in the Wool Follicle

Effects of nutrition on follicle cell numbers, sizes and distribution

With the notable exception of the proportion of cells entering the fibre, all of the follicle-cell parameters are influenced by nutrition. Nutrition alters the size of the follicle bulb, the size and number of cells in the germinative region of the bulb, the rate of bulb cell division and the ultimate size of the cortical cells, which make up the fibre (Table 8.1). Cell turnover time is often, but not invariably, reduced by increased nutrition. The distribution of cells to fibre versus inner root sheath does not appear to be altered by nutrition, but is clearly influenced by the genotype of the animal. Sheep producing coarser and longer wool from larger follicles appear to be more efficient in terms of cell distribution to fibre.

There is a close relationship between the size of the follicle bulb (and associated dermal papilla) and the dimensions of the fibre produced by that follicle (Hynd, 1994a, b). Fibre diameter is closely related to the size of the follicle bulb (width and total volume), while the rate of fibre elongation (fibre length) is related to bulb size, cortical cell length and the proportion of dividing cells entering the fibre proper (Hynd, 1994a, b). The strong relationship between follicle-bulb dimensions and fibre diameter and length may explain the extended period of time required for wool growth to equilibrate with a change in nutrition. While wool growth starts to respond almost instantaneously to a change in nutrient supply, the full extent of the change is not realized for 10–12 weeks. Changes in the number and size of cells in the follicle bulb may occur rapidly, given the high rate of bulb cell division, but other changes that must also occur include a change in the size of the connective-tissue sheath, an increase in the total number of cells in the outer root sheath and a change in the size of the dermal papilla.

Effects of nutrition on cell migration and keratinization

For normal fibre production, there must be synchrony between the two key processes of cell division and keratinization. Indeed, there is evidence that, when the supply of cells from the bulb and the rate of keratinization are out of step, a malformed fibre results. This is the case in deficiencies of copper and zinc, where cell supply is not greatly impaired but the rate and extent of keratinization appear to be reduced. The result is a malformed fibre that is weak. Similarly, when the rate of cell supply is reduced but keratinization continues unabated, as is the case when a lysine-deficient protein is supplied (Hynd, 1989), the fibre is weak and its dimensions are altered dramatically.

The mechanism whereby cysteine or methionine increases wool growth rate is of interest, in that both are presumed to influence fibre growth by supplying the rate-limiting substrate for keratinization. There is no evidence that either amino acid enters the follicle bulb and yet the rate of cell division is increased when they are supplied (Hynd, 1989). This may provide evidence that the rate of keratinization is the rate-limiting process in fibre production and that the rate of cell division increases in response to the increased demand created by more rapid keratinization and hence the distal migration of cells. Follicles may function by 'pull' (keratinization) as well as 'push' (cell division) processes.

Effects of nutrition on wool-fibre composition

An increase in the supply of cysteine to the follicle results not only in increased fibre output (increased diameter and length), but also an increase in the S content of the fibre (Reis, 1979). The increase in wool S level results from an increased expression of genes encoding the high- and ultrahigh-S proteins present in the cortex and cuticle (Fratini *et al.*, 1994). These changes are associated with an increase in the proportion of the fibre occupied by paracortical cells and a decrease in the orthocortical component, suggesting either that there is a greater production of preparacortical cells in the follicle bulb or, more probably, there is a direct effect of cysteine on the differentiation of the migrating cells.

The basic cell type in the wool fibre is the orthocortical cell, containing a lower ratio of IFAP to IF proteins and hence a lower S content. Provision of additional cysteine activates high- and ultrahigh-S genes, with subsequent changes in the IFAP/IF ratio and different packing of the IF proteins to produce paracortical-type cells. There are large differences between sheep in their response to increased cysteine supply. Some sheep increase the cysteine, S and paracortical cell content of their wool to a greater extent than others (Hynd, 1989). It may be that high-producing animals, capable of responding greatly to increased nutrition (see below), do so by continuing to produce relatively low-S proteins, but more of them. Low producers, on the other hand, appear to express more ultrahigh-S proteins and hence less total wool of greater S content.

Effects of Nutrition on Wool Growth Rate

There is a strong positive relationship between feed intake and wool growth rate, although the precise nature of the relationship depends on the composition of the diet, the form of expression of intake (e.g. dry matter, digestible dry matter, digestible organic matter), the genetic wool-growing capacity of the animal and the methodology used to measure wool growth (Allden, 1979; Kempton, 1979). This wool-growth response to dietary intake reflects a response to changes in the supply of amino acids (particularly the S-containing amino acids), energy substrates, minerals and vitamins to the wool follicles.

The wool growth response to protein and energy supply

Figure 8.3 shows the relationship between wool growth rate in Merino sheep and the amount of digestible protein leaving the stomach (DPLS) at four levels of metabolizable energy (ME) intake. It is assumed in this example that the efficiency of utilization of DPLS for wool growth is 11.6%, which was the mean (range 8–15%) for the Merino data reviewed by Hogan *et al.* (1979). It is also assumed that wool growth is linearly related to DPLS until the DPLS : ME ratio exceeds 12 g MJ^{-1} (Kempton, 1979). At low levels of energy intake, therefore, maximum wool growth is reached at low levels of protein supply. Further increases in wool growth then depend on energy intake.

For the majority of diets consumed by grazing sheep (6–11 MJ kg^{-1} dry matter (DM)), consumed at typical rates (800–1500 g DM day^{-1}), wool growth rate will be limited by the supply of protein to the intestines.

The relationships depicted in Fig. 8.3 assume that the composition of the DPLS is 'normal' – that is, largely of microbial origin. Diets containing protein sources that are not only rich in S-containing and other essential amino acids, but also resistant to rumen degradation, would produce a wool growth response greater than that indicated in Fig. 8.3. That is, the efficiency of wool growth would exceed 11.6% and the slope of the line relating wool growth rate to DPLS would be increased.

Effects of nutrition on fibre diameter and length growth rate

The wool-growth responses to nutrition described above contribute to changes in the mean fibre diameter (*D*), the rate of elongation of the fibre (*L*) and, if the nutritional regimen is sufficiently severe, the number of follicles actively producing a fibre (see section on follicle shut-down below). The specific gravity of wool fibres is relatively constant and not influenced by nutrition. Under normal feeding conditions, *L* and *D* respond in the same direction and to approximately the same extent, such that the ratio of *L*/*D* remains approximately constant. For example, a fine-wool Merino might have *L* and *D* values of 320 μm day^{-1} and 17.5 μm, respectively, under a low plane of nutrition, and values of 384 μm day^{-1} and 20.5 μm, respectively, under high nutrition. In this case the *L*/*D* ratio increases slightly (from 18.2 to 18.7) with increased nutrition.

Despite the relative constancy of the *L*/*D* ratio for an individual animal, there are situations in which *L*/*D* can change markedly. For example, the postruminal provision of the lysine-deficient protein zein, from maize, results in a dramatic change in *L*/*D*, with *D* decreasing and *L* increasing. The increase in *L*/*D* can be as much as 100%, resulting from large relative changes in the cellular events discussed above. It remains to be determined whether manipulation of amino acid supply can be used in practical situations (e.g. with shedded sheep producing ultrafine wool) to produce favourable changes in fibre *L* and *D* without detrimental effects on staple strength or other important traits.

Effects of Nutrition on Staple Strength of Merino Wool

Staple strength is second only to mean fibre diameter as a determinant of wool price and is measured as the force (newtons) required to break a staple of wool, corrected for the linear density (weight per unit length) of the staple (kilotex (ktex)). Several features of the fibres within the staple potentially contribute to the staple strength. These are: the mean minimum fibre diameter along the staple (Fig. 8.4); the rate of change in fibre diameter along the staple; variation in diameter between fibres; variation in length between fibres; variation in crimp frequency between fibres; the intrinsic strength of the fibres; and follicle shut-down (Reis, 1992). Nutrition influences a number of these variables.

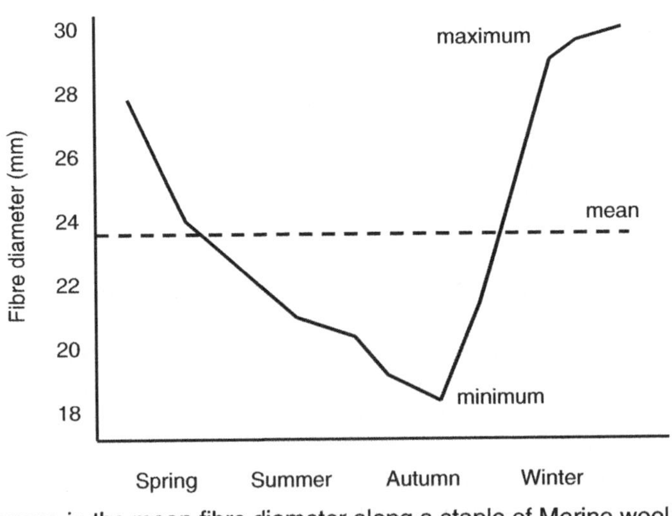

Fig. 8.4. Changes in the mean fibre diameter along a staple of Merino wool from sheep grazing pastures in a Mediterranean environment. Note that the diameter at any point represents the diameter of wool grown on that particular day. Staples break close to the point of minimum diameter, which occurs in autumn in these environments due to a trough in the quantity and quality of feed available.

Effects of nutrition on diameter variations

Changes in nutrient supply throughout the year, as a result of changes in the quantity and quality of forage on offer to grazing sheep, produce variations in wool growth rate and fibre diameter. In highly seasonal environments (e.g. Mediterranean), these variations are substantial (Fig. 8.4). Staples break close to the region of minimum mean fibre diameter and staple strength is often closely related to the minimum fibre diameter of the average staple (Thompson, 1998). There also appears to be some effect of the rate of change in fibre diameter along the staple (Hansford and Kennedy, 1988). This implies that nutritional management to increase staple strength might involve not only increasing the minimum fibre diameter (e.g. by supplementary feeding), but also restricting feed intake when large amounts of feed are available (e.g. by intensive grazing during periods of rapid pasture growth) to prevent rapid change in fibre diameter. Alternatively, one might selectively breed sheep that are more resistant to nutritionally induced fluctuations in fibre diameter (Jackson and Downes, 1979). Sheep with higher mean fibre diameter are more susceptible to diameter variations than animals with a lower mean fibre diameter, regardless of whether variation is measured as absolute or relative values. Selection of sheep with low fibre diameter but high clean-fleece weights would achieve reduced diameter variation without compromising fleece weights.

In contrast to the large effect of nutrition on fibre diameter changes along the staple, there is little, if any, effect of nutrition on variation in diameter, length or crimp frequency between fibres, these being largely dictated by the genotype.

Effects of nutrition on the intrinisic strength of wool fibres

The intrinsic strength of a fibre refers to the strength of the fibre corrected for the cross-sectional area at the point of break. In other words, it is the strength of the basic structure of the fibre. While the protein composition of wool fibres can be markedly altered by nutrition and, in particular, by the S-amino acid supply, there is little evidence that the mechanical strength is altered (Reis, 1992). Gillespie and Marshall (1983) concluded that the IF proteins, some of the high-S proteins and a small component of the high-tyrosine proteins constitute a basic structure of the wool fibre, and that it is the IF proteins that govern the mechanical strength of fibres (Feughelman, 1982). Variations in fibre composition are largely reflected in changes in the IFAP, not the IF, proteins, so there is poor association between fibre composition (e.g. S content) and intrinsic strength (Feughelman and Reis, 1967). Similarly, there is no consistent association between cortical cell type and intrinsic strength (Thompson, 1998). Intrinsic fibre strength is normally much greater than staple strength and has a depressing effect on it only when there is disruption to the oxidative formation of disulphide bonds. This occurs when there is a deficiency of copper (Marston, 1946) or when an unbalanced mix of amino acids is absorbed (Hynd, 1989).

Effects of nutrition on follicle shut-down and fibre shedding

If a restriction in feed intake is sufficiently severe, some follicles cease fibre production and enter a resting or 'shut-down' phase (Schlink and Dollin, 1995; Hynd *et al.*, 1997). This phenomenon occurs in autumn in Mediterranean environments, when nutrient supply is poor. There is also a strong correlation between stocking rate and incidence of shut-down. Both these lines of evidence suggest that shut-down is largely nutritional in origin (Hynd *et al.*, 1997). Discontinuous fibres that result from this inactivity help to reduce staple strength, because they contribute to the amount of material present (the ktex) but not to the load-bearing capacity (newtons) of the staple. Zinc deficiency results not only in impaired keratinization of the fibre, but also in shedding of the fleece (White *et al.*, 1994), with a subsequent reduction in fibre strength. Folic acid deficiency and lysine deficiency similarly cause fibre distortion and degradation (Chapman, 1989).

Effect of Nutrition on Wool Yield

Unwashed wool contains wool fibres, suint, wax, vegetable matter, dust or dirt and detritus (comprising bacterial cells, sloughed epidermal and inner root-sheath cells). Suint consists of water-soluble potassium salts of fatty acids and peptides, urea and pigments. Wax consists of lipids secreted from the sebaceous glands (Fig. 8.1). The Agricultural Research Council (ARC, 1980) summarizes the approximate composition of the fleece as 80% wool fibre, 12% wax and 8% suint, but the proportions of these components of the fleece may vary widely, depending on the genotype of the sheep and the environment. For example, wax content ranges from 3 to 30% of the fleece when different sheep breeds are compared and dirt (which is excluded from the ARC table) may be up to 60% of the weight of the total fleece.

Both wax and suint levels are influenced by nutrition; the important question is: 'Is the change in production of these components proportional to fibre production changes?' In other words, does the ratio of greasy to clean fleece production change with nutrition?

In general, increases in feed intake are accompanied by a simultaneous increase in production of wax and suint, as well as clean fibres, resulting in no change in the yield of clean dry wool. However, there is evidence that an enhanced supply of S-amino acids increases the yield of clean wool fibre (Sherlock *et al.*, 2001). These authors reported increases in yield from 60 to 68% when cysteine was supplied postruminally. They suggested that the increased yield might have resulted from a reduction in the proportion of cells entering the inner root sheath (see above), with a consequent reduction in cell debris in the non-fibre component. Alternatively, there may have been a reduction in wax or suint production. Similar changes have been observed when additional S-amino acids are provided as methionine (G. Mata, 1995, unpublished results) or through feeding rumen-protected canola meal (Masters *et al.*, 1996). In the latter case, a decrease in wax production and an increase in fibre production caused the increase in yield.

Effect of Nutrition on Wool Colour

Unscourable wool yellowness limits the end uses for wool and results in discounted prices. Yellowing arises from several sources, including photo-oxidation of the aromatic amino acids phenylalanine and tyrosine under conditions of high ultraviolet radiation (Goddinger *et al.*, 1994). The breakdown products of these amino acids are precursors to yellow pigments and are part of a complex interaction that involves high temperature and humidity, a low wax-to-suint ratio, high suint pH and potassium content, as well as high numbers of microbes present in the fleece. Under these conditions, the suint forms a detergent, solubilizing the wax and increasing microbial activity. Microbial activity itself will directly result in the production of coloured pigments. Loss of wax then increases the susceptibility of the fibre to pigment infiltration and fibre damage.

The heritability of propensity to yellowing is high (Reid, 1998) and genetics, not nutrition, is the primary determinant. However, Min *et al.* (1998) reported a trend towards reduced yellowness when the S content of wools was increased, possibly due to increased resistance to microbial by-products or a reduction in the aromatic amino acids in the matrix of the cortical cells. In addition, pH and potassium content of suint and the wax/suint ratio are all responsive to changes in either the type or amount of protein in the diet (Crook *et al.*, 2000). Thus, dietary manipulation may also influence susceptibility to wool yellowing.

Reproduction and Wool-growth Responses

The effects of reproduction are likely to influence wool growth directly, as well as indirectly via effects on intake. The process of producing and rearing a lamb results in lower fleece weight, fibre diameter and staple length and may influence staple strength (Corbett, 1979; Masters and Stewart, 1990). Oddy (1985) calculated the deficit in clean wool as the difference between observed wool growth and that expected from the relationship between feed intake and clean wool growth in dry ewes. The resulting deficit ranged from 442 to 548 g over the 5 months of pregnancy (depending on diet), increasing to 613 g in ewes producing twins. There was a further loss of 613–1268 g (up to 2006 g if rearing twins) over 96 days of lactation. These figures are considerably higher than normally reported in field experiments (where feed intakes are variable between parity groups) and represent the true cost of producing lambs.

The effects of pregnancy and lactation are illustrated in Fig. 8.5. Again, wool growth rate responds to an increasing supply of DPLS. In this study, the efficiency of wool growth (i.e. the slope of the line relating wool growth rate to DPLS) for dry ewes was unusually high, at 16.2%, but it was 11.3 % for ewes in late pregnancy and 10.8% for ewes in early lactation. That is, the efficiency of wool growth was reduced by 30 and 33% by pregnancy and lactation, respectively. These changes in wool growth in pregnancy and lactation are partially explained as a passive response to increased competition for nutrients, but, even when a pregnant ewe is fed to maintain conceptus-free live weight, wool growth decreases as pregnancy advances. This reduction is less apparent in ewes consuming poor-quality feed or with low genetic potential to grow wool (Masters and Stewart, 1990). The evidence for hormonal control of wool growth at this time is not convincing. Progesterone, oestrogen, insulin, growth hormone, prolactin, placental lactogen and cortisol all change during pregnancy, but the changes either occur after wool growth is depressed (cortisol, growth hormone and prolactin) and/or there is little evidence that the hormones directly influence wool growth (progesterone, oestrogen, insulin, prolactin and placental lactogen). On the other hand, wool growth in late pregnancy does respond to feeding proteins that are protected from degradation in the rumen, suggesting that reduced wool growth is due to either a lack of or an imbalance in substrate at the follicle (Masters *et al.*, 1996). Changes in blood flow to the skin at this time do not account for this depression in wool growth (Bell *et al.*, 1986) but the wool-growth depression is consistent with the decrease in free amino acids in plasma in late pregnancy (Stewart *et al.*, 1993).

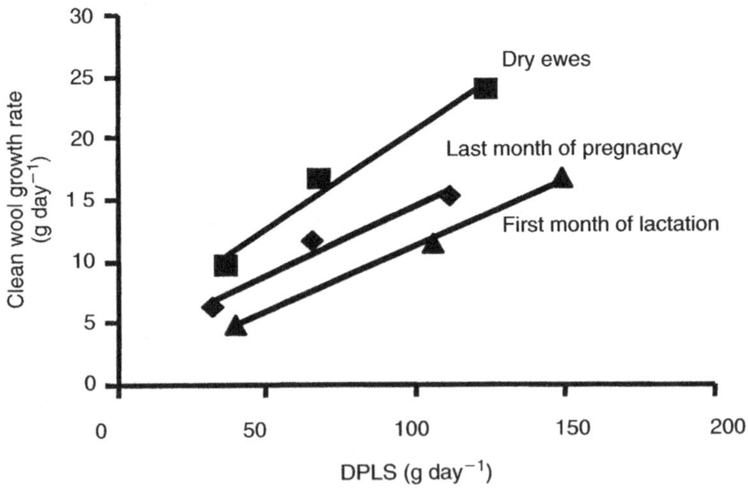

Fig. 8.5. The relationship between digestible protein leaving the stomach (DPLS) and wool growth at different stages of pregnancy and lactation (derived from Oddy, 1985). The efficiency of wool growth is reduced during late pregnancy and lactation.

Although wool growth responds to increased protein entering the small intestine during pregnancy, the primary limitation is not the supply of cysteine. Towards the end of pregnancy, S in wool increases, S-amino acids as a proportion of total free amino acids in plasma increase and infusion of additional cysteine or methionine has little or no effect on wool growth (Williams *et al.*, 1978; Stewart *et al.*, 1993). It is possible that the increased synthesis of the relatively low-S proteins in the fetus and uterus changes the balance of amino acid requirements at this time.

Lactation requires more protein than pregnancy, since 1 kg of milk contains 43–50 g protein (Williams *et al.*, 1976), compared with the approximately 22 g protein day^{-1} deposited into the gravid uterus at the end of pregnancy (Langlands and Sutherland, 1968). To meet this requirement, feed intake increases and the ewe usually enters a catabolic state. Although the efficiency of wool growth of lactating ewes is lower than for either pregnant or dry sheep, wool growth often increases relative to that in late pregnancy, even though the ewe is losing more weight. The combination of catabolism and increased feed intake significantly increases the amino acid flux in the body and provides additional nutrients for both the wool follicle and the mammary gland. There is then direct competition between wool follicles and mammary gland, with a strong negative relationship between wool growth and milk production (Oddy, 1985).

The changes in wool growth rate during pregnancy will change fibre-diameter variability along the fibre and therefore influence staple strength. Whether fibre-diameter variability is increased or decreased during reproduction depends very much on the time of lambing. In a ewe fed to maintain conceptus-free live weight, wool growth and diameter are at a minimum shortly before parturition (Stewart *et al.*, 1993) and at this time are highly sensitive to a reduction in feed availability (Robertson *et al.*, 2000). Under such conditions, feed restriction in late pregnancy will cause large decreases in staple strength (Robertson *et al.*, 2000). However, by lambing during periods of high feed availability, reproduction may decrease maximum fibre diameter and reduce fibre-diameter variability and may even increase staple strength.

In conclusion, the wool-growth response to nutrition is a reflection of changes in the supply of nutrients to the wool follicle, which responds by altering the rate, extent and pattern of its primary processes of cell division, gene expression and protein synthesis. Protein, energy, minerals and vitamins influence these processes, but the precise nature of the wool-growth response to these nutrients is influenced by the genotype of the animal and its reproductive status.

References

Allden, W.G. (1979) Feed intake, diet composition and wool growth. In: Black, J.L. and Reis, P.J. (eds) *Physiological and Environmental Limitations to Wool Growth*. University of New England, Armidale, Australia, pp. 61–78.

ARC (Agricultural Research Council) (1980) *The Nutrient Requirements of Ruminant Livestock*. Commonwealth Agricultural Bureaux, Slough, 351 pp.

Bell, A.W., Hales, J.R.S., Fawcett, A.A. and King, R.B. (1986) Effects of exercise and heat stress on regional blood flow in pregnant sheep. *Journal of Applied Physiology* 60, 1759–1764.

Benevenga, N.J. and Egan, A.R. (1983) Quantitative aspects of methionine metabolism. *Progress in Clinical and Biological Research* 125, 327–341.

Chapman, R.E. (1989) Follicular malfunctions and resultant effects on wool fibres. In: Rogers, G.E., Reis, P.J., Ward, K.A. and Marshall, R.C. (eds) *The Biology of Wool and Hair*. Chapman & Hall, London, pp. 243–256.

Chapman, R.E. and Black, J.L. (1981) Abnormal wool growth and alopecia of artificially-reared lambs. *Australian Journal of Biological Sciences* 34, 11–26.

Chapman, R.E. and Ward, K.A. (1979) Histological and biochemical features of the wool fibre and follicle. In: Black, J.L. and Reis, P.J. (eds) *Physiological and Environmental Limitations to Wool Growth*. University of New England, Armidale, Australia, pp. 193–208.

Chapman, R.E., Downes, A.M. and Wilson, P.A. (1980) Migration and keratinisation of cells in wool follicles. *Australian Journal of Biological Sciences* 33, 587–603.

Corbett, J.L. (1979) Variation in wool growth with physiological state. In: Black, J.L. and Reis, P.J. (eds) *Physiological and Environmental Limitations to Wool Growth*. University of New England, Armidale, Australia, pp. 79–98.

Crook, B.J., Farrell, R.A., Hegarty, R.S. and Purvis, I.W. (2000) Dietary protein and the discolouration of wool from superfine Merino sheep. *Asian–Australasian Journal of Animal Science* 13 (Suppl. C), 164–167.

Downes, A.M., Lyne, A.G. and Clarke, W.H. (1962) Radioautographic studies of the incorporation of [^{35}S] cystine into wool. *Australian Journal of Biological Sciences* 15, 713–719.

Feughelman, M. (1982) The physical properties of alpha-keratin fibres. *Journal of the Society of Cosmetic Chemists* 33, 385–406.

Feughelman, M. and Reis, P.J. (1967) The longitudinal mechanical properties of wool fibers and their relationship to the low sulphur keratin fraction. *Textile Research Journal* 37, 334–336.

Fraser, I.E.B. (1965) Cellular proliferation in the wool follicle bulb. In: Lyne, A.G. and Short, B.F. (eds) *Biology of Skin and Hair Growth*. Angus and Robertson, Sydney, pp. 427–445.

Fratini, A., Powell, B.C., Hynd, P.I., Keough, R.A. and Rogers, G.E. (1994) Dietary cysteine regulates the levels of mRNAs encoding a family of cysteine-rich proteins in wool. *Journal of Investigative Dermatology* 102, 178–185.

Gillespie, J.M. and Marshall, R.C. (1983) A comparison of proteins of normal and trichothiodystrophic human hair. *Journal of Investigative Dermatology* 80, 195–202.

Goddinger, D., Schafer, K. and Hocker, H. (1994) Phenylalanine and tyrosine – two aromatic amino acids involved in photoyellowing of wool. *Wool Technology and Sheep Breeding* 42, 83–89.

Hansford, K.A. and Kennedy, J.P. (1988) Relationship between the rate of change in fibre diameter and staple strength. *Proceedings of the Australian Society of Animal Production* 17, 415.

Hocking Edwards, J.E. and Hynd, P.I. (1992) Cellular characteristics of wool follicles and fibres in Finewool and Strongwool Merinos. *Australian Journal of Agricultural Research* 43, 355–365.

Hogan, J.P., Elliott, N.M. and Hughes, A.D. (1979) Maximum wool growth rates expected from Australian Merino genotypes. In: Black, J.L. and Reis, P.J. (eds) *Physiological and Environmental Limitations to Wool Growth*. University of New England, Armidale, Australia, pp. 43–59.

Hynd, P.I. (1989) Effects of nutrition on wool follicle cell kinetics in sheep differing in efficiency of wool production. *Australian Journal of Agricultural Research* 40, 409–417.

Hynd, P.I. (1994a) Follicular determinants of the length/diameter ratio at two levels of nutrition. *Australian Journal of Agricultural Research* 45, 1137–1147.

Hynd, P.I. (1994b) Follicular determinants of the length and diameter of wool fibres. II. Comparison of sheep differing in thyroid hormone status. *Australian Journal of Agricultural Research* 45, 1149–1157.

Hynd, P.I. (2000) The nutritional biochemistry of wool and hair follicles. *Animal Science* 70, 181–195.

Hynd, P.I. and Nancarrow, M.J. (1996) Inhibition of polyamine synthesis alters hair follicle function and fiber composition. *Journal of Investigative Dermatology* 106, 249–253.

Hynd, P.I., Hughes, A., Earl, C.R. and Penno, N.M. (1997) Seasonal changes in the morphology and activity of wool follicles in Finewool and Strongwool Merino strains at different stocking rates in southern Australia. *Australian Journal of Agricultural Research* 49, 1089–1097.

Jackson, N. and Downes, A.M. (1979) The fibre diameter profile of wool staples from individual sheep. *Australian Journal of Agricultural Research* 30, 163–171.

Kealey, T., Williams, R. and Philpott, M.P. (1991) Intermediary metabolism of the human hair follicle. In: Stenn, K.S., Messenger, A.G. and Baden, H.P. (eds) *The Molecular and Structural Biology of Hair*. Annals of the New York Academy of Sciences, New York, pp. 301–307.

Kempton, T.J. (1979) Protein to energy ratio of absorbed nutrients in relation to wool growth. In: Black, J.L. and Reis, P.J. (eds) *Physiological and Environmental Limitations to Wool Growth*. University of New England, Armidale, Australia, pp. 209–222.

Langlands, J.P. and Sutherland, H.A.M. (1968) An estimate of the nutrients utilized for pregnancy by Merino sheep. *British Journal of Nutrition* 22, 217–227.

Lee, J. and Grace, N.D. (1988) Trace elements and wool. In: McLaren, R.G., Haynes, R.J. and Savage, G.P. (eds) *Trace Elements in New Zealand: Environmental, Human and Animal*. New Zealand Trace Elements Group, Lincoln College, Canterbury, pp. 215–314.

Marston, H.R. (1946) Nutrition and wool production. In: *Proceedings of the Symposium on Fibrous Proteins*. Society of Dyers and Colourists, Leeds, UK, pp. 207–214.

Masters, D.G. and Stewart, C.A. (1990) Wool growth and reproduction. In: Oldham, C.M., Martin, G.B. and Purvis, I.W. (eds) *Reproductive Physiology of Merino Sheep. Concepts and Consequences*. University of Western Australia, Perth, pp. 265–274.

Masters, D.G., Stewart, C.A., Mata, G. and Adams, N.R. (1996) Responses in wool and live-weight when different sources of dietary protein are given to pregnant and lactating ewes. *Animal Science* 62, 497–506.

Min, B.R., Barry, T.N., McNabb, W.C. and Kemp, P.D. (1988) Effect of condensed tannins on the production of wool and on its processing characteristics in sheep grazing *Lotus corniculatus*. *Australian Journal of Agricultural Research* 49, 597–605.

Morel, Y. and Barouki, R. (1999) Repression of gene expression by oxidative stress. *Biochemical Journal* 342, 481–496.

Nattrass, G.N. (2000) Molecular and functional characterisation of a system ASC-like neutral amino acid transporter expressed in the wool follicle. PhD thesis, Adelaide University, Australia.

Oddy, V.H. (1985) Wool growth of pregnant and lactating Merino ewes. *Journal of Agricultural Science, Cambridge* 105, 613–622.

Orwin, D.F.G. (1971) Cell differentiation in the lower outer root sheath of the Romney wool follicles: a companion cell layer. *Australian Journal of Biological Sciences* 24, 989–999.

Philpott, M.P., Green, M.R. and Kealey, T. (1990) Human hair growth *in vitro*. *Journal of Cell Science* 97, 463–471.

Powell, B.C., Nesci, A. and Rogers, G.E. (1991) Regulation of keratin gene expression in hair follicle differentiation. In: Stenn, K.S., Messenger, A.G. and Baden, H.P. (eds) *The Molecular and Structural Biology of Hair*. Annals of the New York Academy of Sciences, New York, pp. 1–20.

Reid, T.C. (1998) Wool yellowing. *Wool Technology and Sheep Breeding* 46, 318–337.

Reis, P.J. (1979) Effects of amino acids on the growth and properties of wool. In: Black, J.L. and Reis, P.J. (eds) *Physiological and Environmental Limitations to Wool Growth*. University of New England, Armidale, Australia, pp. 185–242.

Reis, P.J. (1992) Variations in the strength of wool fibres – a review. *Australian Journal of Agricultural Research* 43, 1337–1351.

Robertson, S.M., Robards, G.E. and Wolfe, E.C. (2000) The timing of nutritional restriction during reproduction influences staple strength. *Australian Journal of Agricultural Research* 51, 125–132.

Schlink, A.C. and Dollin, A.E. (1995) Abnormal shedding contributes to the reduced staple strength of tender wool in Western Australian Merinos. *Wool Technology and Sheep Breeding* 43, 268–284.

Sherlock, R.G., Harris, P.M., Lee, J., Wickham, G.A., Woods, J.L. and McCutcheon, S.N. (2001) Intake and long-term cysteine supplementation change wool characteristics of Romney sheep. *Australian Journal of Agricultural Research* 52, 29–36.

Short, B.F., Wilson, P.A. and Schinckel, P.G. (1965) Proliferation of follicle matrix cells in relation to wool growth. In: Lyne, A.G. and Short, B.F. (eds) *Biology of Skin and Hair Growth*. Angus and Robertson, Sydney, pp. 409–426.

Stewart, C.A., Masters, D.G., Williams, I.H. and Connell, P.J. (1993) Changes in plasma amino acid patterns and wool growth in response to abomasal injections of amino acids during late pregnancy and early lactation. *Australian Journal of Agricultural Research* 44, 959–971.

Taylor, P.M. and Brameld, J.M. (1999) Mechanisms of regulation of transcription and translation. In: Lobley, G.E., White, A. and MacRae, J. (eds) *Protein Metabolism and Nutrition*. Publication No. 96, EAAP, Wageningen, pp. 25–50.

Thompson, A.N. (1998) Intrinsic strength of wool fibres. PhD thesis, Adelaide University, Australia.

White, C.L., Martin, G.B., Hynd, P.I. and Chapman, R.E. (1994) The effect of zinc deficiency on wool growth and skin and wool follicle histology of male Merino lambs. *British Journal of Nutrition* 71, 425–435.

Williams, A.J., Tyrrell, R.N. and Gilmour, A.R. (1978) Effects on wool production during pregnancy and lactation of twice daily abomasal supplementation with casein or methionine and cystine. *Australian Journal of Experimental Agriculture and Animal Husbandry* 18, 52–57.

Williams, A.P., Bishop, D.R., Cockburn, J.E. and Scott, K.J. (1976) Composition of ewe's milk. *Journal of Dairy Research* 43, 325–329.
Wilson, P.A. and Short, B.F. (1979) Cell proliferation and cortical cell production in relation to wool growth. *Australian Journal of Biological Sciences* 32, 317–327.

9 Nutrition for Conception and Pregnancy

J.J. Robinson, J.A. Rooke and T.G. McEvoy

Animal Biology Division, Scottish Agricultural College, Bucksburn, Aberdeen, UK

Introduction

Current knowledge of nutrition for conception and pregnancy in the ewe is based on the results of production trials involving different feeding strategies and of mechanistic studies designed to unravel the underlying control systems and their responses to nutrients. Central to the mechanistic studies is the acquisition of information on how dietary nutrients facilitate the programming and expression of those metabolic pathways that enable ewes to approach their genetic potential for reproduction. In this context nutrition acts directly by providing glucose, amino acids, vitamins and essential chemical elements. It also acts indirectly by modifying the expression of hormonal functions, which, in turn, influence oocyte maturation, ovulation, embryo development, fetal growth and the viability and vigour of the newborn lamb.

This chapter brings together recent observations from the wide range of scientific disciplines that now contribute to our understanding of when and how nutrition affects reproduction. A central theme is the identification of critical windows in development, during which the supply of nutrients to the whole animal, its tissues, organs and cells plays pivotal roles in the expression of immediate and subsequent responses that affect the reproductive processes. There are still many gaps in our knowledge, but new opportunities for developing a more holistic approach to the subject will emerge from the acceptance that, in addition to its fairly immediate effects on adult reproduction, nutrition at earlier stages – indeed, as early as the first trimester of fetal life – may have consequences for lifetime reproductive competence.

Fetal Nutrition and Reproductive Potential

Observations of the reproductive performance of sheep conceived, born and reared under different degrees of nutritional adversity provide evidence that inadequate or inappropriate fetal and/or early postnatal nutrition reduces adult reproductive performance (Gunn *et al.*, 1995; Table 9.1). Mechanistic follow-up studies aimed at identifying when fetal development is vulnerable to undernutrition (Borwick *et al.*, 1997; Rae *et al.*, 2001) have demonstrated that although fetal weight was not affected, the temporal pattern of oogonial development in the fetal ovary was disrupted when Scottish Blackface ewes were restricted to food intakes equivalent to 0.5 × energy maintenance (M) as opposed to 1.0 × M during the first trimester of pregnancy. This degree of undernutrition, despite being below recommended levels, is probably fairly common in ewes kept in harsh hill environments or in arid regions.

The recent appreciation of such an impact of maternal nutrition on a component of the fetal reproductive system is important. The effects may be gonad-specific, since they appear to be independent of any inhibition of the fetal hypothalamopituitary axis (Da Silva *et al.*, 2000). On the available evidence, they have no effect on age at puberty in the female, although they do cause a delay in puberty in the male. Nutritionally compromised ovarian development provides a plausible explanation for the reduction in adult reproductive performance observed by Gunn *et al.* (1995) for ewes conceived under harsh nutritional conditions. However, considerable research is still needed to determine whether the effect is expressed through a reduction in ovulation rate or, as implied by the observations of Gunn *et al.* (1995), an increase in embryo mortality. Limitations in uterine development, as well as inherent weaknesses in the embryo, could contribute to the embryo loss.

Postnatal Nutrition and Reproductive Performance

In commercial sheep-production systems, undernutrition in early postnatal life often follows on from nutritional inadequacies during late preg-

Table 9.1. The effect of fetal and neonatal nutrition on the birth weight and growth of Scottish Blackface ewe lambs and on their subsequent reproductive performance (data from Gunn *et al.*, 1995).

		Lamb weights (kg)			Subsequent reproductive performance (proportion producing multiple births)		
					Lamb crop number		
Feeding level	Stage of development	Birth (April/May)	June	Weaning (August)	1	2	3
Low	Fetal and neonatal	3.51	16.9	30.7	0.30	0.47	0.55
High	Fetal	4.00	17.8	31.9	0.42	0.55	0.68
High	Neonatal	3.48	17.7	31.4	0.44	0.60	0.67

nancy, with the combined periods of food restriction impairing the expression of genetic potential for lamb production. There is very little information on the effect of early postnatal nutrition alone on adult reproductive performance. One study reviewed by Robinson (1990) showed that undernutrition, characterized by a cessation in weight gain for an 8-week period from 6 weeks of age, reduced ovulation rates in ewes for up to 3 years; another by Rhind *et al.* (1998) indicated that a preweaning restriction in growth rate, leading to weaning weights of 23.0 vs. 26.2 kg, significantly reduced lifetime reproductive performance.

In general, studies of postnatal effects of undernutrition on subsequent reproductive performance have concentrated on puberty as an end-point. Across a wide range of domestic species, including sheep, puberty is delayed by feed intakes that restrict growth rates to 50% of an animal's potential. The effects are more pronounced when feed restriction is applied in the early postnatal rather than in the immediately prepubertal phase (Robinson, 1990).

Many sheep are seasonally polyoestrous short-day breeders. Thus spring-born lambs that are well nourished achieve puberty in their first autumn and at younger ages and heavier weights than their poorly nourished contemporaries. An extended period of food restriction during rearing can prevent the occurrence of puberty in the first autumn, with the result that first oestrus is delayed until its induction by the shortening day lengths of the following autumn. This interdependence of nutrition and season in the hormonal control of puberty leads to very wide ranges in pubertal age and size (Adam and Robinson, 1994). Among animals destined for breeding in their first autumn, those reaching puberty at either extreme of the size range are a cause for concern. At the lower end of the range, significant numbers of animals are likely to fall short of the minimum 60% of estimated mature body weight required for satisfactory reproductive performance in their first pregnancy (Meat and Livestock Commission, 1983); for these animals, mating should be delayed until the target weight is achieved. In contrast, pubertal ewe lambs at the upper end of the weight range encountered in practice are likely to display impaired mammogenesis and a reduced lactation potential as a result of rapid growth during the immediate prepubertal phase. These limitations are probably mediated via reduced circulating levels of insulin-like growth factor 1 (IGF-1). There is evidence, however, that they may be avoided by alterations in diet composition. For example, McFadden *et al.* (1990) found that inclusion of rumen-protected polyunsaturated fat in the diet stimulated mammary growth in prepubertal lambs.

Nutrition and Ovulation Rate

In quantitative terms, the nutrients required to fuel ovulation as an event are trivial, and yet the actual number of ova released at oestrus is highly dependent on the nature of the female's long-term nutritional regimens.

Of course, the nutritional status of the ewe immediately prior to ovulation also affects ovulation rate. Here both the ewe's body condition, which reflects long-term food supply, and her current metabolism, which is a function of the immediate availability and quality of food, are important. In addition, as discussed above, both fetal and early postnatal nutrition are involved. So too is nutrition *c.* 6 months before ovulation, when those follicles that go on to ovulate, along with many others that fail to do so, leave the primordial pool and become committed to growth (Fig. 9.1).

Within the 6-month period required for follicle maturation, large numbers of follicles at all stages, from the 'committed' to the 'gonadotrophin-dependent', are lost through atresia (Fig. 9.1). Improved nutrition does not prevent follicle attrition, but it does reduce its magnitude at critical stages, thereby enhancing ovulation rate. Despite considerable effort by many researchers, the mechanisms dictating this nutrition-dependent response are not fully understood. They probably

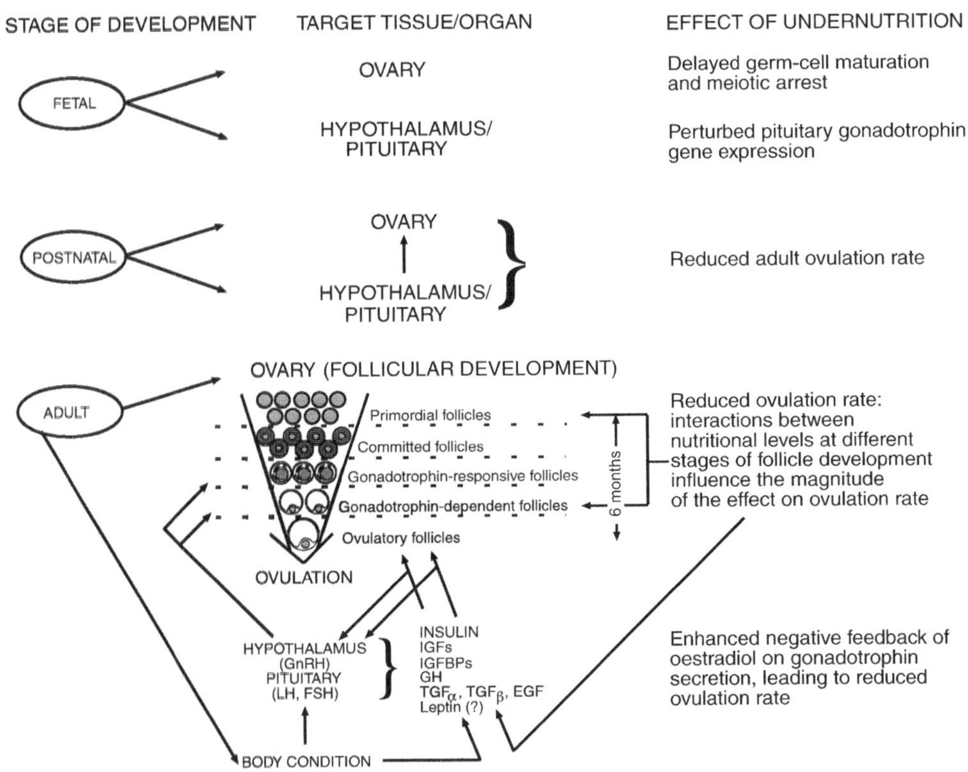

Fig. 9.1. Stages of development during which undernutrition impairs the expression of genetic potential for ovulation rate and the suggested pathways and hormones that are involved at the hypothalamic, pituitary and ovarian levels. IGF, insulin-like growth factor; IGFBP, insulin-like growth factor-binding protein; GH, growth hormone; TGF, transforming growth factor; EGF, epidermal growth factor; GnRH, gonadotrophin-releasing hormone; FSH, follicle-stimulating hormone; LH, luteinizing hormone.

involve direct effects of specific nutrients (volatile fatty acids, glucose, branched-chain amino acids) at the level of the ovarian follicle, together with indirect effects operating through shifts in systemic and intrafollicular concentrations of nutrient-sensitive hormones (Armstrong and Webb, 1997) and via neuroendocrine mechanisms involving gonadotrophin (follicle-stimulating hormone (FSH) and luteinizing hormone (LH)) secretion (Miller *et al.*, 1998; Fig. 9.1). Since responses to nutrition at the gonadal level cannot be explained simply by shifts in the blood concentrations of a specific nutrient, hormone or metabolite, Blache *et al.* (2000) have put forward the hypothesis that there is a central 'sensor–integrator' which processes complex metabolic information on nutritional status and translates it into the appropriate reproductive response.

In the absence of a full understanding of the mechanisms involved in the nutritional control of ovulation, responses to alterations in the quantity and type of food provide the basis for practical feeding recommendations. By way of example, data from the studies of Nottle *et al.* (1997) are used in Table 9.2 to illustrate well-established features of the nutritional effects. These data also introduce the concept that ovulatory responses to improved nutrition in the few weeks before mating (flushing) may be influenced by the plane of nutrition during the period when ovarian follicles leave the primordial pool, approximately 6 months before ovulation. While it has been recognized for many years that poor nutrition at this more remote time can reduce ovulation rate, the suggestion in Table 9.2 (Nottle *et al.*, 1997) that the expression of this adverse effect of earlier limitations of nutrition on ovulation rate can be prevented by preovulatory 'flushing' is both interesting and important. Thus, feed-restricted Merino ewes that lost one-seventh of their body weight between 6 and 4 months before ovulation (Table 9.2, Experiment 1), but recovered this loss over the next 3 months, responded to a 10-day preovulatory lupin-grain supplement (500 g per head day^{-1}) with an average 0.57 extra ovulations per ewe

Table 9.2. Ovulation rates (mean ± SEM) in Merino ewes in relation to time of exposure to an 8-week period of feed restriction and to a daily supplement of 500 g of lupin grain in the 10 days before ovulation (from data presented by Nottle *et al.*, 1997).

	Time of initial exposure to 8-week phase of undernutrition							
	6 months prior to ovulation (Experiment 1)				2 months prior to ovulation (Experiment 2)			
	Feed restricted		Control		Feed restricted		Control	
Lupin supplement	–	+	–	+	–	+	–	+
No. of ewes	50	49	50	49	70	64	72	69
Ovulation rate	1.06 ± 0.07	1.63 ± 0.09	1.28 ± 0.09	1.57 ± 0.08	1.22 ± 0.06	1.38 ± 0.09	1.67 ± 0.08	1.64 ± 0.09
Weight[a] on day 10 pre-ovulation	51		54		48		54	
Direction of weight change before lupin feeding	No change		No change		Gain		Loss	

[a]Weight (kg) estimated from graphs in original publication.

(1.63 vs. 1.06) compared with their previously restricted but 'unflushed' contemporaries. The practical importance of this observation relates to the fact that, 6 months prior to the next season's matings, many adult ewes are in early lactation and experiencing an associated substantial negative energy balance. Thus, in order to overcome the adverse effect of this period of undernutrition on ovulation rate in the following breeding season, it is advisable to make preovulatory 'flushing' an integral part of the ewe's pre-mating management.

Reduced ovulation rates arising from undernutrition that occurs 2 months before ovulation are less amenable to correction by short-term preovulatory flushing (1.38 vs. 1.22: Table 9.2, Experiment 2). This, no doubt, is linked to the reduced body weight and condition of the 'late-restricted' ewes and the inability of the 10-day 'flushing' regimen to return these ewes to a level of body condition more in keeping with the expression of their genetic potential for ovulation rate.

The central role that body condition at mating plays in determining ovulation rate is evident across breeds and management systems and is also apparent in the results presented in Table 9.2. Here the control ewes in Experiment 2 were about 12% heavier (equivalent to approximately 1 extra unit of body condition, using the 5-point scale described by Russel *et al.*, 1969) than their restricted counterparts and, in the absence of 'flushing', their mean ovulation rate was 1.67 compared with 1.22 for those that had been restricted. Such a difference in ovulation rate (0.45) is broadly in line with that anticipated, across a range of genotypes, for a 1 unit difference in body-condition score. Another feature of the data in Table 9.2 that characterizes the consensus view from the scientific literature is the failure of the control ewes in Experiment 2 to respond to flushing (1.64 vs. 1.67). These ewes were already gaining weight and were in good body condition prior to flushing. Thus their current nutrition and their nutritional history would be expected to minimize follicle atresia and maximize ovulation rate, provided no abrupt reduction in nutrition occurred following follicle antrum (cavity) formation, corresponding to the gonadotrophin-responsive and gonadotrophin-dependent stages (Fig. 9.1).

For ewes in suboptimal body condition, increases in ovulation rate have been achieved with an immediate preovulatory period of lupin-grain feeding as short as 4 days. In applying this feeding strategy, however, care must be exercised to ensure that the abrupt increase in feed intake close to ovulation does not become counterproductive through the creation of a metabolic acidosis. For this reason, and despite the fact that lupin-grain feeding for a brief period (6 days) beginning on either day 3 or day 7 of the oestrous cycle has been shown to increase the ovulation rate of Merino ewes by 40%, a longer period of 'flushing' (10–14 days preovulation) is generally recommended (reviewed by Robinson *et al.*, 1999a). On a flock basis, the natural spread in the timing of ovulation also makes this a more relevant practical option.

The preceding description of the ovulatory response to feeding clearly demonstrates the importance of short-term nutritional inputs. For the most part, however, benefits accrue only because of earlier inadequacies when ovarian follicles were leaving the primordial pool or because later undernutrition led to suboptimal body condition at ovulation. Following the lactational depletion of body reserves, achieving the target condition score (3–3.5 on the 5-point scale described by Russel *et al.*, 1969) for maximum ovulation rate can be a slow process. It often requires, in the first instance, repletion of body protein, followed by a gain of up to 1.5 units of body condition. For a 70 kg ewe, this equates to *c.* 8 kg of body fat. At energy intakes equivalent to twice maintenance, replacing this amount of fat requires realimentation periods of *c.* 90 and 65 days in ewes consuming forages with 8 and 12 MJ of metabolizable energy (ME) kg^{-1} dry matter (DM), respectively. In view of the importance of body condition to ovulation rate, the overall aim should be to achieve a uniform level of body condition on a flock basis that is as close as possible to the optimum. This may mean grouping ewes after weaning according to their body condition and allocating forage and, if necessary, supplementary feed according to needs. It may even require feed restriction of overfat ewes (condition score $\geq$ 4) in order to bring them into the 3–3.5 condition-score range, thereby minimizing the adverse effect of overfatness on early embryo survival (Rhind *et al.*, 1984).

Throughout the period of nutritional control for optimum ovulation and immediately thereafter, care must also be taken to ensure that other dietary factors do not impair normal ovarian function. Most notable among these are the phyto-oestrogens, which, in the 'Great Southern' region of Western Australia alone, are estimated to cause permanent subclinical infertility in *c.* 4 million ewes (Adams, 1995). Phyto-oestrogens occur in subterranean clover (*Trifolium subterraneum*), red clover (*Trifolium pratense*), Berseem clover (*Trifolium alexandrinum*) and bird's-foot trefoil (*Lotus corniculatus*) and in legumes such as *Vicia americana* and *Astragalus serotinus* (see Waghorn *et al.*, Chapter 15, this volume). Factors that accentuate their adverse effects on various components of fertility (ovulation, sperm transport, fertilization and embryo survival) are *in situ* fungal attack, resulting in the production of the oestrogenic compounds coumestrol and sativol, and conservation of forage in the form of hay or silage. For example, the conservation process increases concentrations of the oestrogen precursor formononetin, which is converted in the rumen into the phyto-oestrogen equol (7,4-dihydroxyisoflavin).

Nutrition for Optimum Embryo Survival

Both pre- and postovulatory nutrition affect embryo survival; the former via its effects on oocyte quality and the latter via its influence on the composition of the oviductal and uterine secretions that nourish the embryo during its early cell divisions. While improved nutrition during the immediate preovulatory period usually enhances the quality and viability of embryos arising from a naturally occurring oestrus, this is not so when ewes are superovulated with exogenous gonadotrophins prior to donation of embryos (McEvoy *et al.*, 2001). Under these conditions, high-plane feeding (≥ 2 × M) can result in embryos of reduced viability, with associated alterations in metabolism and gene expression that are indicative of cellular stress. Although the causal mechanisms are not fully understood, they appear to be linked to suboptimal oocyte quality arising from inadequate progesterone concentrations during oocyte maturation, mainly because there is a highly significant inverse relationship between feeding level and systemic progesterone concentrations in the ewe. This was the reasoning behind the initial recommendation of a maintenance level of feeding for superovulated embryo-donor ewes. On the basis of experience, this feeding strategy is now widely adopted by breeders using multiple ovulation and embryo transfer (MOET) for genetic improvement.

Despite the tiny size of the fertilized egg (diameter *c.* 150 μm) and its minute requirement for nutrients, high feeding levels are often recommended during early pregnancy. Results from numerous recent experiments, however, demonstrate that high feed intakes post-mating decrease pregnancy rates and litter sizes by reducing blood progesterone to concentrations that compromise embryo survival, with 11- and 12-day-old embryos being particularly vulnerable. Thus, for ewes of body condition score 3–3.5 at mating, it is now accepted that for maximum embryo survival the optimal feeding level during the first month of pregnancy is maintenance. At the experimental level, diets fortified with fatty acids (palmitic, stearic and oleic) in the form of calcium soaps, to ensure their passage to the small intestine without adverse effects on rumen function, have been used successfully in ewes to enhance luteal progesterone production (Kuran *et al.*, 1999). So too have dietary supplements of fish oils, which are rich in the fatty acids eicosapentaenoic (EPA; C20:5n-3) and docosahexaenoic (DHA; C22:6n-3) acid, which partially resist biohydrogenation by the rumen microbes. In addition, linoleic acid (C18:2n-6) and some n-3 fatty acids (e.g. EPA and DHA) may confer further benefits in situations where the natural signal from the embryo for the maintenance of pregnancy, interferon tau (IFN-τ), is weak, by suppressing the synthesis of its main antagonist, uterine prostaglandin $F_{2\alpha}$ (reviewed by Robinson *et al.*, 1999a).

Trace elements and vitamins play important roles in embryo survival through their effects on steroid hormone synthesis, expression of growth factors and gene transcription, all of which influence cell proliferation and differentiation. While new insights into micronutrient involvement at the molecular level reveal the nature of the damaging effects of their deficiencies on the embryo (Ashworth and Antipatis, 2001), excesses can also cause problems (McEvoy *et al.*, 2001). Emerging from these studies is the realization that, in addition to the well-recognized adverse effects of imbalances of micronutrients, such as selenium and vitamins A and E, on embryo survival, there are more subtle effects of 'micronutrient programming' during early pregnancy that only become apparent at birth. For example, cobalt inadequacy leads to deficiencies in folate as well as vitamin B_{12} and also to elevated plasma concentrations of homocysteine and methylmalonic acid. While the importance of folate for embryo development is well established, there is now evidence that high concentrations of homocysteine *per se* can interfere with the normal development of the neural tube and neural crest of the embryo by inhibiting the function of *N*-methyl-D-aspartate receptors in its neural epithelium (Rosenquist and Finnell, 2001). These findings perhaps provide an explanation for the observation by Fisher and MacPherson (1991) that subclinical cobalt deficiency during early pregnancy had an adverse effect on the vigour of newborn lambs, as indicated by significant increases in the times taken by them to find the udder and suck and reductions in their serum immunoglobulin G (IgG) concentrations and survival rates.

In addition to micronutrient imbalances, a wide range of naturally occurring plant and forage toxicants affect the development and viability of embryos. These have been the subject of a recent comprehensive review (McEvoy *et al.*, 2001) and will not be considered here. Suffice it to say that current research on the subject involves both *in vivo* and *in vitro* approaches designed to identify those critical times when the embryo is vulnerable to the toxins, the mechanisms of action of the toxins and the possibilities for developing effective antidotes.

Placental Size and Function

Nutritional imbalances, such as vitamin E and selenium deficiencies, which lead to sibling embryo mortality during implantation, decrease the subsequent fetal growth and birth weight of survivors by restricting placental size. Apart from this example, there is little evidence in practical production systems (Kelly, 1992) for effects of ewe nutrition on placental growth during early pregnancy (up to 6 weeks). Very rapid weight gain (*c.* 300 g day^{-1}) in adolescent pregnant ewes will reduce placental size and fetal growth but, even so, the effect is much greater during the second than the first trimester (Wallace *et al.*, 1999). However, in those studies, when daily injections of progesterone were given between days 5 and 55 of pregnancy to reverse the suppressive effects of high-plane feeding on this hormone, singleton lamb birth weights increased by *c.* 30%, but did so in the absence of an increase in placental size. This progesterone-mediated effect on fetal growth appears to be initiated prior to trophoblast elongation, i.e. before day 11 of pregnancy. It therefore implies that there can be early programming effects of nutrition that operate via shifts in progesterone concentration to cause alterations in placental function (e.g. its vascularity and its glucose and amino acid transporter abundance) and/or the expression of genes within the embryo that control subsequent fetal growth. Evidence that the nutritional environment of the pre-implantation embryo can alter gene expression and distort what has been generally regarded as a fairly close relationship between the size of the fetus and its placenta comes from the oversize fetuses arising from the transfer of embryos cultured *in vitro* from the zygote to blastocyst stage. Their oversize, which can occur in the absence of a proportional increase in placental size (Robinson *et al.*, 1999c), is associated with a doubling of their circulating concentrations of IGF-binding protein 2 (IGFBP2) and reduced methylation and expression of the imprinted *insulin-like growth factor 2 receptor* (*IGF2R*) gene (Young *et al.*, 2001).

Undoubtedly, the most sensitive period for nutritional modification of placental growth with an associated effect on lamb birth weight is between 50 and 90 days of gestation, the period of rapid proliferative growth of the placenta. In reviewing the literature, Kelly (1992) found that, of 16 experiments comparing high- and low-plane feeding during this period, all but two demonstrated an effect on placental weight. High-plane feeding increased placental size in nine of those 14 experiments and decreased it in three. In the other two experiments, the direction of the nutritional response was influenced by ewe body weight and condition score, with sub-maintenance feeding decreasing placental size in light/low condition-score ewes and increasing it in heavy/high condition-score ewes. These observations are confirmed by more recent data sets included in the review of Heasman *et al.* (1999). They reinforce the recommendation (Meat and Livestock Commission, 1983) that, for mature ewes of good body condition at mating (condition score 3.5), a mild degree of undernutrition from 30 to 90 days of gestation, leading to the gradual loss of half a unit of condition score, enhances placental growth. For those in poor body condition at mating (condition score 2.0), undernutrition has the opposite effect.

The degree of maturity of the ewe also interacts with plane of nutrition in mid-pregnancy to affect placental and fetal growth. This is well illustrated by the recent data of Wallace *et al.* (1999), in which daily liveweight gains by pregnant adolescent ewes (weight at conception *c.* 40 kg; projected mature weight *c.* 75 kg) of *c.* 300 g from days 50 to 104 of gestation gave mean (± SEM) placental cotyledon weights of only 120 (± 27) g on day 104, compared with 234 (± 30) g for those restricted to the recommended (Meat and Livestock Commission, 1983) daily growth rates of *c.* 80 g day^{-1}. These adverse effects on the placenta were reflected in reduced birth weights of singleton lambs (3.1 (± 0.24) vs. 4.9 (± 0.47) kg) and, despite intensive care, a fivefold increase in lamb mortality. Although these observations are from an extreme nutritional model, they illustrate the importance for successful reproduction in growing/reproducing ewes of establishing and achieving targets for both body weight at conception and weight gains during pregnancy. The concept of 'targets' was established in the 1970s, albeit with limited information compared with what is now available, and included feeding recommendations in the form of stylized weight-change curves, augmented with supporting information on body condition (Meat and Livestock Commission, 1983). A modified composite version of these stylized curves that captures the preceding nutritional principles and translates them into suggested targets for optimum lifetime reproductive performance of ewes with a mean adult litter size of two is illustrated in Fig. 9.2.

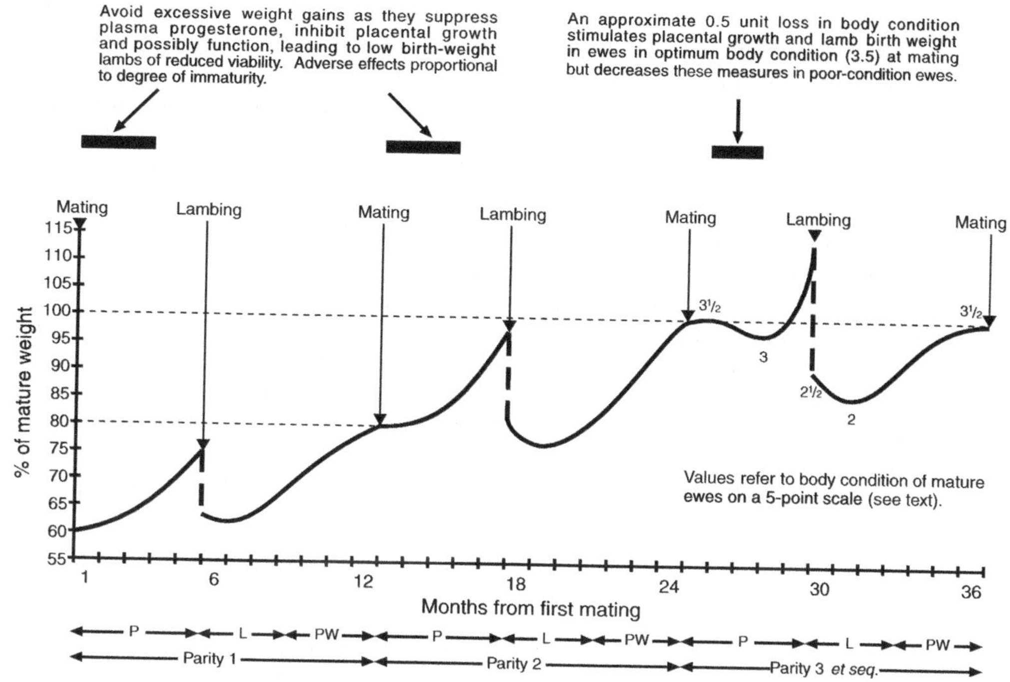

Fig. 9.2. Live weight and body condition score targets for optimum lifetime reproductive performance (P, pregnancy; L, lactation; PW, postweaning), with summary information on the effects of plane of nutrition on placental and fetal growth.

Partition of Nutrients during Pregnancy

While easily monitored targets, such as those in Fig. 9.2, are extremely valuable in improving nutritional management for conception and pregnancy, significant deviations from these targets often occur in practice. These lead to alterations in body condition during late pregnancy, which, in the absence of effects on placental size, interact with current nutrition to influence nutrient partitioning and neonatal viability. For example, when fat ewes are fed a diet supplying inadequate energy, they mobilize body energy reserves and, provided the magnitude of the energy deficit is not so large or so acute as to induce pregnancy toxaemia, they are better at sustaining fetal growth than their thinner counterparts. On the other hand, when allowed free access to food, thin ewes eat more than fat ones but partition the extra nutrients to maternal rather than conceptus tissues. When the effects of body condition *per se* are tested by feeding both fat and thin ewes to requirements (AFRC, 1993), birth weights are not affected, but the fat content of the lamb is positively correlated with the fat content of its dam (McNeill *et al.*, 1997a). In view of the beneficial and sometimes critical role of the newborn lamb's adipose tissue in heat production, this observation has important implications for lamb survival.

In the preceding examples of different forms of nutrient partitioning, there is clear evidence that the ability of ewes to sustain fetal growth during energy undernutrition is positively correlated with their intake of metabolizable protein (Fig. 9.3). As well as providing quantitative information on the response in lamb birth weight to protein, the data in Fig. 9.3 add another dimension to nutrient partitioning in late pregnancy by demonstrating that it also involves redistribution of protein between the components of the maternal body. This is best illustrated in the data for the intermediate level of protein, which could be regarded as marginal to requirements in that it caused a small reduction in lamb birth weight. In this situation, the protein content of the maternal organs (empty digestive tract, liver, kidneys, heart, lungs, etc.) increased by an amount that was similar to the loss of protein from the maternal carcass. This redistribution of protein presumably reflects the important functional roles of the maternal organs during late pregnancy, perhaps made possible, when dietary protein is inadequate, by the pregnancy-induced susceptibility of maternal muscles to proteolysis.

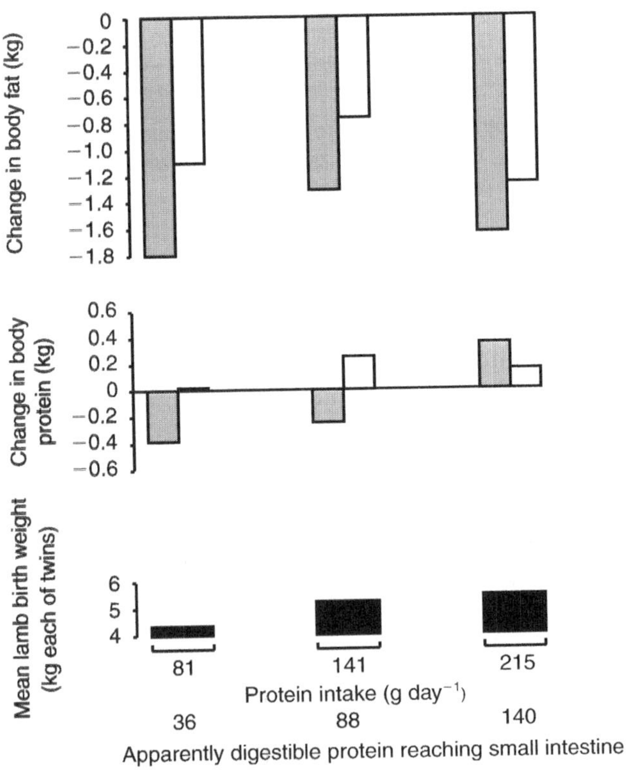

Fig. 9.3. Lamb birth weights and the changes between days 110 and 140 of gestation in the amounts of protein and fat in the carcasses (shaded columns) and maternal organs (open columns) of twin-bearing pregnant ewes (*c.* 62 kg) receiving different levels of dietary protein, and the SCA (1990) requirements for energy (based on data presented by McNeill *et al.*, 1997b).

Muscle proteolysis is only one of many pregnancy-induced metabolic adaptations in maternal tissues, the expression of which is accentuated or modified by undernutrition. Others, which are the subject of a recent comprehensive review (Bell and Ehrhardt, 2000), are included in Fig. 9.4. For some of the adaptations, the endocrine effectors remain unknown and are the subject of speculation, whereas, for others, progress has been made in their identification. In the case of fetal calcium requirements, for example, the evidence is that when the maternal diet is inadequate, fetal IGF-2 and a fetal parathyroid hormone-related protein (PTHrP) act to ensure provision of calcium from the maternal skeleton. Of the hormones of pregnancy, placental lactogen is attracting renewed research interest, in that, along with progesterone and oestradiol, it is probably involved in reducing the sensitivity of maternal tissues to insulin. It also stimulates fetal growth, mammary development and milk production (Leibovich *et al.*, 2000).

A pregnancy-induced adaptation of the maternal body not included in Fig. 9.4, but potentially important in the nutrition of the ewe during late pregnancy, is the increase of *c.* 15% in the amount of amino nitrogen reaching the abomasum (reviewed by Robinson *et al.*, 1999a). This increase occurs in the absence of changes in either diet quality or intake and is the result of a reduction in rumen retention time, leading to an increase in the rumen undegraded protein fraction that more than compensates for an associated reduction in the yield of microbial protein. Clearly, quantitative

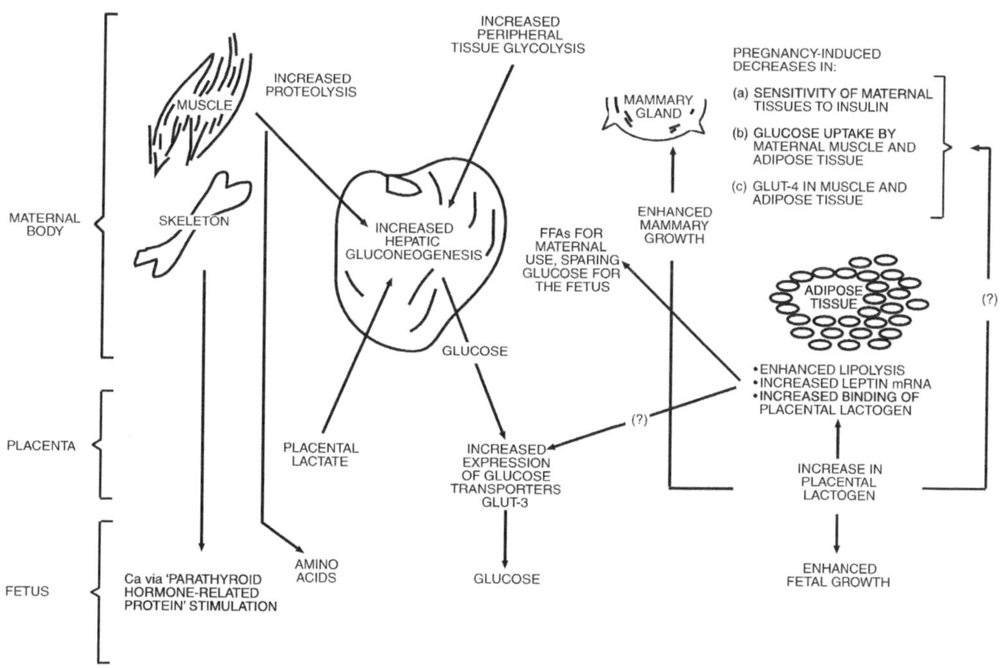

Fig. 9.4. Pregnancy-induced metabolic adaptations in maternal tissues. FFAs, free fatty acids; mRNA, messenger RNA.

data for a much wider range of diet types are needed before these observations can be used, with confidence, to modify existing feeding standards for protein. Information is also required to verify or refute the suggestion (Ngongoni *et al.*, 1987) that the pregnancy-induced increase in rumen outflow is, in common with similar increases in outflow rate that occur following cold exposure or winter shearing of pregnant ewes, the result of a change in maternal thyroid function. If further investigation reveals that the phenomenon occurs widely in practical production systems, it could signal an opportunity for nutritionists to exploit further the beneficial effects of the rumen-undegraded dietary protein (UDP) fraction by increasing the inclusion rate of highly digestible UDP supplements in the diet. This is particularly relevant in many extensive systems, where low energy intakes inevitably lead to low yields of microbial protein, which fail to meet the amino acid requirements for normal fetal growth and the production of the amount of colostrum required to maximize neonatal viability.

Macronutrient Recommendations and their Limitations

Estimates of the rates of accretion of the macronutrients in the conceptus form the basis for the widely adopted factorial method of determining dietary needs. It is not our purpose to retabulate these estimates or, indeed, to compare the various published standards (Agricultural and Food Research Council (AFRC), 1993; Standing Committee on Agriculture (SCA), 1990; Institut National de la Recherche Agronomique (INRA), 1989; National Research Council (NRC), 1985), as this has been done for energy and protein by Sinclair and Wilkinson (2000). Anyway, the consequence for fetal growth of the differences between feeding standards is largely nullified by the metabolic and compositional changes in maternal tissues and organs referred to earlier. Rather, it is important to identify problems encountered in the implementation of current recommendations. In this regard, the recent findings of Donaldson *et al.* (2001) are relevant. They show that current recommendations (AFRC, 1993) for metabolizable protein during late pregnancy fail to meet the additional protein needs of ewes for acquisition of immunity to gastrointestinal parasites and would have to be increased by 20% to help achieve maximum immunity (see also Coop and Sykes, Chapter 14, this volume). While it can be argued that the provision of nutrients to ensure full expression of the immune system should not be considered within the nutrient requirements for reproduction, the counter-arguments appear more compelling: first, a competent immune system is essential in many environments for the overall success of the reproductive process; and, secondly, late pregnancy is a critical window for the dietary control of immune expression. Of course, there is still a need to bring greater precision to the understanding of the nutritional stimulation of the immune response by identifying the specific nutrients that are required for its expression. At present, these remain elusive but may involve the sulphur-containing amino acids, notably cysteine, high concentrations of which occur in the leukotrienes, which play a central role in the acquisition of cell-mediated immunity, which typifies the development of resistance to intestinal parasitism.

In addition to its possible involvement in the development of maternal immunity, cysteine becomes one of the first limiting amino acids for fetal growth during late pregnancy (Robinson *et al.*, 1999a) in ewes that are not receiving supplements of high-quality UDP and are therefore dependent on microbial protein for most of their amino acids. The reason for this is the high concentration of cysteine, present as cystine, in the lamb's birth coat, the normal development of which is important for thermoregulation and survival. The priority of the fetus for amino acids is such that, if necessary, maternal wool growth is impaired in order to sustain fetal needs. However, undernutrition during the last trimester of pregnancy in Merino ewes can also impair the development of secondary wool follicles in the fetus, leading to subsequent depressions in the quantity and quality of their wool as adults (Kelly *et al.*, 1996). While there is the potential to meet some of the cysteine requirements in late pregnancy through interconversion from microbial methionine, methionine itself becomes limiting when its microbial production is constrained by low intakes of rumen-fermentable energy; so too does the essential amino acid histidine. This reinforces the importance of providing twin- and triplet-bearing ewes with undegradable protein supplements rich in the sulphur-containing amino acids and histidine during the last 3–4 weeks of their pregnancies.

Of the amino acids once regarded as 'non-essential', glycine is particularly interesting in that it is a precursor in the synthesis of a range of compounds of physiological importance and is now regarded as a 'conditionally essential' amino acid. It has a high rate of accretion in the fetus, making its supply from microbial protein during late pregnancy marginal to requirements (Robinson *et al.*, 1999a). Its production via interconversion from serine within the placenta helps to alleviate its microbial protein deficit, with the added benefit of providing active carbon units for purine synthesis, DNA methylation and the control of gene expression. In terms of diet formulation, the fact that fish meal is rich in glycine, in addition to its high content of sulphur-containing amino acids, may further contribute to its high nutritional value as a dietary protein supplement during late pregnancy.

The limitation of tabulated nutrient requirements is not restricted to protein but extends to energy and the mineral elements, notably calcium. In the case of energy, Hutchings (1997) points out that in the AFRC (1993) calculation of ME requirements for pregnancy, greater clarity is required in defining the value to use for ewe weight. To illustrate the relevance of this point, Hutchings (1997) carried out simulations of the total energy demands during pregnancy for a ewe with a fasted non-pregnant weight of 37.6 kg, carrying a single lamb. Graphical presentation by Hutchings of these demands provides estimates of 830 and 740 MJ for diets with ME concentrations (M/D) of 7.5 and 13 MJ kg^{-1} DM, respectively. Simulations for the same ewe, but allowing for conceptus gain by using fasted pregnant weight, gave corresponding estimates of 890 and 795 MJ (i.e. *c.* 7%

higher). Going beyond AFRC (1993) by making an allowance for the effect of the ME content of the diet on the efficiency of ME utilization for fetal growth (0.11 for M/D = 7.5, rising to 0.18 for M/D = 13) in the simulations that used the non-pregnant ewe weight, the total ME requirement increased from 830 to 865 MJ at M/D = 7.5 and decreased from 740 to 705 MJ at M/D = 13. While this increase and decrease in energy requirements at low and high metabolizabilities, respectively, are fairly minor in single-bearing ewes, they are significantly accentuated as litter size increases and thus the energy costs of conceptus growth comprise an increasing proportion of the total ME demands for pregnancy.

For calcium (Ca), the limitation of tabulated requirements is different from that for either protein or energy. Here, a deficiency in late pregnancy, expressed by overt symptoms of hypocalcaemia, is almost always the result of a failure in the endocrine mechanism that promotes Ca absorption and its skeletal mobilization, rather than an inadequate dietary intake of the element (Sykes and Russel, 2000). Central to the endocrine control of Ca absorption is parathyroid hormone (PTH), which promotes the conversion of vitamin D-derived 25-hydroxycholecalciferol to 1,25-dihydroxycholecalciferol. The latter stimulates the active intestinal Ca absorption system that is required to meet the increased Ca demands for fetal growth, by promoting the production of a Ca-binding protein in the alimentary tract; it also stimulates Ca resorption from bone. The stimulus for the rise in PTH is a fall in extracellular fluid Ca. The prevention of clinical symptoms of hypocalcaemia therefore involves the controlled 'awakening' of these homoeostatic control mechanisms by creating a small deficit in extracellular-fluid Ca that is sufficient to increase PTH and yet avoids a metabolic crisis. In practice, this can be achieved by feeding a diet that is relatively low in Ca well before the rapid increase in demand for Ca in late pregnancy, and then following up with an increase in dietary concentration as parturition approaches (Sykes and Russel, 2000). Low dietary cation–anion (Na + K)–(Cl + S) balances also help to maintain Ca homoeostasis by stimulating bone Ca resorption. There also appears to be an intermediate optimum concentration of magnesium in plasma (*c.* 0.9 mM) for stimulating the activities of 1,25-dihydroxycholecalciferol and PTH and therefore maximizing the efficiency of Ca resorption from bone (Sykes and Russel, 2000).

The Importance of Vitamin E, Selenium and Iodine for Neonatal Viability

Improvements in the energy and protein nutrition of the pregnant ewe in the absence of adequate intakes of essential trace elements and vitamins invariably lead to lack of vigour and reduced viability in the newborn lamb. The reason for this is that improved nutrition reduces maternal tissue catabolism and thus decreases the release of essential nutrients, such as, for example, vitamin E from the mobilized adipose tissue where it is stored. This vitamin and the selenium-containing glutathione peroxidases operate in the lipid membranes and cytosol of the cell, respectively, to prevent oxidative damage and cell dysfunction and to enhance immune function. Selenium crosses the placenta into the fetus and also the mammary barrier, particularly during the colostrum-production phase. Thus the selenium status of both the newborn lamb and its colostrum supply reflect that of the ewe. In contrast, vitamin E does not cross the placenta in significant amounts; rather, it is concentrated in the colostrum, on which the newborn lamb is dependent for its supply. Thus, newborn lambs with presuckling serum vitamin E (α-tocopherol) concentrations of approximately 0.4 μg ml^{-1} exhibited increases to 1.4, 1.8, 2.4 and 4.5 μg ml^{-1} at 3 days of age when they were suckled by ewes supplemented during the final 28 days of pregnancy with 0, 15, 30 and 60 mg day^{-1}, respectively, of α-tocopheryl acetate (McDowell *et al.*, 1996). In view of the variable and sometimes suboptimal intakes of colostrum and the importance of the vitamin E status of the lamb in the development of immune function, 100 mg per head day^{-1} of supplementary α-tocopheryl acetate is commonly advocated in the UK for ewes during their last 4 weeks of pregnancy.

The importance of the antioxidant roles of vitamin E and selenium is accentuated in ewes grazing spring grass rich in polyunsaturated fatty acids or where the energy density of late-pregnancy concentrate supplements is boosted by polyunsaturated fatty acid-enriched supplements. Alkali treatment of cereal grains to reduce their fermentation rate in the rumen causes a deterioration in their vitamin E status. So too does cereal-grain storage at high moisture contents without or with propionic acid as a preservative. Failure to correct such deficiencies when cereals treated in these ways are included in concentrate supplements for pregnant ewes leads to the birth of lambs of low vigour and viability.

Selenium also interacts with iodine to influence thyroid function via a membrane-bound selenoprotein, type I iodothyronine deiodinase, which converts thyroxine (T_4) to the active thyroid hormone, tri-iodothyronine (T_3), in extrathyroidal tissues, including the brown adipose tissue of the newborn lamb. Thus selenium deficiency in the newborn lamb is characterized by high T_4 and low T_3 concentrations. The low T_3 results in a failure of transcription of the uncoupling protein gene required to induce the heat-generation capacity of brown adipocyte mitochondria that is essential for maintaining prefeeding body temperature and viability in cold environments. An overview of the preceding interrelationships between vitamin E, selenium and iodine, augmented with additional information relating to their important physiological roles and their relevance to feeding practice, is presented in Fig. 9.5.

Nutrition and Colostrum Production

Despite its essential role in the provision of the newborn lamb with an immediate supply of vitamin E, immunoglobulins and metabolic fuel, there is little information on dietary means to optimize colostrum production.

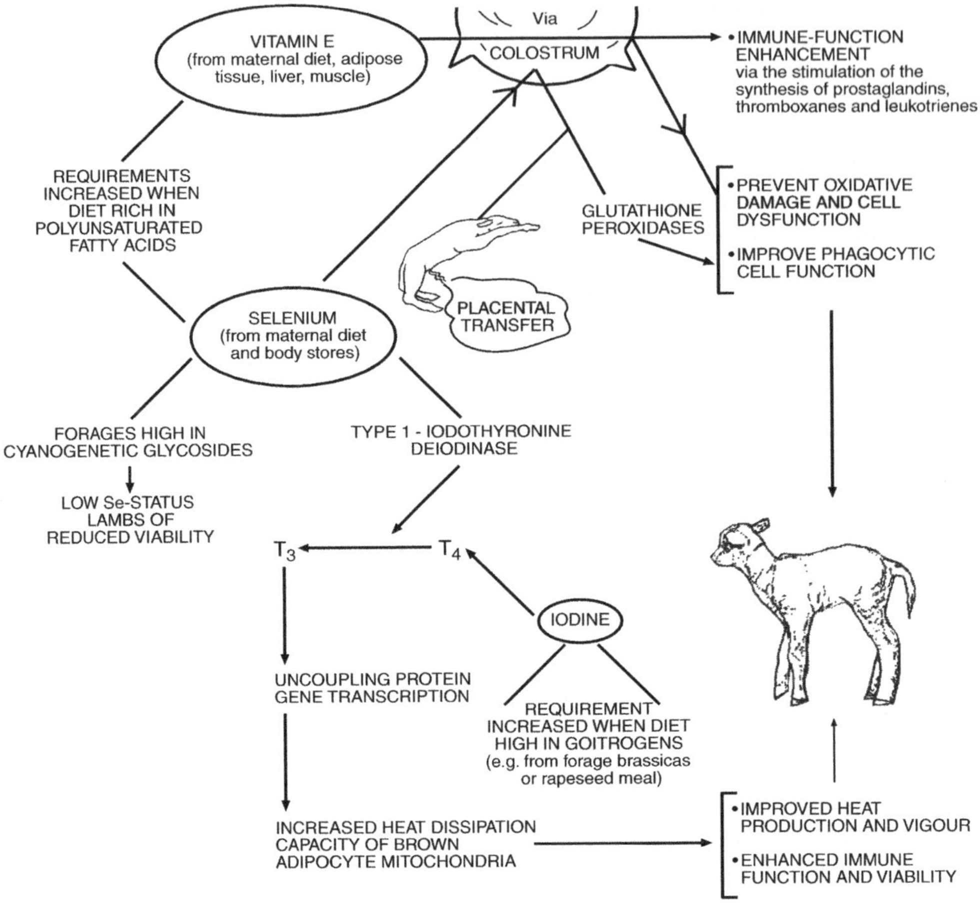

Fig. 9.5. Interrelationships between vitamin E, selenium and iodine in the metabolism and viability of newborn lambs (from data reviewed by McDowell *et al.*, 1996; Robinson *et al.*, 1999a, b; Underwood and Suttle, 1999).

Undernutrition delays the late-pregnancy fall in the ewe's systemic progesterone concentrations, probably as a result of reduced hepatic clearance by those enzymes (cytochromes b_5 and P450) involved in the oxidative metabolism of steroids. This delays the late-pregnancy increase in blood flow to the udder, depriving it of important metabolic substrates for colostrum production. With an immediate requirement at birth for 50 ml of colostrum per kg lamb birth weight, it is important that the maternal nutrient supply meets this target. At present, there are insufficient data in the literature to quantify the separate effects of dietary energy and protein *per se* during late pregnancy on colostrum yields. None the less, the data in Fig. 9.6 for a range of basal feeds given *ad libitum*, either alone or with a protein supplement in the form of soybean meal, provide a basis on which to build. In addition to the clear relationship between the ewe's ME intake over the

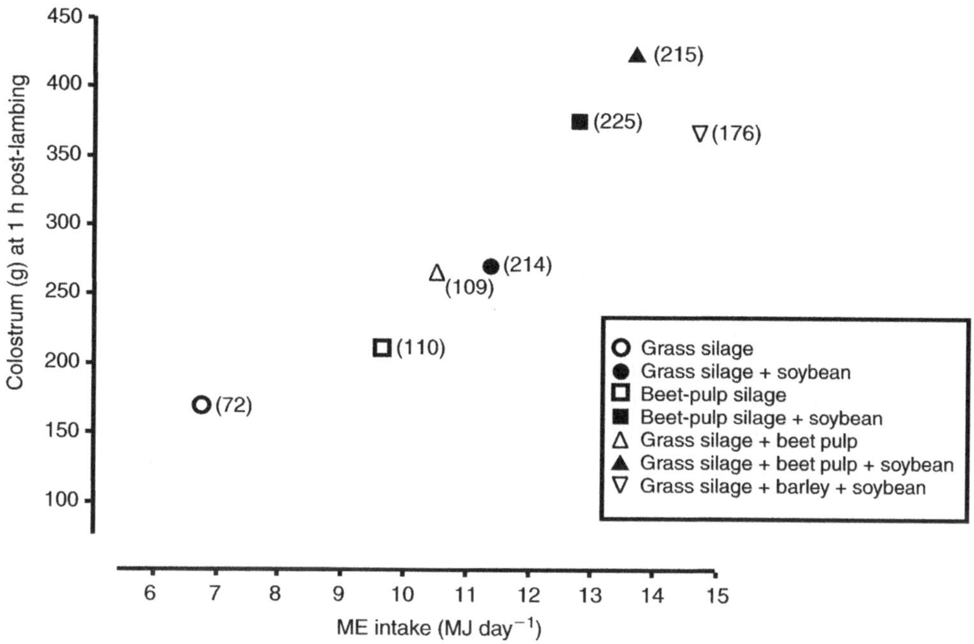

Fig. 9.6. Mean colostrum yields at 1 h post-lambing by twin-bearing crossbred ewes (*c.* 75 kg live weight) in relation to mean daily ME intake during the last 3 weeks of pregnancy; values in parentheses are daily intakes of crude protein (g) (plotted from data of O'Doherty and Crosby, 1997).

last 3 weeks of pregnancy and colostrum yield (Fig. 9.6), O'Doherty and Crosby (1997) found that pre-lambing protein supplementation significantly increased the efficiency of absorption of colostral IgG by lambs, reflecting a similar observation in cattle.

An important feature of the data in Fig. 9.6 is the stimulatory effect of a protein supplement (215 g of soybean DM; equivalent to *c.* 2.5 MJ of ME) on total energy intake. For the grass-silage diet the increase in mean daily ME intake as a result of including the protein supplement was 4.6 MJ and for the 'beet-pulp silage' and 'grass silage + beet pulp' diets the increases were each 3.2 MJ, a clear demonstration of the enhancing effect of the protein on forage intake.

In interpreting the data in Fig. 9.6 in relation to feeding standards for energy and protein provision during late pregnancy, it is important to note that ewes were in excellent body condition (mean score 3.24) on day 91 of their pregnancies, but, by lambing, those on the lowest energy intake had lost almost a complete unit of condition score, a loss that could not have been tolerated by ewes in body-condition score of 2.5 or less at day 91. In contrast, those on the three highest levels of ME intake had acceptable body-condition score losses, ranging from zero for those producing the largest amount of colostrum ('grass silage + beet pulp + soybean' diet) to means of *c.* 0.33 units for the other two.

Conclusions

- The role of nutrition in the expression of the reproductive potential of sheep involves long-term programming, as well as contemporary effects.
- Improvements in energy and protein nutrition enhance reproductive efficiency, but care is required lest they expose the oocyte, embryo and fetus to deficiencies of specific minerals and vitamins that would otherwise be supplied by the catabolism of maternal tissues.
- Current recommendations for protein during late pregnancy may require upward revision in the light of recent findings on the beneficial effects of higher protein levels in the acquisition of immunity to gastrointestinal parasites.
- Fetal amino acid requirements are still a matter of speculation and yet, with more information regarding their metabolic and functional roles, greater precision could be brought to supplementary feeding regimens.
- Major improvements in nutrition will come from enhanced understanding of how dietary nutrients alter hormone concentrations and facilitate the programming and expression of the biochemical pathways involved in oocyte maturation, the development of the embryo and fetus, the viability of the newborn lamb and the secretion of colostrum. An example is the recent advance in understanding the interactions among vitamin E, selenium and iodine, which is proving beneficial in the formulation of diets for improved lamb survival. (See Plate 9.1.)

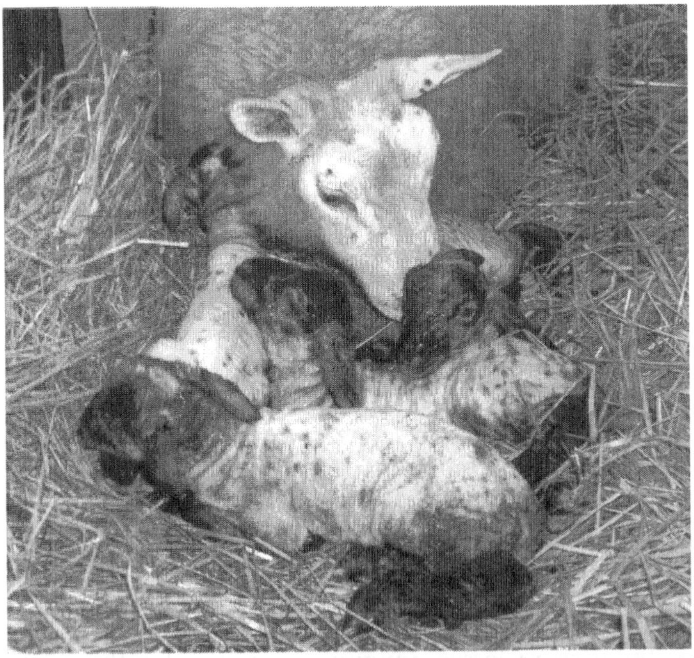

Plate 9.1. A cross-bred British Milksheep ewe with her Suffolk-sired lambs. Multiple births of this size place great nutritional demands on the ewe during late pregnancy and throughout lactation (see Chapter 10).

Acknowledgements

The authors express their gratitude to research colleagues for helpful discussions in the preparation of this chapter. Original research from our laboratory referred to in this review was funded by the Scottish Executive Environment and Rural Affairs Department and by the UK Department for Environment, Food and Rural Affairs.

References

Adam, C.L. and Robinson, J.J. (1994) The role of nutrition and photoperiod in the timing of puberty. *Proceedings of the Nutrition Society* 53, 89–102.

Adams, N. (1995) Detection of the effects of phyto-oestrogens on sheep and cattle. *Journal of Animal Science* 73, 1509–1515.

AFRC (Agricultural and Food Research Council) (1993) *Energy and Protein Requirements of Ruminants. An Advisory Manual Prepared by the AFRC Technical Committee on Responses to Nutrients*. CAB International, Wallingford, UK, 159 pp.

Armstrong, D.G. and Webb, R. (1997) Ovarian follicular dominance: the role of intraovarian growth factors and novel proteins. *Reviews of Reproduction* 2, 139–146.

Ashworth, C.J. and Antipatis, C. (2001) Micronutrient programming of development throughout gestation. *Reproduction* 122, 527–535.

Bell, A.W. and Ehrhardt, R.A. (2000) Regulation of macro-nutrient partitioning between maternal conceptus tissues in the pregnant ruminant. In: Cronjé, P.B. (ed.) *Ruminant Physiology, Digestion, Metabolism, Growth and Reproduction*. CAB International, Wallingford, UK, pp. 275–293.

Blache, D., Chagas, L.M., Blackberry, M.A., Vercoe, P.E. and Martin, G.B. (2000) Metabolic factors affecting the reproductive axis in male sheep. *Journal of Reproduction and Fertility* 120, 1–11.

Borwick, S.C., Rhind, S.M., McMillan, S.R. and Racey, P.A. (1997) Effect of undernutrition of ewes from the time of mating on fetal ovarian development in mid-gestation. *Reproduction, Fertility and Development* 9, 711–715.

Da Silva, P., Aitken, R.P., Rhind, S.M. and Wallace, J.M. (2000) The effect of nutritionally-mediated placental growth restriction on fetal pituitary gonadotrophin gene expression and gonadal morphology at Day 104 of gestation. *Journal of Reproduction and Fertility Abstract Series* 25, 95.

Donaldson, J., van Houtert, M.F.J. and Sykes, A.R. (2001) The effect of dietary fishmeal supplementation on parasite burdens of periparturient sheep. *Animal Science* 72, 149–158.

Fisher, C.E.J. and MacPherson, A. (1991) Effect of cobalt deficiency in the pregnant ewe on reproductive performance and lamb viability. *Research in Veterinary Science* 50, 319–327.

Gunn, R.G., Sim, D.A. and Hunter, E.A. (1995) Effects of nutrition *in utero* and in early life on the subsequent lifetime reproductive performance of Scottish Blackface ewes in two management systems. *Animal Science* 60, 223–230.

Heasman, L., Clarke, L., Stephenson, T.J. and Symonds, M.E. (1999) The influence of maternal nutrient restriction in early to mid-pregnancy on placental and fetal development in sheep. *Proceedings of the Nutrition Society* 58, 283–288.

Hutchings, N.J. (1997) Estimating the metabolizable energy requirement for pregnancy in sheep. *Animal Science* 64, 463–467.

INRA (Institut National de la Recherche Agronomique) (1989) *Ruminant Nutrition: Recommended Allowances and Feed Tables*. INRA, Paris.

Kelly, R.W. (1992) Nutrition and placental development. *Proceedings of the Nutrition Society of Australia* 17, 203–211.

Kelly, R.W., MacLeod, I., Hynd, P. and Greeff, J. (1996) Nutrition during fetal life alters annual wool production and quality in young Merino sheep. *Australian Journal of Experimental Agriculture* 36, 259–267.

Kuran, M., Onal, A., Robinson, J.J., Mackie, K., Speake, B.K. and McEvoy, T.G. (1999) A dietary supplement of calcium soaps of fatty acids enhances luteal function in sheep. *Animal Science* 69, 385–393.

Leibovich, H., Gertler, A., Bazer, F.W. and Gotwine, E. (2000) Active immunization of ewes against ovine placental lactogen increases birth weight of lambs and milk production with no adverse effect on conception rate. *Animal Reproduction Science* 64, 33–47.

McDowell, L.R., Williams, S.N., Hidiroglou, N., Njeru, C.A., Hill, G.M., Ochoa, L. and Wilkinson, N.S. (1996) Vitamin E supplementation for the ruminant. *Animal Feed Science and Technology* 60, 273–296.

McEvoy, T.G., Robinson, J.J., Ashworth, C.J., Rooke, J.A. and Sinclair, K.D. (2001) Feed and forage toxicants affecting embryo survival and fetal development. *Theriogenology* 55, 113–129.

McFadden, T.B., Daniel, T.E. and Akers, R.M. (1990) Effects of plane of nutrition, growth hormone and unsaturated fat on growth hormone, insulin and prolactin receptors in prepubertal lambs. *Journal of Animal Science* 68, 3180–3189.

McNeill, D.M., Kelly, R.W. and Williams, I.H. (1997a) The partition of nutrients in ewes maintained in a moderate compared with a lean body condition in late pregnancy. *Australian Journal of Agricultural Research* 48, 743–752.

McNeill, D.M., Slepetis, R., Ehrhardt, R.A., Smith, D.M. and Bell, A.W. (1997b) Protein requirements of sheep in late pregnancy: partitioning of nitrogen between gravid uterus and maternal tissues. *Journal of Animal Science* 75, 809–816.

Meat and Livestock Commission (1983) *Feeding the Ewe*. MLC Sheep Improvement Services, Milton Keynes, UK, 78 pp.

Miller, D.W., Blache, D., Boukhliq, R., Curlewis, J.D. and Martin, G.B. (1998) Central metabolic messengers and the effects of nutrition on gonadotrophin secretion in sheep. *Journal of Reproduction and Fertility* 112, 347–356.

Ngongoni, N.T., Robinson, J.J., Kay, R.N.B., Stephenson, R.G.A., Atkinson, T. and Grant, I. (1987) The effect of altering the hormone status of ewes on the outflow rate of protein supplements from the rumen and so on protein degradability. *Animal Production* 44, 395–404.

Nottle, M.B., Kleemann, D.O. and Seamark, R.F. (1997) Effect of previous undernutrition on the ovulation rate of Merino ewes supplemented with lupin grain. *Animal Reproduction Science* 49, 29–36.

NRC (National Research Council) (1985) *Nutrient Requirements of Sheep*, 6th edn. National Academy Press, Washington, DC.

O'Doherty, J.V. and Crosby, T.F. (1997) The effect of diet in late pregnancy on colostrum production and immunoglobulin absorption in sheep. *Animal Science* 64, 87–96.

Rae, M.T., Palassio, S., Kyle, C.E., Brooks, A.N., Lea, R.G., Miller, D.W. and Rhind, S.M. (2001) Effect of maternal undernutrition during pregnancy on early ovarian development and subsequent follicular development in sheep fetuses. *Reproduction* 122, 915–922.

Rhind, S.M., Gunn, R.G., Doney, J.M. and Leslie, I.D. (1984) A note on the reproductive performance of Greyface ewes in moderately fat and very fat condition at mating. *Animal Production* 38, 305–307.

Rhind, S.M., Elston, D.A., Jones, C.R., Rees, M.E., McMillan, S.R. and Gunn, R.G. (1998) Effects of restriction of growth and development of Brecon Cheviot ewe lambs on subsequent lifetime reproductive performance. *Small Ruminant Research* 30, 121–126.

Robinson, J.J. (1990) Nutrition in the reproduction of farm animals. *Nutrition Research Reviews* 3, 253–276.

Robinson, J.J., Sinclair, K.D., Randel, R.D. and Sykes, A.R. (1999a) Nutritional management of the female ruminant: mechanistic approaches and predictive models. In: Jung, H.-J.G. and Fahey, G.C. (eds) *Nutritional Ecology of Herbivores. Proceedings of the Vth International Symposium on Nutrition of Herbivores*. American Society of Animal Science, Savoy, Illinois, pp. 550–608.

Robinson, J.J., McEvoy, T.G. and Sinclair, K.D. (1999b) Nutritional effects on foetal growth. *Animal Science* 68, 315–331.

Robinson, J.J., McEvoy, T.G. and Sinclair, K.D. (1999c) Maternal nutrition and foetal growth. *Reproduction in Domestic Animals*, Suppl. 6, 14–19.

Rosenquist, T.H. and Finnell, R.H. (2001) Genes, folate and homocysteine in embryonic development. *Proceedings of the Nutrition Society* 60, 53–61.

Russel, A.J.F., Doney, J.M. and Gunn, R.G. (1969) Subjective assessment of body fat in live sheep. *Journal of Agricultural Science, Cambridge* 72, 451–454.

SCA (1990) *Feeding Standards for Australian Livestock. Ruminants*. Standing Committee on Agriculture, CSIRO Publications, Melbourne, 266 pp.

Sinclair, L.A. and Wilkinson, R.G. (2000) Feeding systems for sheep. In: Theodorou, M.K. and France, J. (eds) *Feeding Systems and Feed Evaluation Models*. CAB International, Wallingford, UK, pp. 155–180.

Sykes, A.R. and Russel, A.J.F. (2000) Deficiency of mineral macro-elements. In: Martin, W.B. and Aitken, I.D. (eds) *Diseases of Sheep*, 3rd edn. Blackwell Science, Oxford, pp. 318–331.

Underwood, E.J. and Suttle, N.F. (1999) *The Mineral Nutrition of Livestock*, 3rd edn. CAB International, Wallingford, UK, 614 pp.

Wallace, J.M., Bourke, D.A. and Aitken, R.P. (1999) Nutrition and fetal growth: paradoxical effects in overnourished adolescent sheep. *Journal of Reproduction and Fertility*, Suppl. 54, 385–399.

Young, L.E., Fernandes, K., McEvoy, T.G., Butterwith, S.C., Gutierrez, C.G., Carolan, C., Broadbent, P.J., Robinson, J.J., Wilmut, I. and Sinclair, K.D. (2001) Epigenetic change in IGF2R is associated with fetal overgrowth after embryo culture. *Nature Genetics* 27, 153–154.

10 Nutrition during Lactation

T.T. Treacher[1] and G. Caja[2]

[1]51 Western Road, Oxford, UK; [2]Facultad de Veterinaria, Universidad Autonoma de Barcelona, Bellaterra, Spain

Introduction

In the majority of sheep production systems, sheep are kept for meat or wool production and ewes rear their lambs until weaning, at 3 or 4 months of age. During this period, lamb growth is largely determined by milk intake. Early lactation is the period of highest nutrient requirements in the ewe's whole productive cycle, and failure of management at this time has a major impact on lamb growth. This generally affects the profitability of the system and, in lambs retained as flock replacements, can reduce lifetime performance.

In a number of countries, mainly in Asia and Europe, ewes' milk is an important direct source of animal protein in the human diet. In Afghanistan, Greece, Iraq, Somalia and Syria, more than 30% of the total production of milk, from cows, buffalo, sheep and goats, comes from ewes. In France, Greece, Italy and Spain, large numbers of dairy sheep are kept to produce milk for high-quality, expensive cheeses. In dairy systems, ewes generally rear their lambs before milking is started. The length of both suckling and milking periods varies widely, from 1 month of suckling and 5 or 6 months of milking, in the traditional Mediterranean system, to 3 months suckling and a month of milking in, for example, central Europe. The various dairy systems are discussed in Treacher (1987).

Composition of Ewes' Milk

Typical figures for the mean composition of ewes' milk (g kg^{-1} liquid milk) are: fat 71, protein 57, lactose 48, ash 9 and solids-not-fat 115 (Ashton *et al.*, 1964). At the start of lactation, the contents of fat and protein are high. They decrease to the peak of lactation and then increase through the remainder of lactation, as yield decreases. Lactose content shows little variation, as the amount of lactose synthesized determines milk yield. The negative relationship between yield and the contents of fat and protein is more general and applies also when differences in yield arise from genotype, individual variation or selection within a breed (see review by Bencini and Pulina, 1997). Change in composition during lactation has a large effect on the gross energy of milk, which may vary from 3.8 to 5.5 MJ kg^{-1} (Brett *et al.*, 1972). Equation (1) (Brett *et al.*, 1972), based on data from 92 samples taken from Merino (mean fat 72 g kg^{-1}) and Border Leicester (mean fat 105 g kg^{-1}) ewes, predicts gross energy, E (MJ kg^{-1}), from fat, F (g kg^{-1}), and day of lactation, D:

$$E = 0.0328F + 0.0025D + 2.20 \qquad \text{RSD} = \pm 0.14 \qquad (1)$$

Milk fat consists almost entirely of triglycerides, with most of the fatty acids being monounsaturated and containing even numbers of carbon atoms in the range 14 to 18. However, about 22% of the lipid consists of fatty acids in the C4 to C10 range (Yousef and Ashton, 1967). The major constituent of milk protein is casein in a number of variant forms, all of which are characterized by a high content of proline and are present in complexes with calcium and phosphate. In addition, milk protein contains β-lactoglobulin and α-lactalbumin and traces of immunoglobulins. Colostrum, secreted in the first day or two of lactation, contains high concentrations of lipid and protein – in particular, immunoglobulins. These are absorbed directly through the gut of the young lamb and are crucial to its survival, giving it passive immunity to diseases to which the ewe has immunity. They also provide protection against gut infections.

The mean metabolizability of the gross energy (GE) in ewe's milk is 0.94 and the efficiency of use of the resultant metabolizable energy (ME) is 0.85 for the maintenance of the lamb and 0.7 for growth (ARC, 1980). If the GE of the milk were 4.5 MJ kg^{-1}, then a daily intake of 1 kg in excess of the lamb's maintenance requirement would sustain a daily growth rate of between 330 g and 270 g as the energy value of the live weight gain increased, with the lamb's growth, from 9 MJ kg^{-1} to 11 MJ kg^{-1}.

The Mammary Gland

Milk is secreted from alveoli laid down in the fat pad of the udder in the period between mid-pregnancy and just after parturition, under the control of a large number of hormones. These include oestrogen, progesterone, adrenal corticoids, somatotrophin, prolactin, placental lactogen, insulin and thyroid hormones, and, in addition, there are numerous growth factors produced by the fat pad itself. Each alveolus is spherical, with a central lumen that is lined with a single layer of secretory cells. The bases of these cells are covered by a layer of myoepithelial cells and a basement membrane. A capillary network supplies each alveolus with the milk precursors. The alveoli discharge into fine ducts leading to larger ducts and the gland cistern. Full milk secretion starts when progesterone secretion falls at parturition. The milk is ejected from the alveoli when the myoepithelial cells contract in response to the release into the bloodstream of oxytocin from the posterior pituitary gland. At weaning, the secretory tissue undergoes involution through cell death, leaving only the myoepithelial layer.

Synthesis of Milk

The main pathway for the synthesis of the fatty acids in milk fat is through the condensation of 2-carbon units (molecules of malonyl-coenzyme A (CoA)) originating from the microbial breakdown of carbohydrate to acetate in the rumen. Fatty acids are also derived directly from the diet or from the breakdown of adipose tissue. The esters of the fatty acids are incorporated into triglycerides, the glycerol being derived either from the hydrolysis of plasma lipids or by glycolysis. The milk fat is released from the epithelial cells as globules, each enclosed in a membrane.

Lactose, a carbohydrate found only in milk, is synthesized from glucose, via galactose. The secondary stage, the combination of glucose and galactose to form the disaccharide, is facilitated by the milk protein α-lactalbumin. β-Lactoglobulin, α-lactalbumin and the milk caseins are synthesized from circulating amino acids, whereas the immunoglobulins are transferred directly into the epithelial cells from the bloodstream. Milk protein and lactose move together through the secretory cells in micelles and the osmotic pressure exerted by lactose draws water into the secretion, which, at the surface of the cell, is discharged into the duct, together with the mineral components of the milk. For greater detail on the synthesis of milk in the ewe, refer to Thomas and Rook (1983).

Estimation of Milk Production

Accurate estimates of milk production (by the ewe) or intake (by the lamb) are difficult, as all methods interfere to some extent with the natural behaviour of ewes and lambs. Three methods have been used to measure yield directly: weighing before and after suckling; measuring milk secretion rate; or tracer-based techniques. In addition, milk production in early lactation can be estimated indirectly, with reasonable accuracy, from the growth rate of lambs. Although the gross efficiency of conversion of milk to liveweight gain increases as intake increases above maintenance, the curvilinearity is not great over the first few weeks and a linear relationship can be assumed. Published relationships of this kind (e.g. Dove and Freer, 1979; Dove, 1988) indicate that lambs consuming only milk gain 160–170 g day^{-1} per kg of liquid milk, which is equivalent to about 6.0 kg of milk kg^{-1} of gain or about 1 kg gain kg^{-1} milk dry matter (DM) consumed. Beyond 4–6 weeks of age in most management systems, the slope of relationships between liveweight gain and milk intake declines markedly, indicating the intake of nutrients from herbage.

Estimating milk intake by weighing before and after suckling

This method is very laborious, as the lambs are weighed before and after suckling on four to six occasions in 24 h (e.g. Wallace, 1948) or, less commonly, on three occasions in 12 h. Between sucklings, the lambs are separated from their mothers or the udder is covered. The daily yield is the total of the weight increments of the ewe's offspring during suckling. Errors can arise from disturbance affecting suckling behaviour or milk ejection, the incomplete emptying of the udder by single lambs, the difficulty of measuring small weight increments as the lambs get larger and defecation or urination between the first and second weighings.

Estimating milk production rate using oxytocin

Milk production can be estimated by milking the ewe until the udder is empty, after an intravenous injection of approximately 2 iu of oxytocin to achieve ejection of the milk. This procedure is done at the beginning and end of a period of approximately 4 h, during which the lambs are prevented from sucking. Production rate is calculated as the weight of milk at the second milking divided by the exact time in minutes between the two milkings and then extrapolated to a daily milk production (e.g. Doney *et al.*, 1979). This method can lead to overestimates of milk intake if the degree of emptying of the udder by milking is greater than would be achieved by the lambs. Doney *et al.* (1979) found that this method gave higher estimates of yield than the lamb-weighing method in the first week of lactation, especially in ewes with single lambs, but, by the third week of lactation, the differences between the two methods were not significant and were unaffected by the number of lambs suckled or by ewe genotype.

Tracer-based methods

The third approach to measuring milk intake is to estimate the dilution, by a component of the milk consumed by the lamb, of a marker or tracer introduced into a known body pool. Most commonly, the body-water pool is labelled by the administration to the lamb of either tritiated water (TOH) (Dove and Freer, 1979) or deuterium oxide (D_2O) (Dove, 1988). The turnover of the tracer is monitored in water extracted from blood samples taken 4–7 days apart, during which period the animals are left undisturbed. The procedure is based on two assumptions: that milk is the only source of water for the lamb and that the amount of water in the lamb does not change over the period of measurement. Before peak lactation in the ewe, lambs consume negligible amounts of drinking water and solid food and single markers have been used successfully to estimate milk intake (e.g. Dove and Freer, 1979). The second assumption is clearly not met, because weight gain in the lamb contains at least 65% water and estimates of milk intake have to be corrected for the increase in body-water content (Dove and Freer, 1979).

In older lambs, the overestimation of milk intake resulting from the ingestion of drinking water or solid food, especially herbage, is overcome by using a 'double-isotope' procedure, in which D_2O is injected into the lamb to estimate its total water turnover, while the proportion of this coming from milk is estimated by injecting the ewe with TOH and monitoring the transfer of TOH to the offspring (Dove, 1988).

The major disadvantages of the tracer-based methods are the possible environmental and regulatory consequences of administering radioisotopes (TOH) to animals and the difficulty and cost of D_2O analysis. Nevertheless, these methods are the most accurate for estimating milk intake and have a further advantage in nutritional studies in that changes in the protein and fat content of both ewe and lamb can be estimated from their body-water contents.

Factors Affecting Milk Production

Effect of genotype of ewe

Variation in milk yield between and within breeds is very wide. In meat breeds selected for lamb production, yield at the peak of lactation varies between 2.0 and 4.0 kg day^{-1}, with total yields in 3 months of lactation varying from 150 to 200 kg in ewes with twin lambs and from 90 to 160 kg in ewes with singles. In small local breeds and some wool breeds, notably Merinos, yields are lower. Differences between dairy breeds are larger. Unselected local breeds may produce less than 100 kg during 6 months of milking, after rearing a lamb for about 1 month, while highly selected breeds, such as the East Friesland and Assaf, which are milked throughout a longer lactation, have yields of 600–1000 kg. Between these extremes are a number of European dairy breeds, including Lacaune, Manchega, Churra, Latxa, Manech and Sarde, which now have significant numbers of ewes in selection schemes and have yields, after rearing a lamb for a month, of 150–250 kg in approximately 200 days of milking.

Nutrition in pregnancy

Almost all the development of secretory tissue in the ewe's udder occurs in the last third of pregnancy, with a very small amount – approximately 5% – occurring in the first month of lactation. Severe undernutrition in the last weeks of pregnancy results in a small udder, which has little colostrum present at lambing, and a delay of several hours in the initiation of full lactation. This may have a major effect on lamb survival, especially as the lambs are likely to be small and lacking body reserves at birth. Experiments in which underfeeding was severe (reduction of 17–32% in twin birth weight) found reductions of 7–35% in milk yield over the whole lactation (Wallace, 1948; Treacher, 1970).

Nutrition earlier in pregnancy (see Robinson *et al.*, Chapter 9, this volume), before the period of mammary development, may affect milk production via placental size and secretion of placental lactogen. Growth of the placenta, which is completed by 90 days of pregnancy, can be affected by severe underfeeding. If nutrition in late pregnancy is good, this does not lead to a reduction in lamb birth weight, but Davis *et al.* (1980) and Dove *et al.* (1988) found effects of mid-pregnancy feeding on milk yield and lamb growth, even when birth weight was not reduced. This may be related to nutritional effects on placental size and hence placental lactogen concentrations. In sheep, plasma lactogen concentrations increase until close to the end of pregnancy and are affected by placenta size and by the number of fetuses carried.

If there is underfeeding in early lactation, milk production may be affected by the amount of body reserves available for utilization after lambing. Although undernutrition in pregnancy increases the utilization of body reserves before lambing, the level of reserves is also affected by deposition and utilization of fat occurring before mating and in early and mid-pregnancy. The effects of body reserves at lambing on feed intake and on the level and efficiency of milk production are discussed below.

Effect of number of lambs suckled

Ewes suckling twins generally produce 40% more milk than ewes with singles at the same level of nutrition (Treacher, 1983). Differences reported in the literature range from negligible to increases of 70%, with the majority in the range of 30–50%. In ewes with twins, the peak of lactation is not only higher but is reached sooner – in the second or third week of lactation, compared with the third to fifth week in ewes with singles (Wallace, 1948). Yield decreases slightly more rapidly in ewes with twins and, by week 12 of lactation, the difference in yield between ewes with twins and singles is negligible (Fig. 10.1).

The small amount of information on yields from ewes suckling larger litters of three or four lambs shows wide differences, which may, in part, reflect the small numbers of ewes studied. Differences between ewes suckling triplets and those suckling twins range from negligible (Wallace, 1948) to increases of 30% (Loerch *et al.*,1985). This occurs almost entirely in the first month of lactation, with little difference, or even slightly lower yields, in mid- and late lactation (Peart *et al.*, 1975), possibly related to problems with sore teats and lamb rejection (Gallo and Davies, 1988).

Increases in milk production in ewes suckling twins or larger litters result mainly from the number of lambs suckled. This reflects the increased stimulus resulting from the increased frequency and duration of suckling by two or more lambs. It is not affected by the number of fetuses carried in pregnancy. For example, Loerch *et al.* (1985) found that ewes suckling triplets produced 28% more milk than ewes allowed to suckle only two lambs after carrying triplets in pregnancy. The potential milk yield of ewes suckling singles is not expressed and their production

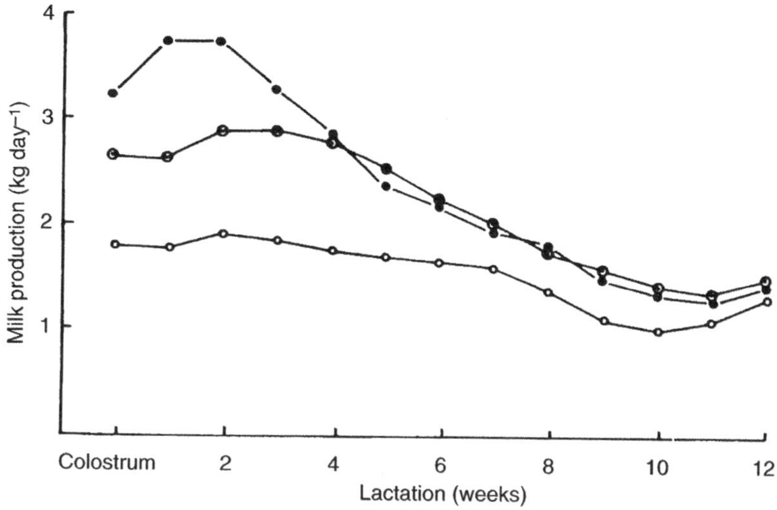

Fig. 10.1. Mean lactation curves of ewes: ●, triplet-suckled; ⊖, twin-suckled; ○, single-suckled (reproduced from Peart *et al.*, 1975, by courtesy of the editor and publishers, *Journal of Agricultural Science, Cambridge*).

reflects the voluntary intake of milk by the lamb. This is supported by differences in yields in ewes suckling lambs of different genotypes, as a result of mating with different breeds of ram or of cross-fostering of lambs at birth between ewes of different breeds. This response may be mediated through initial differences in lamb birth weight (e.g. Moore, 1966), but, in other cases (e.g. Peart *et al.*, 1975), the increase appears to result from differences in appetite between lamb genotypes. Although Slen *et al.* (1963) suggested that the yield of ewes suckling twins reflected their potential, increases in yield in ewes suckling triplets show that the potential may be slightly greater.

All the information discussed above relates to management systems where lambs have continuous access to ewes, except when this is altered during measurements of milk yield. In dairy systems, management during the suckling period, before milking is started at about 1 month after lambing, may be different, with lambs separated from the ewes for some part of the day. Gargouri *et al.* (1993) found a reduction of 20% in yield in the first month of lactation when suckling was restricted to two periods of 15 min compared with unrestricted access (see Fig. 10.2). The restricted suckling regime also reduced fat content and increased crude protein content of the milk.

Effect of milking

In dairy systems, the start of milking at the end of approximately 1 month of suckling results in a dramatic reduction in milk yield, which persists for the remainder of the lactation (Labussière and Pétrequin, 1969). Figure 10.2 shows reductions of 55% and 29% between the fourth week of suckling and the first week of milking in ewes with previously unrestricted and restricted access of lambs, respectively. In the period of machine milking, yields in both groups were almost identical.

Pattern and Level of Intake in Lactating Ewes

Voluntary intake of feed by ewes normally increases rapidly at the start of lactation and then continues to rise for several weeks. Foot and Russel (1979) measured intakes of a high-quality chopped, dried grass (DM digestibility (DMD) 70%) over the full cycle of pregnancy, lactation and dry periods. Intake in the first week of lactation was 10% higher than the intake 2 weeks before lambing. Intake increased rapidly in weeks 2 and 3 of lactation and then continued to rise at a slower rate to a maximum in week 8, approximately 4 weeks after the peak of lactation. In ewes suckling twins and singles, maximum daily intakes were 3.0 and 2.5 kg DM, respectively (44 and 37 g DM kg^{-1} of weight post-lambing, respectively), 85% and 47% above their intakes in week 1 of lactation. Thereafter intake decreased slowly until weaning, after which it declined by 20%.

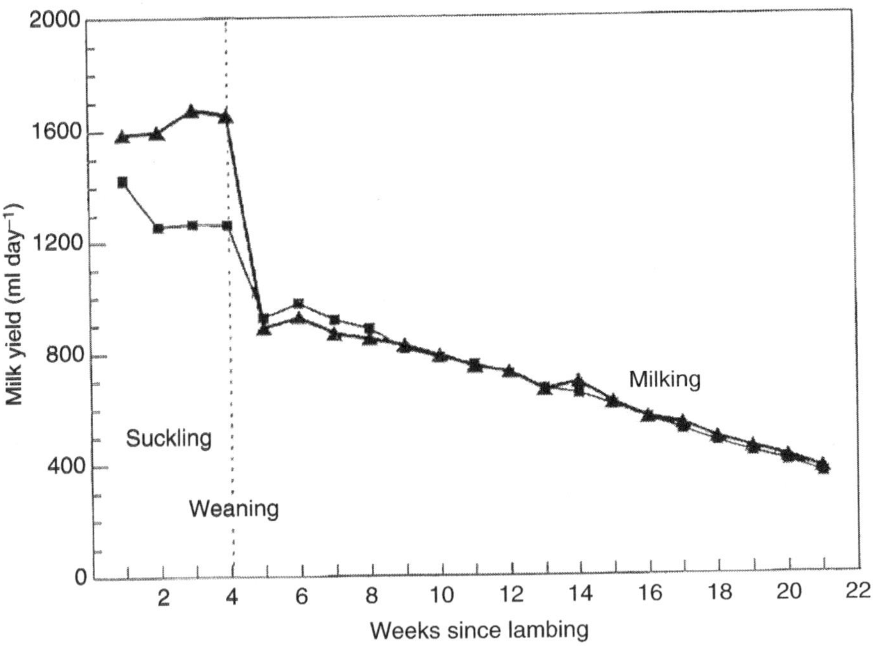

Fig. 10.2. Effects of extent of access by lambs to the ewe: ▲, unrestricted access; ■, access restricted to two 15 min periods per day, on the milk yield of Manchega ewes during suckling and subsequent machine milking (adapted from Gargouri *et al.*, 1993).

These large increases in intake in early lactation, as a result of the great increase in metabolic demand for milk production, are accompanied by major effects on the digestive system. The weight, size, nitrogen content and enzyme activity of reticulorumen, abomasum and small intestine increase. The small intestines reach a maximum weight 30 days after lambing and the rumen and abomasum later, at about 50 days. These changes enable the lactating ewe to maintain the same diet digestiblity in spite of large increases in intake. If food intake is restricted in early lactation, these changes to the digestive tract are reduced.

While the pattern of intake described above is typical of ewes offered high-quality long forage, it is clear that on other diets and at pasture different patterns and levels of intake may occur. On a low-quality forage, intake rises slowly and may not peak before weaning occurs 3 or 4 months after lambing (Hadjipieris and Holmes, 1966). At pasture, grazing pressure, availability of herbage and changes in pasture digestibility and sward structure, which are often rapid, all affect the level and pattern of intake. Generally, peak intakes by lactating ewes at pasture in spring occur within 4 weeks of lambing, unless herbage availability is very restricted by either poor pasture growth or high grazing pressures. Gibb *et al.* (1981), for example, found that a peak daily intake of 3.75 kg organic matter (OM) (44 g OM kg^{-1} live-weight (LW) post-lambing) occurred in week 3 of lactation in ewes suckling twins and grazed at a daily herbage allowance of 60 g DM kg^{-1} LW of ewe, while at an allowance of 30 g DM kg^{-1} LW a lower peak intake of 2.30 kg OM (27g OM kg^{-1} LW) was delayed to week 5 (see Plate 10.1).

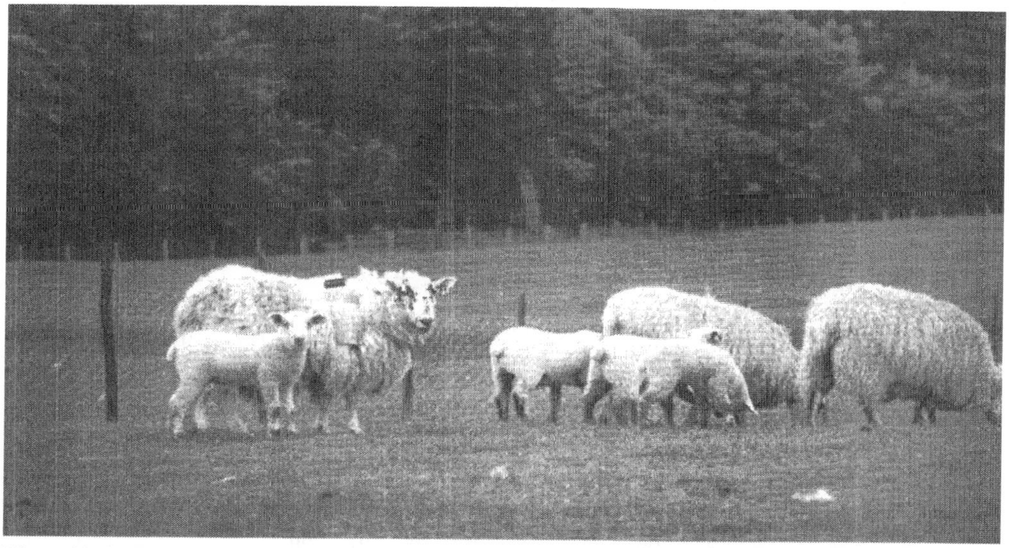

Plate 10.1. Border Leicester × Scottish Blackface ewes and their lambs grazing perennial ryegrass pastures in Lanarkshire, central Scotland. The ewe on the left is carrying equipment that allows the estimation of the intake and nutritive value of the pasture in relation to the nutrient requirements for lactation.

Penning *et al.* (1991) and Morris *et al.* (1994) found that lactating ewes grazing swards with surface height in the optimum range (4.5–12 cm) for maintaining near-maximal intakes reached peak intakes of 2.6–3.0 kg OM (38–46 g kg^{-1} LW) in week 4 of lactation, approximately 20% higher than the intake in the first week of lactation. On shorter swards, the patterns of intake varied from a peak at 8 weeks to an almost constant intake over this period.

Body condition at lambing does not have a major effect on absolute intake by lactating ewes. Peart (1970), Foot and Russel (1979) and Gibb and Treacher (1980) found that non-significant differences in intake occurred in ewes differing in live weight at lambing by 10–15 kg or by 1.0–2.0 units of body-condition score (on a scale of 1–5).

Requirements in Lactation

Responses to intake of energy and protein

The model described by Robinson (1980) provides a useful starting-point for considering responses in milk production by the ewe to intake of energy and protein and hence nutrient requirements of the ewe during early lactation. Figure 10.3 demonstrates three important principles relating to the response to variation in intake of ME and metabolizable protein (MP):

1. For a particular level of ME intake there is a critical protein intake, below which milk yield will decrease.
2. The minimum ratio of crude protein (CP) to ME increases with increasing level of milk yield.

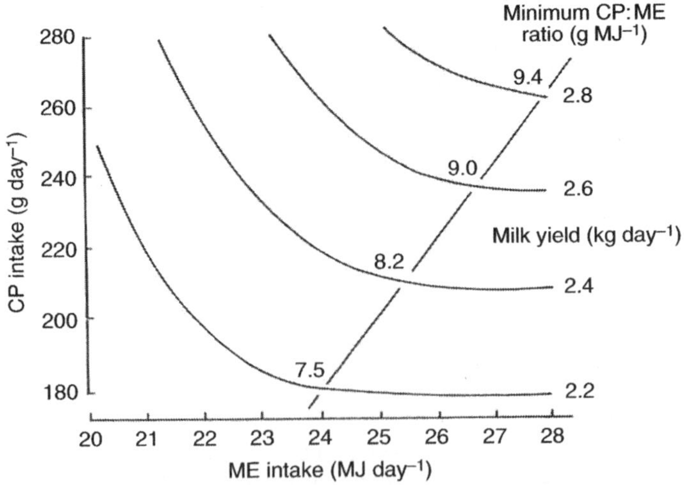

Fig. 10.3. Response in milk yield to alterations in dietary CP and ME for 70 kg ewes suckling twin lambs (reproduced with permission from Treacher, 1983).

3. An increase in MP intake without a change in ME intake will result in an increase in milk production and mobilization of body reserves, if the ewe has not reached her potential yield.

This model demonstrates that, in early lactation, when energy requirements are high and voluntary intake has not reached its peak, protein intake is likely to have a critical effect on milk production. The extent of the response to protein intake, however, depends on the level of body reserves in the ewe in early lactation. This is discussed further below.

Although this model was derived from data from a single experiment, there are many experiments that confirm its principles. Figure 10.4 from Robinson (1990) shows responses of milk yield in a series of experiments in which increasing amounts of soybean meal and fish meal were added to low-protein basal diets while maintaining a constant intake of energy. At each energy level, the addition of protein to the basal diet increased milk production. At an ME intake of 18.3 MJ day^{-1}, the maximum response occurred with an intake of CP of 300 g day^{-1} and was not increased by a greater intake of protein. At intakes of 22.5, 25.0 and 28.3 MJ ME day^{-1}, the maximum response occurred at protein intakes of 350, 450 and 450 g CP day^{-1}, respectively.

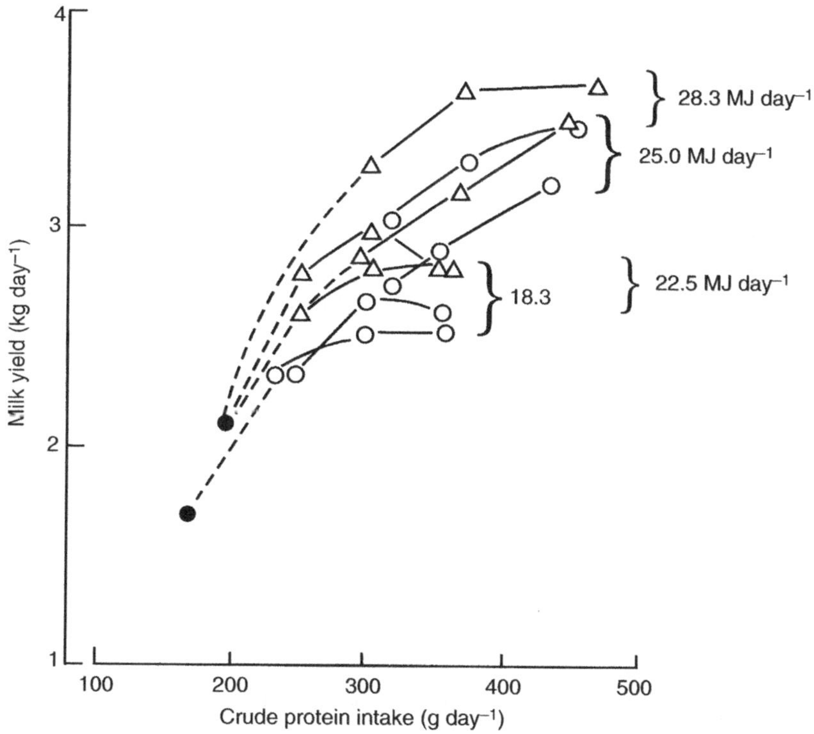

Fig. 10.4. The effect of metabolizable energy intake (18.3, 22.5, 25.0 and 28.3 MJ day^{-1}) and protein sources on the milk yield of Finn Dorset ewes in early lactation: ●, basal diet of hay and barley; ○, basal diet with different proportions of barley replaced by soybean meal; △, basal diet with different proportions of barley replaced by fish meal. (Adapted from Robinson, 1990.)

Requirements for lactating ewes

The Agricultural and Food Research Council (AFRC, 1993) system uses the following procedures for calculating the ME and MP requirements for lactating ewes. Systems in other countries (e.g. SCA, 1990) generally follow a similar process.

Metabolizable energy

The requirement for adult ewes, ME_{mp} (MJ) is derived from Equation (2), which sums the requirements for maintenance of a ewe of weight W kg, producing Y kg day^{-1} of milk with a GE content of V MJ kg^{-1} and changing in weight by G kg day^{-1}. For each fraction, the net energy (NE) requirement, E, is divided by the efficiency, k, with which ME is used; each of the appropriate k values is a function of the quality of the diet, calculated either as q_m (NE/GE) or M/D (ME kg^{-1} DM). The total is adjusted, C, for the level of feeding (for an alternative approach to this adjustment, as used in the Australian system (SCA, 1990), see Corbett and Ball, Chapter 7, this volume). In the examples shown in Table 10.1, a 5% safety margin has been included.

$$ME_{mp} = C(E_m/k_m + E_l/k_l + E_g/k_g) \quad (2)$$

where:

$$C = 1 + 0.018((ME_{mp}/ME_m) - 1)$$
$$E_m = 0.23(W/1.08)^{0.75} + E_a$$
$$k_m = 0.35q_m + 0.503$$
$$E_l = VY$$
$$k_l = 0.35q_m + 0.420$$
$$E_g = \begin{cases} (26.0G/1.09) & \text{for weight gain} \\ -(26.0G/1.09)0.84 & \text{for weight loss} \end{cases}$$
$$k_g = 0.95k_l$$

Table 10.1. Daily requirements based on AFRC (1993) for metabolizable energy (MJ ME) and metabolizable protein (g MP) for housed[a] lactating ewes, weighing 70 kg, producing 5 g clean wool per day, yielding 1, 2 or 3 kg of milk per day and either maintaining weight or losing 100 g per day when fed a diet with an energy concentration of 11.5 MJ ME kg^{-1} DM (q_m = 0.61).

	Milk yield (kg per day)					
Weight change	1		2		3	
(g per day)	ME	MP	ME	MP	ME	MP
0	16.6	152	24.6	228	33.0	303
–100	13.0	140	21.1	215	29.5	291

[a]For ewes on lowland and on hill pasture, ME requirements are increased by 0.35 and 1.30 MJ day^{-1}, respectively.

In Equation (2), the activity allowance, E_a, depends on the distance walked and the steepness of the terrain and may range from $0.0096W$ MJ for housed ewes to $0.024W$ MJ for ewes grazing hills. The energy content of milk may be adjusted to suit a specific analysis.

Metabolizable protein

In a similar way, the requirement for MP (Table 10.1) is calculated as the sum of the requirements for maintenance (MP_m), wool growth (MP_w), lactation (MP_l) and weight change (MP_g). The efficiency of utilization of absorbed amino acids for these four purposes is 1.0, 0.26, 0.68 and 1.0, respectively, so the total requirement for a ewe of weight W kg, producing F g wool and Y kg milk (containing 48.9 g true protein kg^{-1}) and retaining P kg protein as body tissue is as shown in Equation (3).

$$MP = 2.1875W^{0.75} + F/0.26 + 48.9Y/0.68 + P \quad (3)$$

The ewe's requirement for MP is met from the digestible fractions of the microbial CP synthesized in the rumen in proportion to ME intake and the dietary CP that escapes degradation in the rumen (see Annison *et al.*, Chapter 5, this volume). Calculations of MP supply, using the AFRC (1993) system are shown in Table 10.2 for one of the feeding situations set out in Table 10.1. It should be noted that, although microbial protein provides by far the largest part of the MP requirements, the effective rumen degradability of dietary protein (ERDP) may be critical in determining whether the MP needs of the lactating ewe are met by a particular diet.

Table 10.2. The supply of metabolizable protein (AFRC, 1993) from a diet with an energy concentration of 11.5 MJ ME kg^{-1} DM and a crude protein content of 200 g kg^{-1}, at two levels of protein degradability in the rumen, when used to maintain the weight of a 70 kg housed lactating ewe that is producing 5 g wool and 2 kg milk day^{-1} and is estimated to require 228 g MP day^{-1} (see Table 10.1).

Intake of dry matter (DMI) (kg)		2.14	
Intake of ME (MJ)		24.6	
Intake of crude protein (CPI) (g)	200 × DMI	428	
Fermentable ME (FME)[a] (MJ)	10.8 × DMI	23.1	
Microbial crude protein (MCP) (g)	11 × FME	254	
Effective rumen degradability of protein (ERDP)[b]		0.75	0.85
Undegraded dietary protein (UDP) (g)	CPI(1-ERDP)	107	64
Digested undegraded protein (DUP)[c] (g)	0.7 × UDP	75	45
Metabolizable protein (g)	0.6375 × MCP + DUP	237	207

[a]FME = ME intake (MEI) – (ME in fat and silage acids; here assumed to total 0.7 MJ kg^{-1} DM).
[b]ERDP is a measure, expressed as a decimal proportion, of rumen degradability weighted for the speed of degradation and adjusted for rumen outflow rate (AFRC, 1993).
[c]Digestibility of the undegraded protein is predicted from the content of acid-detergent insoluble protein and is here assumed to be 70%.

Efficiency of use of body reserves for milk production

Energy requirements in early lactation are high and, because of the slow increase in voluntary intake following parturition (see above), are unlikely to be met from the ewe's diet. As a result, ewes generally utilize body reserves in the first weeks of lactation, even when offered feed *ad libitum* (Cowan *et al.*, 1980) or when grazing at high herbage allowances (e.g. Gibb and Treacher, 1980). Although energy allowances for ewes in early lactation include adjustments for the energy derived from mobilization of fat reserves, they are calculated, as discussed above, assuming constant values for both the energy content of liveweight loss and the efficiency of its use for milk production. Both these assumptions are simplifications, as both the energy value of weight change and the efficiency of its use for milk production vary.

Cowan *et al.* (1980, 1981) and Geenty and Sykes (1986) found that the apparent energy content of weight change in the first 6 weeks of lactation varied widely, from 24 to 90 and from 43 to 100 MJ kg^{-1} of liveweight loss, in pen-fed and grazing ewes, respectively. These large differences in the energy values of weight change arise from the effect of two processes: an increase in body water, as fat is mobilized, and an increase in the weight of digesta and of the alimentary tract, which accompanies the increase in voluntary intake in early lactation. Both these processes lead to an underestimation of the energy content of live weight lost in early lactation.

Estimates of the efficiency of use of energy derived from body reserves for milk production vary widely but decline as the rate of loss of reserves from the body increases (Robinson, 1987). The reserves utilized in early lactation are mainly fat, as the labile reserve of protein in the body is small. Cowan *et al.* (1979) found that a loss of fat of 6.9 kg between days 12 and 41 of lactation was accompanied by a non-significant reduction in protein of only 0.4 kg, approximately 14 g day^{-1}. Energy from the fat was sufficient to produce approximately 50 kg of milk, while the body protein contributed protein for synthesis of approximately 6 kg of milk. Bocquier *et al.* (1987) suggested that the maximum rate of mobilization of protein from body reserves is 25 g day^{-1} in lactating ewes. Geenty and Sykes (1986) comment that, although the mobilization of protein in early lactation is small, it may have an important metabolic effect in ewes that are well fed in late pregnancy. In their study, there was a positive relationship between efficiency of milk production and body protein, which contributed between 2 and 10% of the total energy mobilized in the first 6 weeks of lactation.

The extent of losses of reserves in early lactation is affected not only by nutrient intake, but also by the level of body reserves. Thin ewes with poor reserves mobilize less energy and produce less milk than fatter ewes subjected to the same level of undernutrition. Figure 10.5, from Robinson (1990), shows the response of yield in 70 kg ewes with 5, 10, 15 or 20 kg of body fat, equivalent to body-condition scores in the range 1.0–3.5, to intakes of 20, 25 and 30 MJ ME day^{-1}. The highest intake supplied the energy requirements with all ewes producing 3.5 kg milk day^{-1} and almost main-

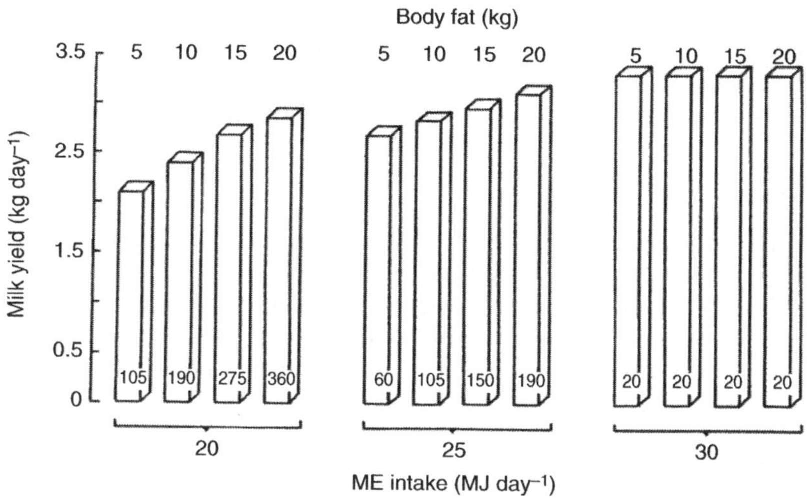

Fig. 10.5. The effect on milk production in twin-suckling ewes of 70 kg body weight of metabolizable energy (ME) intake (20, 25 or 30 MJ day^{-1}) and body fatness (5, 10, 15 or 20 kg of body fat equal to body-condition scores ranging from 1 to 3.5). The values in each histogram are the rates of fat loss (g day^{-1}) from the body. (Reproduced with permission from Robinson, 1990.)

taining weight (20 g day^{-1} loss). At lower intakes, yield was reduced to a greater extent in the ewes with lower reserves, as ewes with larger reserves mobilized more fat and produced more milk, although they were unable to compensate in full for the reduction in energy intake. Ewes with 20 kg of fat reserves and daily intakes of 20 and 25 MJ ME produced 2.9 and 3.0 kg of milk day^{-1} and lost 360 and 190 g LW, respectively. At the same intakes, the thinnest ewes, with 5 kg of fat, produced 2.1 and 2.8 kg of milk and lost 105 and 60 g LW, respectively. This model demonstrates that intakes below requirements inevitably lead to some reduction in milk yield. In the case of ewes in good body condition, however, the reduction is small.

Protein requirements and periparturient rise in faecal egg counts

Recent work in New Zealand suggests that protein requirements derived by the factorial method outlined above may underestimate the requirements for lactating ewes exposed to nematode parasite infection. This is because the immune system has a relatively low priority for nutrients, compared with other physiological requirements, and may need additional protein. The periparturient rise in worm burdens and faecal egg counts is attributed to a temporary relaxation of the immune response of the ewe to nematode parasites (see Coop and Sykes, Chapter 14, this volume). Donaldson *et al.* (2001) showed that, in lactating ewes fed just below their full requirements for ME, worm burdens were inversely related to protein intake in the range 85–145% of AFRC (1993) requirements for MP. The reduction in the parasite burden was caused by an increase in the ability of the ewes to reject ingested larvae. The authors suggest that a daily intake of MP of approximately 350 g, 20% above the AFRC (1993) requirement, is necessary to maintain maximum immunity against nematode parasites in ewes with milk yields of more than 3.0 kg day^{-1} rearing rapidly growing twins.

Effects of poor nutrition in early lactation

Restricted nutrition for periods of 7–14 days in early lactation has little lasting effect on milk yield, which returns to a normal level within a few days of feeding being increased. If, however, low-plane feeding is continued for 28 days, there is either no response to an increase in feeding (Peart, 1970) or only a slow return to a normal level of yield over a period of 2 weeks.

Mineral nutrition

The most important mineral disorders in lactating ewes are hypomagnesaemia and, to a lesser extent, hypocalcaemia.

Hypomagnesaemia

The incidence of hypomagnesaemia (grass tetany or staggers) is generally low in sheep, but can be a problem in individual flocks at pasture at the peak of lactation, in the first 4–6 weeks after lambing. It is more common in older ewes rearing twin lambs, particularly if the ewes are underfed, as is the case with grass tetany in beef cattle. It is most likely to occur in spring on heavily fertilized, improved pastures, especially where fertilizers containing high levels of potassium have been applied in early spring. High levels of potassium in herbage reduce the absorption and utilization of magnesium by the animal.

Onset of hypomagnesaemia is generally very rapid and will result in death unless treated. An outbreak usually starts with the death of a ewe that appeared normal a few hours earlier. Before tetany occurs, ewes appear nervous or excited, with trembling, particularly in the facial muscles. These symptoms may be induced by transportation, exercise, rapid diet change or the presence of strange dogs or people.

Underwood and Suttle (1999) suggest that a mean serum magnesium concentration below 0.60 mmol l^{-1} indicates that a flock will probably respond to supplementation with magnesium. Response to supplementation may possibly occur at serum levels in the range 0.60–0.75 mmol l^{-1}. The disorder can be diagnosed in dead animals by analysing the vitreous humour of the eye, where values below 0.75 mmol l^{-1} indicate hypomagnesaemia. Dietary requirements for magnesium specified by Underwood and Suttle (1999) for lactating ewes are given in Table 10.3.

Ewes in the early stages of hypomagnesaemia can be treated by intravenous injection with magnesium hypophosphite. This is always given with calcium, as 50 ml of a 250 g l^{-1} solution of calcium borogluconate contain-

Table 10.3. Dietary requirements for magnesium for lactating ewes weighing 75 kg (Underwood and Suttle, 1999).

Milk yield (kg day^{-1})	Dry-matter intake[a] (kg day^{-1})	Dietary requirement (g kg^{-1} DM)	
		At pasture	Indoors
1	1.5	1.4	0.70
2	2.2	1.3	0.65
3	2.9	1.3	0.65

[a]Energy concentration of diet (q) = 0.6.

ing 25 g of magnesium hypophosphite. Although ewes often show a rapid response to injection and may resume grazing within minutes, relapses are frequent. In intensive systems, treated ewes may be moved indoors and fed hay and concentrates. No additional magnesium is required in the diets of housed ewes but supplementation may be needed for lactating ewes at pasture in early spring. This is normally given as calcined magnesite in concentrates or in free-access mineral blocks or feed blocks. Individual intakes of blocks, however, vary widely (see Dove, Chapter 6, this volume) and a significant proportion of ewes may be inadequately supplemented (Underwood and Suttle, 1999).

Hypocalcaemia

Hypocalcaemia is not common in lactating ewes. It is more likely to occur in late pregnancy, when the highest requirements for calcium are found in twin-bearing ewes. In pregnancy, hypocalcaemia may be associated with pregnancy toxaemia resulting from low feed intake or a sudden change in feed. Hypocalcaemia itself generally results from the poor mobilization of Ca from bone, rather than from low Ca intake. Excess phosphorus in the diet, relative to its Ca content, reduces bone resorption and is a predisposing factor. The Ca : P ratio of the diet should, if possible, be maintained in the range 1.4 : 1.0 to 1.0 : 1.0. Inadequate protein intake in early lactation also affects Ca metabolism. Chrisp *et al.* (1989) found that a dietary protein supplement increased milk yield, with the resulting increase in Ca demand being met by increased absorption from the alimentary tract, rather than from increased bone resorption.

The symptoms of hypocalcaemia are uncoordinated movement, tremors and rapid breathing. The animal falls, rapidly becomes paralysed, with the head and legs extended, and finally goes into a coma. Death is not generally as rapid as in hypomagnesaemia and the ewe may survive for 4–48 h.

The Ca requirements in Table 10.4 were derived using a coefficient of absorption of 0.68 (AFRC, 1991). As skeletal mobilization occurs and dietary requirements do not have to be met each day, Underwood and Suttle (1999) suggest that a diet with an average concentration of 3 g Ca kg^{-1} DM throughout the year is unlikely to reduce performance.

Table 10.4. Dietary requirements for calcium for lactating ewes weighing 75 kg (AFRC, 1991).

Physiological state	Diet quality	Dry-matter intake (kg day^{-1})	Weight change	Dietary requirement (g kg^{-1} DM)
End of pregnancy	L	2.4		3.2
	H	1.6		4.3
Lactation	L	2.8–3.7	M	2.8
	L	2.3–3.2	N	3.1
	H	1.8–2.4	M	3.8
	H	1.5–2.1	N	4.3

L, poorly digestible diet ($q = 0.5$); H, highly digestible diet ($q = 0.7$); M, maintenance; N, weight loss of 0.1 kg day^{-1}.

In the early stages of hypocalcaemia, treatment by intravenous injection of calcium borogluconate is generally effective and ewes will stand and eat within about an hour of treatment. Calcium intake in late pregnancy should be restricted to a level close to requirement, as high intake of Ca reduces the ability of the ewe to maintain Ca levels in the blood by mobilizing bone Ca in early lactation.

Nutritional Management for Lactation

Management at pasture

Management in lactation is critical. Within the constraints of other management operations, lambing is usually timed to coincide with the start of herbage growth, so that the peak of herbage production coincides, as far as possible, with the period of greatest feed requirements of the flock.

In many northern-hemisphere temperate pasture areas, spring lambing is constrained quite narrowly by winter cold. In intensively grazed systems, operations aimed at achieving particular sward heights have been shown to form a sound basis for management, in concert with supplementation, N fertilization and herbage conservation (Treacher, 1990). The use of decision rules based on sward height results from studies on grazed swards showing that, although gross herbage production is lower on short swards, greater amounts of leaf are harvested and less dies. Key guidelines relate to the use of supplementation in early spring, until the sward maintains a target height of 3–4 cm. Thereafter, until the flowering season ends, in about mid-June, grazing pressure may be increased by closing areas for conservation in order to maintain sward height at below 6 cm, and nearer to 4 cm on mixed-grass swards. This prevents deterioration in sward structure and a decline in herbage digestibility.

In many southern-hemisphere temperate pasture areas, winters are milder but pastures senesce in late spring and there is often a pressing need to minimize supplementary feeding. In such areas, lambing in winter rather than spring may be more appropriate. This allows sufficient time for lambs to be marketed or to reach a survival weight before the end of the pasture season, although it may reduce early growth rates in the lambs. Management based on sward height is less common in these systems and management is concerned, rather, with selecting a year-round stocking rate that strikes the best balance between individual ewe nutrition, especially at lambing, and profit per hectare of pasture.

Diet composition

Concentrate : forage ratio

A low proportion of long forage in the diet of lactating ewes results in a reduction in the fat content of the milk, as it does in dairy cows. Goodchild *et al.* (1999) found that, from day 60 to 120 of lactation, when milk yields were low (*c.* 420 g day^{-1}), feeding a diet with a concentrate to straw ratio of 92 : 8 and an acid-detergent fibre (ADF) content of 170 g kg^{-1} DM, compared with a diet with a ratio of 47 : 53 and 385 g ADF kg^{-1} DM, decreased the fat content (73 vs. 65 g kg^{-1}) but did not affect the milk yield. This problem of low fat is common in some intensive dairy systems in Mediterranean countries, where forages are expensive and it is economic to feed high levels of concentrates. It can be overcome, at least partially, by feeding buffers in high-concentrate diets to correct the rumen pH.

Protected fat

In experiments with dairy ewes, the inclusion in the diet of calcium soaps of long-chain fatty acids (CSFA), which are protected from hydrolysis in the rumen, did not affect milk yield or weight change of the ewes (e.g. Casals *et al.*, 1999). Fat content, however, increased, particularly in early lactation, while protein content declined throughout lactation. The few experiments on suckling ewes generally show that, although milk composition was altered, lamb growth rates did not increase.

The increase in milk fat is accompanied by changes in the proportions of fatty acids, which could potentially affect the organoleptic characteristics of cheese made from the milk. In general, the proportion of short- and medium-chain fatty acids (C4:0–C14:1) is reduced and that of palmitic (C16:0) and oleic (C18:1) acids is increased, but initial studies in Spain have shown little difference in the quality of cheese at the end of the maturation period. These results suggest that supplementation with concentrates containing CSFA may be used to increase milk fat in early lactation, where penalties are imposed by cheese manufacturers for milk with a low fat content.

Protein sources and protected protein sources

In general, supplementing diets of lactating ewes with protein sources of low degradability in the rumen has given variable results. Responses are most likely in early lactation, when voluntary intake is low and the ewes are in negative energy balance. Figure 10.6 from Robinson (1983) shows that the responses of milk yield to supplements of approximately 70 g day^{-1} of groundnut, soybean, meat and bone, linseed, fish and blood meal are broadly related to the degradability of the protein in the rumen. Urea, a non-protein nitrogen source that is completely degraded in the rumen, had a negligible effect on milk production. In the case of the less degradable protein sources of fish and blood meal, but not linseed, there was a response to feeding an additional increment of approximately 60 g day^{-1} of supplement. Although 75–80% of the variation in yield resulted from differences in the amount of amino acid nitrogen reaching the abomasum, the remaining variation probably results from differences in the amino acid composition of the protein. Dove *et al.* (1985) supplemented ewes

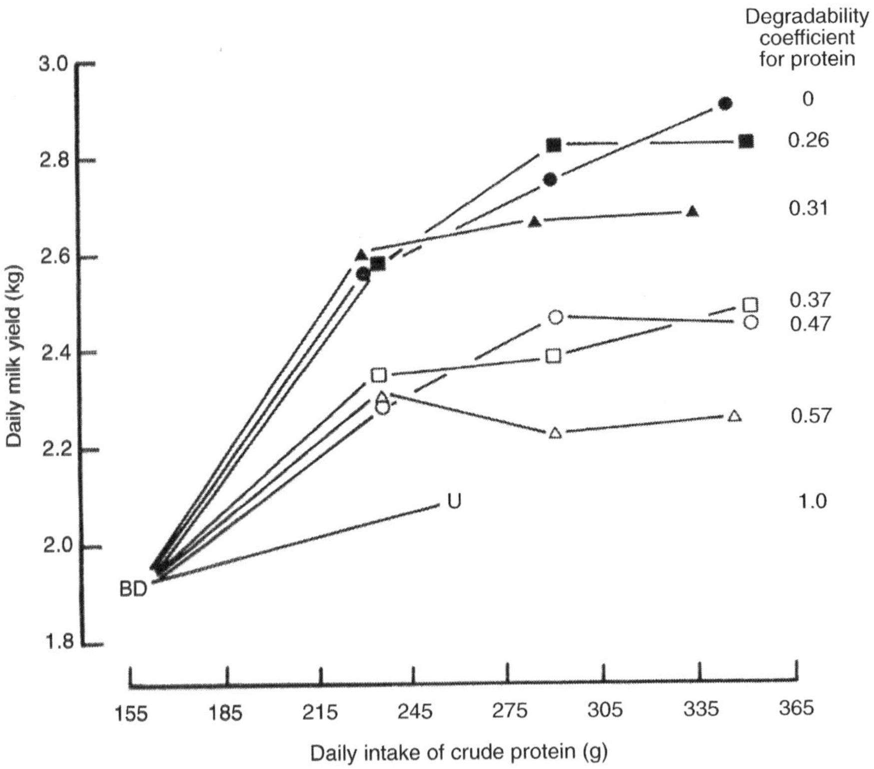

Fig. 10.6. The effect of supplementing a basal diet (BD) of hay and barley with: urea (U); groundnut meal (△); soybean meal (○); meat and bone meal (□); linseed meal (▲); fish meal (■) or blood meal (●), together with the degradability coefficient for each protein source. (Reproduced with permission from Robinson, 1983.)

grazing short pasture with an energy source, with or without formaldehyde-treated soybean meal, and the presence of the protected protein increased milk yield by 33%. Bocquier *et al.* (1994) increased the protein content of milk by feeding 3 or 6 g day^{-1} of protected methionine to dairy ewes already fed more than their energy and protein requirements. Lynch *et al.* (1991) and Baldwin *et al.* (1993), however, found no significant response in either yield or protein content to feeding protected lysine and/or methionine.

These and other similar results must be seen within the context of the overall protein requirements of the ewe; a partially protected protein supplement may be satisfying a need for ERDP. For example, Wilkinson *et al.* (2000) found that supplements differing in digestible undegradable protein content had no effect on the yield of dairy ewes at pasture. The ratio of ERDP to fermentable ME (FME) was, however, below the optimum for rumen function and milk yield increased in response to an increased intake of ERDP resulting from feeding urea.

Conclusion

Ewe milk production has a major impact on the performance and profitability of many sheep systems. The slow increase in voluntary intake in early lactation, when nutrient requirements are at their peak, means that ewes are invariably in negative balance for a few weeks after lambing, although weight change may conceal the energy loss, due to tissue hydration. In the absence of supplementary feeding, this will result in a reduction in milk yield unless the ewe had sufficient body reserves at lambing. The main areas of doubt with current recommendations on nutrient requirements are the energy value of body reserves utilized during lactation and the minimum energy intakes required in early lactation to prevent reduction in milk production throughout the remainder of the lactation.

References

AFRC (1991) A reappraisal of the calcium and phosphorus requirements of sheep and cattle. Technical Committee on Responses to Nutrients, Report Number 6. *Nutrition Abstracts and Reviews (Series B)* 61, 573–612.

AFRC (1993) *Energy and Protein Requirements of Ruminants. An Advisory Manual Prepared by the AFRC Technical Committee on Responses to Nutrients.* CAB International, Wallingford, UK.

ARC (1980) *The Nutrient Requirements of Ruminant Livestock.* Commonwealth Agricultural Bureaux, Farnham Royal, UK, 351 pp.

Ashton, W.M., Owen, J.B. and Ingleton, J.W. (1964) A study of the composition of Clun Forest ewe's milk. *Journal of Agricultural Science, Cambridge* 63, 85–90.

Baldwin, J.A., Horton, G.M.J., Wholt, J.E., Palatini, D.D. and Emanuele, S.M. (1993) Rumen protected methionine for lactation, wool and growth in sheep. *Small Ruminant Research* 12, 125–132.

Bencini, R. and Pulina, G. (1997) The quality of sheep milk: a review. *Australian Journal of Experimental Agriculture* 37, 485–504.

Bocquier, F., Thériez, M. and Brelurut, A. (1987) Recommendations alimentaires pour les brebis en lactation. *Bulletin Technique du Centre de Recherche Zootecnie et Veterinaire, Theix, Institute National de la Recherche Agronomique* 70, 199–211.

Bocquier, F., Delmas, G., Sloan, B.K., Vacaresse, C. and Van Quackebeke, E. (1994) Effets de la supplémentation en méthionine protégée sur la production et la composition du lait de brebis Lacaune. *Rencontres Recherche Ruminants* 1, 101–104.

Brett, D.J., Corbett, J.L. and Inskip, M.W. (1972) Estimation of the energy value of ewe milk. *Proceedings of the Australian Society of Animal Production* 9, 286–291.

Casals, R., Caja, G., Such, X., Torre, C. and Calsamiglia, S. (1999) Effects of calcium soap and rumen undegraded protein on the milk production and composition of dairy ewes. *Journal of Dairy Research* 66, 177–191.

Chrisp, J.S., Sykes, A.R. and Grace, N.D. (1989) Kinetic aspects of calcium metabolism in lactating sheep offered herbages with different Ca concentrations and the effect of protein supplementation. *British Journal of Nutrition* 61, 45–58.

Cowan, R.T., Robinson, J.J., Greenhalgh, J.F.D. and Pennie, K. (1979) Body composition changes in lactating ewes estimated by serial slaughter and deuterium dilution. *Animal Production* 29, 81–90.

Cowan, R.T., Robinson, J.J., McDonald, I. and Smart, R. (1980) Effects of body fatness at lambing and diet in lactation on body tissue loss, feed intake and milk yield of ewes in early lactation. *Journal of Agricultural Science, Cambridge* 92, 123–132.

Cowan, R.T., Robinson, J.J., McHattie, I. and Pennie, K. (1981) Effects of protein concentration in the diet on milk yield, change in body composition and efficiency of utilisation of body tissue for milk production in ewes. *Animal Production* 33, 111–120.

Davis, S.R., Hughson, G.A., Farquhar, P.A. and Rattray, P.V. (1980) The relationship between the degree of udder development and milk production from Coopworth ewes. *Proceedings of the New Zealand Society of Animal Production* 40, 163–165.

Donaldson, J., van Houtert, M.F.J. and Sykes, A.R. (2001) The effect of dietary fishmeal supplementation on parasite burdens of periparturient sheep. *Animal Science* 67, 523–533.

Doney, J.M., Peart, J.N., Smith, W.F. and Louda, F. (1979) A consideration of the techniques for estimation of milk yield by suckled sheep and a comparison of estimates obtained by two methods in relation to the effect of breed, level of production and the stage of lactation. *Journal of Agricultural Science, Cambridge* 92, 123–132.

Dove, H. (1988) Estimating the intake of milk by lambs, from the turnover of deuterium- or tritium-labelled water. *British Journal of Nutrition* 60, 375–387.

Dove, H. and Freer, M. (1979) The accuracy of tritiated water turnover rate as an estimate of milk intake in lambs. *Australian Journal of Agricultural Research* 30, 725–739.

Dove, H., Milne, J.A., Lamb, C.S., McCormack, H.A. and Spence, A.M. (1985) The effect of supplementation on non-ammonia nitrogen flows at the abomasum of lactating grazing ewes. *Proceedings of the Nutrition Society* 44, 63A.

Dove, H., Freer, M. and Donnelly, J.R. (1988) Effects of nutrition in early pregnancy on ewe and lamb performance in the subsequent lactation. *Proceedings of the Nutrition Society of Australia* 13, 111.

Foot, J.Z. and Russel, A.J.F. (1979) The relationship between voluntary intake food intake during pregnancy and forage intake during lactation and after weaning. *Animal Production* 28, 25–39.

Gallo, C.B. and Davies, D.A.R. (1988) Rearing twin and triplet lambs on the ewe. *Animal Production* 47, 111–121.

Gargouri, A., Such, X., Caja, G., Casals, R., Ferret, A., Vbergara, H. and Peris, S. (1993) Estrategias de cria-ordeño en ovino lechero: 1. Efecto del tipo de cria (Libre o Restringida) y número de ordeños diarios (2 ó 3) sobre la producción de leche de ovejas de raza Manchega. *Información Tecnica Economica Agraria (ITEA)* Volumen Extra Número 12, 30–32.

Geenty, K.G. and Sykes, A.R. (1986) Effect of herbage allowance during pregnancy and lactation on feed intake, milk production, body composition and energy utilisation of ewes at pasture. *Journal of Agricultural Science, Cambridge* 106, 351–367.

Gibb, M.J. and Treacher, T.T. (1980) The effect of ewe body condition at lambing on the performance of ewes and their lambs at pasture. *Journal of Agricultural Science, Cambridge* 95, 631–640.

Gibb, M.J., Treacher, T.T. and Shanmungalingum, V.S. (1981) Herbage intake and performance of grazing ewes and their lambs when weaned at 6, 8, 10 or 14 weeks of age. *Animal Production* 33, 223–232.

Goodchild, A.V., El-Awad, A.I. and Gursoy, O. (1999) Effect of feeding level in late pregnancy and early lactation and fibre level in mid lactation on body mass, milk production and quality. *Animal Science* 68, 231–241.

Hadjipieris, G. and Holmes, W. (1966) Studies on feed intake and feed utilisation by sheep. 1. Voluntary intake by dry, pregnant and lactating ewes. *Journal of Agricultural Science, Cambridge* 66, 217–223.

Labussière, J. and Pétrequin, P. (1969) Relations entre l'aptitude à la traite des brebis et la perte de production laitière constatée au moment du sevrage. *Annales de Zootechnie* 18, 5–15.

Loerch, S.C., McClure, K.E. and Parker, C.F. (1985) Effects of number of lambs suckled and supplemental protein source on lactating ewe performance. *Journal of Animal Science* 60, 7–13.

Lynch, G.P., Elsasser, T.H., Jackson, C., Rumsey, T.S. and Camp, M.J. (1991) Nitrogen metabolism of lactating ewes fed rumen-protected methionine and lysine. *Journal of Dairy Science* 74, 2268–2276.

Moore, R.W. (1966) Genetic factors affecting the milk intake of lambs. *Australian Journal of Agricultural Science* 17, 191–199.

Morris, S.T., McCutcheon, S.N., Parker, W.J. and Blair, H.T. (1994) Effect of sward surface height on herbage intake and performance of lactating ewes lambed in winter and continuously stocked on pasture. *Journal of Agricultural Science, Cambridge* 122, 471–482.

Peart, J.N. (1970) The influence of liveweight and body condition on the subsequent milk production of Blackface ewes following a period of undernutrition in early lactation. *Journal of Agricultural Science, Cambridge* 75, 459–469.

Peart, J.N., Edwards, R.A. and Donaldson, E. (1975) The yield and composition of the milk of Finnish Landrace × Blackface ewes II. Ewes and lambs grazed on pasture. *Journal of Agricultural Science, Cambridge* 85, 315–324.

Penning, P.D., Parsons, A.J., Orr, R.J. and Treacher, T.T. (1991) Intake and behaviour responses by sheep to changes in sward characteristics under continuous grazing. *Grass and Forage Science* 46, 15–28.

Robinson, J.J. (1980) Energy requirements of ewes during late pregnancy and early lactation. *Veterinary Record* 106, 282–284.

Robinson, J.J. (1983) Nutrient requirements of the breeding ewe. In: Haresign, W. (ed.) *Recent Advances in Animal Nutrition*. Butterworths, London, pp. 143–161.

Robinson, J.J. (1987) Energy and protein requirements of the ewe. In: Haresign, W. and Cole, D.J.A. (eds) *Recent Advances in Animal Nutrition*. Butterworths, London, pp. 187–204.

Robinson, J.J. (1990) Nutrition over the winter period – the breeding female. In: Slade, C.F.R. and Lawrence, T.L.J. (eds) *New Developments in Sheep Production*. Occasional Publication No. 14, British Society of Animal Production, Edinburgh, pp. 55–69.

SCA (1990) *Feeding Standards for Australian Livestock. Ruminants*. Standing Committee on Agriculture and CSIRO, Melbourne, 266 pp.

Slen, S.B., Clark, R.D. and Hironaka, R. (1963) A comparison of milk production and its relation to lamb growth in five breeds of sheep. *Canadian Journal of Animal Science* 43, 16–21.

Thomas, P.C. and Rook, J.A.F. (1983) Milk secretion and its nutritional regulation. In: Rook, J.A.F. and Thomas, P.C. (eds) *Nutritional Physiology of Farm Animals*. Longman, London, pp. 314–368.

Treacher, T.T. (1970) Effects of nutrition in late pregnancy on subsequent milk production in ewes. *Animal Production* 12, 23–36.

Treacher, T.T. (1983) Nutrient requirements for lactation in the ewe. In: Haresign, W. (ed.) *Sheep Production*. Butterworths, London, pp. 133–153.

Treacher, T.T. (1987) Milk. In: Marai, I.F.M. and Owen, J.B. (eds) *New Techniques in Sheep Production*. Butterworths, London, pp. 25–33.

Treacher, T.T. (1990) Grazing management and supplementation for the lowland sheep flock. In: Slade, C.F.R. and Lawrence, T.L.J. (eds) *New Developments in Sheep Production*. Occasional Publication No. 14, British Society of Animal Production, Edinburgh, pp. 45–54.

Underwood, E.J. and Suttle, N.F. (1999) *The Mineral Nutrition of Livestock*, 3rd edn. CAB International, Wallingford, UK.

Wallace, L.R. (1948) Growth of lambs before and after birth in relation to the level of nutrition. *Journal of Agricultural Science, Cambridge* 38, 93–153.

Wilkinson, R.G., Sinclair, L.A., Powles, J. and Minter, C.M. (2000) Response of lactating ewes grazing grass to variations in effective rumen degradable protein and digestible undegradable protein supply from concentrate supplements. *Animal Science* 71, 369–379.

Yousef, I.M.K. and Ashton, W.M. (1967) A study of the composition of Clun Forest ewe's milk III. Ewe's milk fat: a preliminary note. *Journal of Agricultural Science, Cambridge* 68, 103–107.

11 Nutrition for Sheep-meat Production

V.H. Oddy[1] and R.D. Sainz[2]

[1]*Meat and Livestock Australia, North Sydney, New South Wales, Australia;*
[2]*Department of Animal Science, University of California, Davis, California, USA*

Introduction

In most developed countries, food production exceeds the demand. Affluent consumers become more selective about their purchase and consumption choices, and these depend as much on ethical and emotional considerations as on strict nutritional grounds. The perception that dietary fat, in general, and saturated fat, in particular, are linked to obesity, circulating cholesterol and cardiovascular disease is common. This perception has dramatically affected the demand for animal products, especially for red meat. This trend is expected to continue, so that the challenge facing the sheep-meat industry is to produce lean, healthy meat under humane, ecologically sound conditions. This will require a solid scientific and technical foundation in the biology underlying animal production.

In response to consumer preferences, processors require lambs that meet criteria for age, carcass weight, carcass fat cover and meat-quality attributes. Processors traditionally achieve these specifications by purchasing lambs produced in a diverse range of extensive-production environments. Increasingly, producers are attempting to achieve specifications within the constraints of their production environments, mainly by combining improved genotypes with a practical knowledge of grazing management, animal nutrition and parasite control. The supply of nutrients is most readily affected by management practices and has arguably the greatest effect on the supply of lambs that meet market specifications. Management of the production system depends on an understanding of the relationships between intake of pastures and their nutrient yield, animal genotype and product (meat) output and quality. Here we describe and discuss how some of these factors affect efficiency of feed use by lambs, their body composition in terms of lean and fat content and aspects of carcass quality (principally fat content and meat yield).

Growth and Metabolism

Growth is an increase in size and encompasses both structural and functional development. In terms of body components, the accretion of protein rather than fat is the major indicator of growth. One objective of understanding growth physiology is to maximize the utility of livestock for humans, in terms of productive performance (i.e. growth rate), efficiency (i.e. output : input) and product quality (relative to market requirements). In general terms, the ideal animal is one that grows rapidly and efficiently to the desired weight, at which its body contains a minimum of bone, a maximum of muscle and the optimal amount of fat.

Animal growth is a function of the animal's genetic potential and the extent to which the environment allows this potential to be expressed. Among the main environmental variables that affect animal performance, nutrition is the most important. Clearly, production of meat requires the accumulation of skeletal muscle, i.e. a large difference between the rates of synthesis and degradation of myofibrillar and sarcoplasmic proteins. This in turn requires the provision of adequate amounts and appropriate balances of amino acids and other nutrients. Therefore, the amount and composition of the feed available to the animal will dictate its growth pattern, within the constraints imposed by its genetic potential and climatic and pathogenic stresses.

As an animal grows, its form changes to suit different functions, such as exchange with the environment, locomotion, feeding and reproduction. Initially, cells proliferate through mitotic division until, under the influence of local physical, chemical and neural factors, they differentiate into specialized cells, which become 'locked in' to a specific function and form. Because of differential timing of cell differentiation and proliferation and subsequent cell enlargement, different tissues grow at different times and at different rates. Growth occurs in 'waves', beginning cranially and running caudally and from distal limbs towards the torso (Palsson, 1955). In addition to changes in tissue and organ cellularity and function, which affect conformation, the chemical composition of the animal body also changes during development, with the proportion of fat increasing at an increasing rate as the animal approaches maturity (Fig. 11.1). The concept of maturity is of considerable significance and, for many purposes (including genetic selection), maturity has been defined as that stage when the animal's body contains, say, 25% fat. The degree of maturity can then be specified in relation to mature weight (Taylor, 1980). It follows that, at any given weight, an animal with a greater mature weight will be less mature and leaner than one with a smaller mature weight.

Growth pattern

The pattern of development of the major chemical (and industrially valuable) components of the lamb (protein and fat) has been described elsewhere. For example, in his comprehensive review, Black (1983) noted the

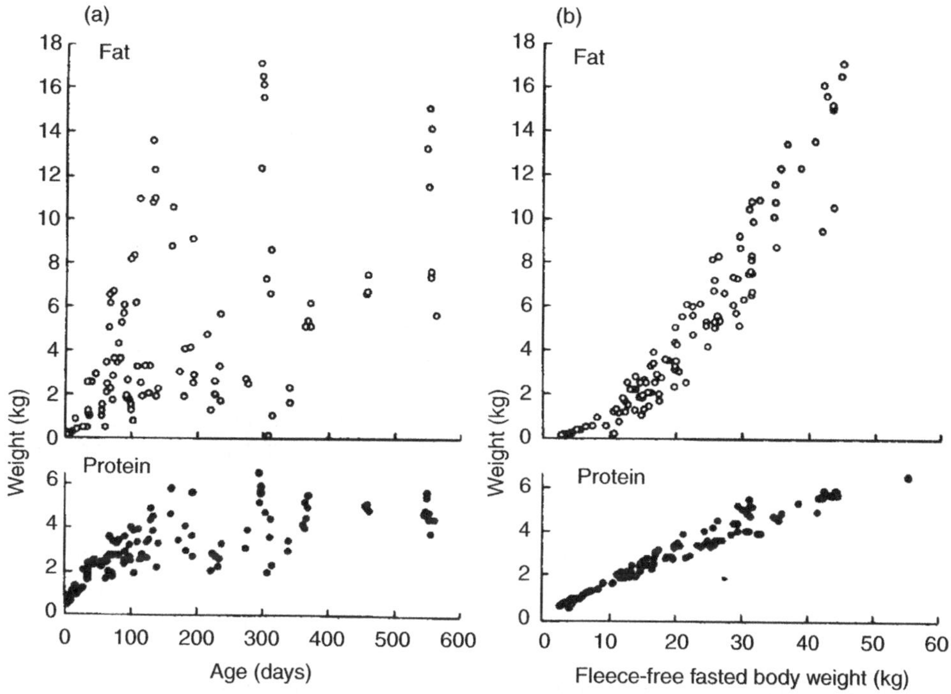

Fig. 11.1. The relationship between weight of protein and fat in lambs and (a) age and (b) fleece-free fasted body weight (FFFBW) (diagram from Black, 1983). Note the lack of relationship between chemical composition of the body and age, particularly after 100 days, and the comparatively close relationship between protein content and FFFBW.

general lack of relationship between the age of the lamb and its protein and fat content, but noted a substantially closer relationship between protein and fat content and the fleece-free fasted weight of lambs (Fig. 11.1). This apparently simple relationship masks a more complex pattern of development when viewed at the level of individual organs. Butterfield (1988) has detailed the pattern of development of the organs (including individual muscle and fat depots) of lambs and sheep. Where feed intake is unrestricted, the proportion of growth in early postnatal life is greater for the brain, intestine, liver, heart and muscle than for body weight and the fat depots contribute a lesser proportion of body-weight gain (Black, 1983; Butterfield, 1988; Fig. 11.2).

Where feed intake is restricted, particularly in the period before about 30% maturity, the proportion of organs change, relative to the unrestricted case shown in Fig. 11.2. The response is complex. The weights of very early-maturing organs, such as the brain and eyes, are not affected by feed restriction, and their proportion of body weight may be greater than shown in Fig. 11.2 (Palsson and Verges, 1952). Organs that are particularly sensitive to feed intake, such as the intestine and liver, may have proportional weights somewhat less than those indicated

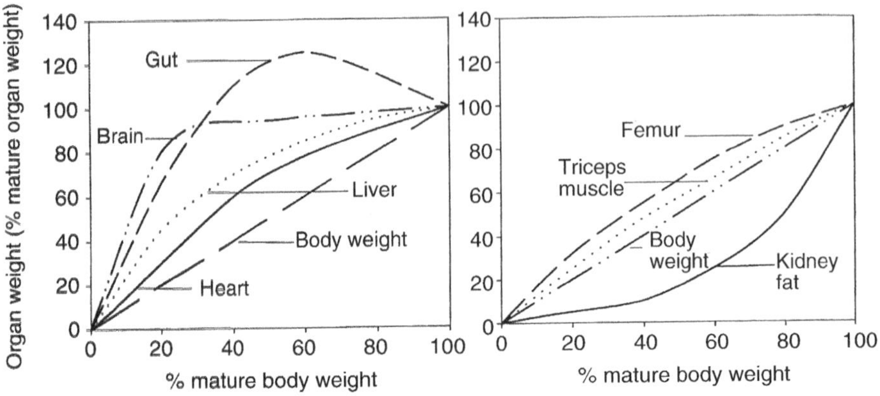

Fig. 11.2. Pattern of postnatal growth of organs of Merino sheep relative to their live weight as a percentage of their weight at maturity (adapted from Black, 1983, and Butterfield, 1988).

by Fig. 11.2. The proportion of fat in the body will be reduced at low degrees of maturity, but may increase at high degrees of maturity. This comes about because of a lower proportion of feed energy intake available for deposition in adipose tissue, and also because low levels of nutrition early in life may reduce the capacity of muscles to reach their mature size (Tulloh *et al.*, 1986).

Utilization of feed energy for maintenance

The idea of a maintenance requirement for energy or individual nutrients has little relevance to growing animals other than as a useful way of calculating that part of the energy intake not used for growth. The conventional definition of maintenance is that point at which energy intake is the same as energy expenditure, i.e. retained energy (RE) equals zero (see Fig. 7.1a, Corbett and Ball, Chapter 7, this volume). Note that retained energy is synonymous with energy balance (EB) – that is, RE = EB. At maintenance, the metabolizable energy (ME) intake (MEI) is exactly balanced by heat production. There is no requirement that body composition should remain unaltered when RE = 0; indeed, in most cases, sheep will continue to grow wool (i.e. deposit protein) and will variously gain or lose fat and/or protein in the body. The efficiency of ME use for maintenance (k_m) is then defined as the slope of the line relating RE to MEI.

However, the relationship between RE and MEI is actually curvilinear (Blaxter and Boyne, 1978), rather than discontinuous, as in Fig. 7.1c, implying that efficiency of energy retention is also a continuous function of RE and MEI (see Corbett and Ball, Chapter 7, this volume).

The conventional nutritional view is that the principal determinant of efficiency of energy use for maintenance is the ME density of the ingested feed dry matter (M/D) (MJ kg^{-1}). Efficiency of ME utilization for maintenance (k_m defined as in Fig. 7.1) lies in the range 0.65–0.72, when calculated from calorimetric measurements of heat production, or in the range 0.54–0.60, when calculated from comparative slaughter studies. The reasons for the difference are discussed by Corbett and Ball (Chapter 7, this volume). One method for calculating the efficiency of energy use for maintenance from M/D is that used by the Agricultural Research Council (ARC, 1980):

$$k_m = 0.55 + 0.016\mathrm{M/D}$$

However, as noted below, there is also considerable other variation, possibly genetic, in the efficiency of feed use for maintenance (Herd *et al.*, 1993).

The difficulty of defining maintenance in growing sheep has long been recognized. Lines and Pierce (1931) described the effects of previous level of feeding on fasting heat production, and recommended a standard procedure for time without feed and amount of feed before such measurements. Such an approach to the problem of defining a dynamic biological variable has been used to great effect in the development of practical feeding systems (Corbett *et al.*, 1987). In the future, it is likely that attempts will be made to add further factors (perhaps for differences between breeds, effects of internal and external parasites) to generalized maintenance equations (SCA, 1990). However, the problem remains that these factors are contributors to an arbitrary separation of energy expenditure for maintenance from that for growth and other bodily functions, whereas, in reality, energy expenditure at zero energy retention (i.e. maintenance) is dynamic. Current attempts to develop mathematical frameworks that can accommodate variable energy cost at energy balance are discussed below.

Utilization of feed energy for growth

Leaving aside the small cost of growing wool, the energy retained in the tissues of the young growing sheep (RE) is defined as the difference between MEI and total heat production, H. Note that in the National Research Council (NRC, 1985) system, net energy for growth is equivalent to retained energy, that is, NE_g = RE. Total heat production is that generated by maintenance and the heat produced during growth (Equation (1)). To calculate NE_g, the ME available for gain, ME_g, is multiplied by the net efficiency of energy use for growth, k_g (Equation (3)). The energy content of gain is calculated from total energy retention, which is the sum of energy retained in fat and protein (protein 23.8 kJ g^{-1}, fat 39.6 kJ g^{-1}). The small amount of carbohydrate deposited, principally as glycogen and glycoproteins (< 2% of total weight and < 1% of energy), is usually ignored. The major terms related to energy utilization in domestic animals were defined by the NRC (1981):

$$NE_g = MEI - (H_e + H_d + H_r) \quad (1)$$

$$ME_g = MEI - ME_m = MEI - (H_e + H_d) \quad (2)$$

$$NE_g = ME_g - H_r = k_g ME_g \quad (3)$$

where:

H_e = endogenous heat energy (i.e. fasting heat production or basal metabolism)
H_d = heat of digestion, absorption and assimilation
H_r = heat produced during growth (cost of product synthesis)
k_g = efficiency of energy retention = $1 - H_r/ME_g$

From a nutritional perspective, the variation in k_g is influenced mainly by the ME density of the feed. An empirical relationship often used to calculate efficiency of gain (ARC, 1980) is:

$$k_g = 0.0435M/D$$

Given the expected range in M/D, predicted values of k_g would vary from 0.30 to 0.57. In reality the range of efficiency of gain is greater. As with maintenance, estimates of efficiency of energy use calculated from studies in which energy deposition in the body was measured directly tend to be lower compared with measurement of heat production in a calorimeter. For example, Rattray *et al.* (1974) report an estimate of k_g of 0.41 in young growing sheep compared with 0.48 calculated by the above equation. Sainz *et al.* (1990) report, for a diet with M/D 10.6, values for k_g of 0.42–0.44 for wethers and 0.39–0.42 for ewes and, for a diet of M/D 8.7, k_g values of 0.25–0.27 for wethers and 0.17–0.21 for ewes. These compare with predicted values from the ARC equation of 0.46 and 0.38, respectively. Similarly, it can be calculated from Hegarty *et al.* (1999), who fed castrated male lambs a diet with M/D of 10, that k_g was 0.37 if maintenance was derived from the EB of the control group or 0.43 if maintenance was adjusted for additional MEI (SCA, 1990). These data highlight the difficulty in determining maintenance and the consequences of incorrect estimation.

Estimates of k_g are amalgamated estimates of rate of gain of different tissues, each with different rates of gain of chemical components. These are mainly protein and fat, each with its own efficiency of energy accretion. The energetic efficiency of protein deposition in ruminants is reported to be 0.2 (Owens *et al.*, 1995), compared with 0.45 in pigs (Kielanowski, 1965), and the efficiency of deposition of energy in fat is 0.75. However, fat and protein accretion are so highly correlated that it is difficult to estimate efficiency of energy retention in both protein and fat with precision from data collected in serial slaughter studies (Bernier *et al.*, 1987). We therefore need alternative methods for estimating energetic efficiency of fat and protein deposition. One of these methods involves direct measures of protein deposition and energy expenditure in lambs eating different amounts of the same feed (Oddy, 1999). Such studies suggest that, at least in muscle, the efficiency of protein deposition depends on the rate of protein synthesis relative to the rate of protein accretion (i.e. synthesis minus degradation (see below)).

A consequence of different energetic efficiencies of deposition of protein and fat is that, if the composition of gain varies, either due to level of feeding, and thus rate of gain, or due to stage of development of the animal, then the overall energetic efficiency of gain should also vary. Present feeding systems make no adjustment for efficiency as affected by rate and composition of gain or animal maturity.

Effect of protein turnover on efficiency of metabolism

Protein accretion in skeletal muscle and other tissues results whenever the rate of synthesis exceeds the rate of degradation (see Fig. 11.3). Mechanisms of protein synthesis have been well understood for some time (Pain and Clemens, 1980), and involve transcription, amino acid transport and acylation to transfer RNA (tRNA), translation and post-translational modification. Protein synthesis is subject to control by various endocrine, autocrine and paracrine hormones, including insulin, insulin-like growth factor 1 (IGF-1), cortisol and sex steroids, and responds dramatically to nutrition (Fig. 11.3). In contrast, protein breakdown is poorly understood. Mechanisms for degrading cellular proteins reside in lysosomes (e.g. cathepsins) or in the cytosol (such as the calpains and a multicatalytic protease) (see Goll *et al.*, 1992).

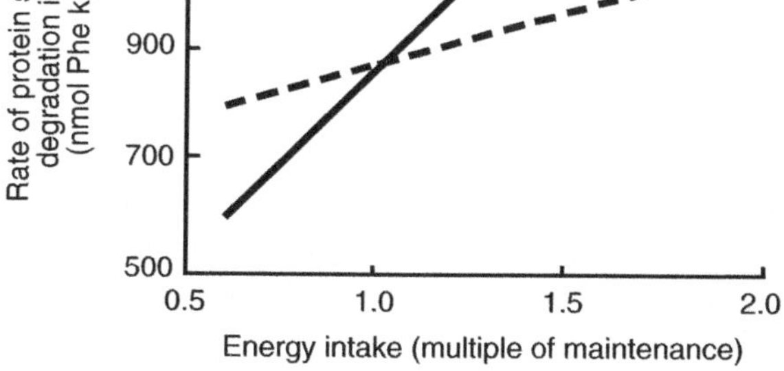

Fig. 11.3. Effects of feed intake (expressed as multiples of calculated maintenance energy requirement) on hind-limb protein synthesis (solid line) and degradation (dashed line) in sheep (data from Thomson *et al.*, 1997). Protein synthesis and degradation were measured using an arteriovenous difference technique; the units refer to flux of the marker amino acid, phenylalanine, across the hind limb.

It has been recognized for some time that heat production is closely related to whole-body protein mass (Waterlow *et al.*, 1978) and to the rate of protein synthesis (for a summary, see Webster, 1984). Why does this occur?

The key determinant of efficiency of protein deposition is the rate of protein synthesis relative to the rate of protein gain. Since protein gain = protein synthesis – protein degradation, it follows that, when protein gain = 0, protein synthesis = protein degradation. At low rates of protein accretion, it would be expected that the energetic efficiency of protein gain would approach 0. The theoretical maximum energetic efficiency of protein gain (0.94, calculated as described in Fig. 11.4) occurs when protein synthesis equals protein gain, i.e. protein degradation = 0.

Protein degradation is an important process for remodelling cell structure and recycling of amino acids within and between cells. Protein degradation always occurs, so the theoretical maximal efficiency of protein gain is never attained. Because of temporal differences in the rates of protein synthesis and degradation within and between organs, such as those related to the pattern of feed intake, stage of animal development, disease state and genotype, the relative rate of protein accretion is very much less than the rate of protein synthesis. Accordingly, the theoretical energetic efficiency of protein accretion, k_p, depends upon the rate of protein synthesis relative to accretion, and the relationship is not linear (Fig. 11.4). The calculated value of k_p in growing non-ruminants (0.44)

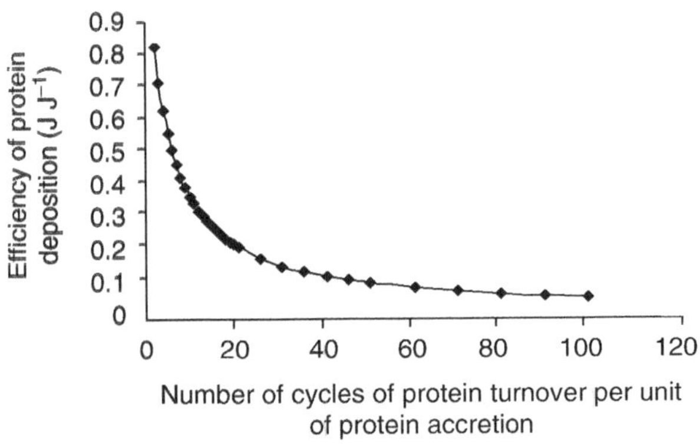

Fig. 11.4. Theoretical efficiency of energy use for protein gain as affected by the rate of protein synthesis relative to the rate of protein gain.* Calculated efficiency based on energy cost of protein synthesis of 4.5 kJ g^{-1} protein deposited (Buttery and Annison, 1973) and protein energy content of 23.8 kJ g^{-1}.
*Consider the following equality:

Protein gain = protein synthesis – protein degradation

For each 1 g of protein gain, then it is possible to have *n* g of protein synthesis and (*n* – 1) g of protein degradation. The diagram considers the energetic consequences of increasing *n*, the number of g of protein synthesis per g of protein gained.

suggests that, on average, the rate of protein synthesis exceeds accretion by a factor of 7 : 1. In ruminants, where the reported k_p is 0.2, the rate of protein synthesis relative to accretion may be closer to 20 : 1. However, the actual rate of protein synthesis is notoriously difficult to measure, and the estimates of energy cost of protein synthesis may be too low. None the less, the implications are clear: reduction in the relative proportion of protein synthesis relative to accretion affects the efficiency of protein and total energy gain.

All this discussion would be academic if there were no systematic variation in the rates of protein synthesis relative to accretion. Figure 11.5 shows that age and growth rate (rate of protein gain) affect the relative proportion of protein synthesis to accretion in (milk-fed) lambs. Lambs selected for weaning weight differ in their responses of protein synthesis and degradation to feed intake (see Fig. 11.6 below). On this basis it would be expected that the energetic efficiency of protein deposition is variable and subject to systematic change due at least to age, growth rate (level of feed intake) and genotype.

Current feeding systems consider the efficiency of retention of energy in gain to be affected only by the ME density of a feed. Clearly there is scope for further refinement in our understanding. An outstanding practical application may include the development of genotypes of lambs with relatively high efficiency of energy utilization for protein accretion. Given the observation that heat production is proportional to lean mass and protein synthesis, identification of genotypes that differ in protein synthesis and associated heat production has the potential to reduce significantly the amount of feed used to achieve a particular weight and body composition. One undesirable consequence of this strategy, however, is that animals with lower rates of muscle-protein degradation may also have impaired proteolysis post-mortem, which would result in tougher meat (McDonagh *et al.*, 1999).

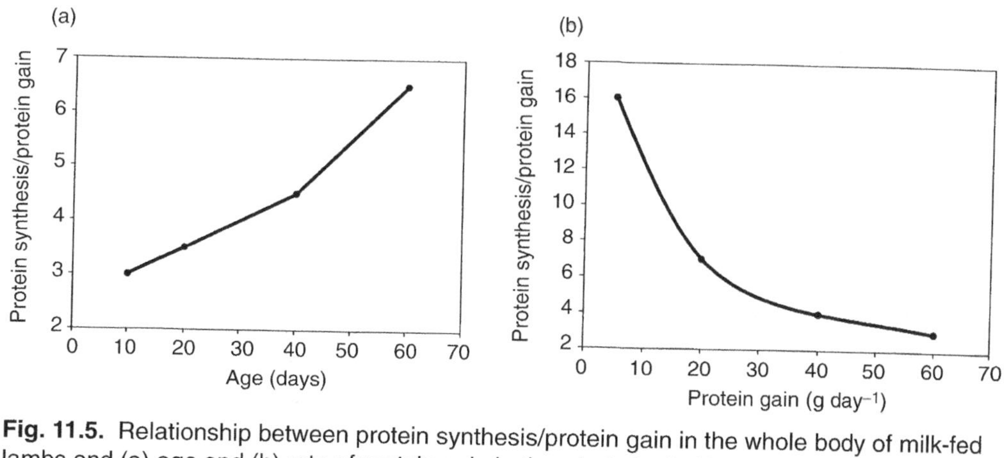

Fig. 11.5. Relationship between protein synthesis/protein gain in the whole body of milk-fed lambs and (a) age and (b) rate of protein gain in the whole body (data from Oddy, 1986).

Fat metabolism

Fat deposition is the balance between the relative rates of anabolism (i.e. lipogenesis) and catabolism (i.e. lipolysis) (Vernon, 1986). Most body fat is laid down as triacylglycerols (TAG), through the processes of lipogenesis from acetyl-coenzyme A (CoA) (derived from acetate) and esterification of fatty-acyl-CoA (FA-CoA) to α-glycerol phosphate (derived from glucose). Lipolysis is carried out mainly by hormone-sensitive lipase (HSL), yielding free (non-esterified) fatty acids (NEFA) and glycerol. NEFA may be reactivated to FA-CoA and re-esterified to form TAG, or they may enter the circulation. Since released glycerol cannot be reutilized in adipose tissue, it is released into the bloodstream and taken up by the liver for gluconeogenesis.

Fat metabolism and deposition are controlled by hormonal and nutritional factors, and depend to a large extent on the age of the animal and its energy status. The rate of fat deposition is more clearly related to the amount of energy available in excess of requirements for maintenance and lean growth than to specific metabolic changes in adipose tissue (Sainz and Wolff, 1990).

Effects of Genotype

We now understand (in broad terms) that both the pattern and extent of growth are regulated through expression of specific genes. The principal determinant of the timing and extent of gene expression is an innate 'programme' within the genome itself. However, the extent and timing of expression of specific genes that regulate development are also controlled by nutrient supply. The pattern of nutrient supply, and thus gene expression, is influenced by what Dawkins (1983) describes as the 'extended phenotype' – that is, the inherited relationship between the genome and the environment in which it is expressed. For example, a lamb is affected by maternal factors that influence uterine and preweaning nutritional environment and which, from a nutritional perspective, represent effects of the mother's genome. In crossbred lambs, this (maternal) half of the genome has both direct (additive genetic) and indirect (maternal) effects. Maternal effects may include effects on fetal development of the lamb due to placental insufficiency or lactational capability less than the intake potential of the progeny. The dominant perinatal nutritional influence is the capability of lambs to maximize their mothers' lactational capacity and hence the relative contribution of milk to the ingested nutrient supply. After weaning, nutrient supply is provided by ingestion and digestion of predominantly cellulose-based feeds. The ability of the lamb to ingest and to digest these feeds are both significantly influenced by inherited characters (genes). As a lamb becomes older, and in particular after weaning, feed intake is often constrained by the quality and quantity of available pasture or supplement. Accordingly, knowledge about the nutritional response of sheep of different genotypes will almost certainly be required in future feeding systems.

Growth and composition of growth

The pattern of deposition of fat and protein in sheep of different genotypes is remarkably similar when scaled as a proportion of mature size, although small but commercially significant breed differences remain (Butterfield, 1988). In the breeds of sheep commonly used in meat-production systems, between-breed variation in the proportion of dissected muscle, bone and fat (expressed on a % maturity basis) is not significant – with the exception that the Texel breed has approximately 2% more lean meat and less fat (Kempster *et al.*, 1987). The only genetic difference that may be large and significant is the so-called Callipyge mutation, in which the mass of selected hind-limb muscles (e.g. m. biceps femoris) may increase to 40% more than the weight of the same muscle in control animals at 6 months post-partum (Koohmaraie *et al.*, 1995). This occurs as a consequence of hypertrophy of muscle fibres.

Realized responses to long-term selection for growth rate at weaning in sheep include an increase in feed intake both pre- and postweaning (Oddy *et al.*, 1995). In the preruminant lamb from weaning-weight selection lines, lambs differ predominantly in propensity for feed intake rather than capacity for rate of deposition of lean tissue (Oddy, 1993), the reverse of what is observed in pigs. Selection for weight in Merino sheep is also associated with differences in partitioning between body and wool. Although the relationship between N (and energy) intake and N balance does not change with selection, the site of protein deposition does, i.e. more protein is deposited in the body and less in the wool of lambs selected for increased weaning weight (Oddy *et al.*, 1989).

Protein metabolism

Growth rate may be improved by a reduction in the rate of protein degradation. For example, fast-growing genetic lines of sheep have lower rates of muscle-protein breakdown than slow-growing lines (Oddy *et al.*, 1989). Similar results have been observed with other species. At least in cattle and sheep, there appears to be a genotype × nutrition interaction in the response of protein turnover (Oddy, 1999). In comparing sheep from lines selected for high or low growth rates, Oddy *et al.* (1995) found that low-growth-line sheep displayed the expected response to different levels of feeding (Fig. 11.6a). On the other hand, sheep from the high-growth line exhibited a qualitatively different response to nutrition (Fig. 11.6b). In those animals, protein synthesis did not increase with feeding level and protein degradation showed a marked decrease in response to improved nutrition. This genotype-specific response confirms the importance of protein degradation in genetic growth potential, but is inconsistent with the current view of nutritional control of protein accretion.

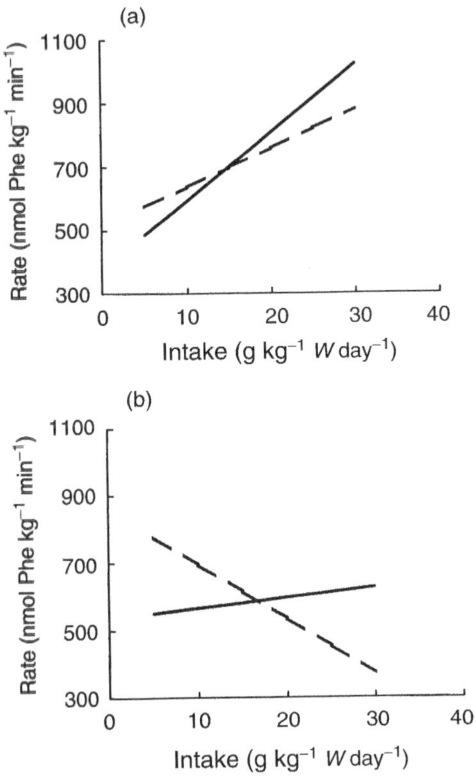

Fig. 11.6. Effects of feed intake on hind-limb protein synthesis (solid line) and degradation (dashed line) in sheep selected for low weaning weight (*W*–) (a) and high weaning weight (*W*+) (b) (data from Oddy *et al.*, 1995). Protein synthesis and degradation were measured using an arteriovenous difference technique; the units refer to flux of the marker amino acid, phenylalanine, across the hind limb.

Residual feed intake

There is considerable variation in calculated maintenance requirement within lines of sheep selected for and against weaning weight (Herd *et al.*, 1993). Similar observations of deviation in estimated maintenance requirement in cattle (Herd, 1992) were used to establish lines of beef cattle that differ in residual feed intake (RFI) (Arthur *et al.*, 1998). RFI is defined as the difference between the actual intake by an individual animal and intake predicted from the animal's own weight and weight gain but compared within a contemporary group. The heritability of RFI is about 35% in cattle (Arthur *et al.*, 1998), similar to equivalent measures in mice (Nielsen, 1998). These recent observations indicate that an additional source of variation in the response of animals to nutrition is variation in maintenance requirement and, as we suggest later, efficiency of feed deposited as body gain.

There is as yet no clear understanding of the effects of genetic variation on nutritional requirements and responses in lambs. Animals from selection lines, by definition, differ in their response to the same nutritional environment. This may occur through changes in patterns of nutrient utilization, as in the examples above, or there may be variation in the amounts and proportions of nutrients available to the animal from the same amount of feed eaten. Genetic selection of sheep for weaning weight has been shown to affect the digestion of feed (Herd *et al.*, 1993) and, in sheep selected for wool growth, the amount of microbial protein (Kahn, 1996) and absorbed amino acids (Lush *et al.*, 1991) relative to feed intake have also been altered. Given the wide variety of available genotypes and the opportunities for selection and genetic manipulation, the interactions between genotypes and nutritional environment will certainly require much further study.

Effects of Diet on Composition of Gain

At any given stage of maturity, the relative contribution of protein and fat to retained energy in response to increased feed intake follows the general pattern shown in Fig. 11.7. The absolute rates and relative proportions of protein and fat accretion in response to nutrient input are influenced by the stage of maturity. Briefly, less-mature lambs have potentially higher rates of protein accretion in the body and relatively higher proportions of

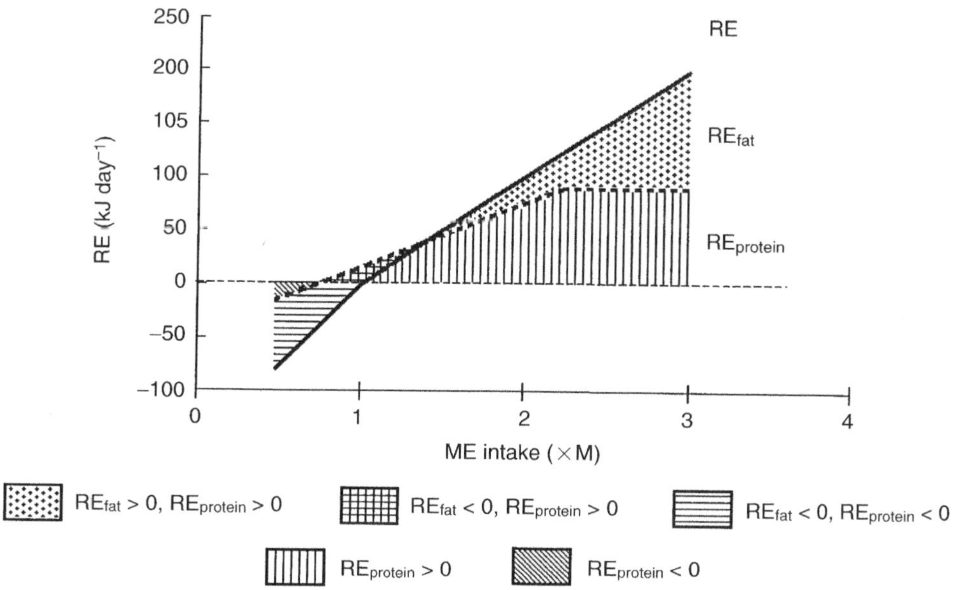

Fig. 11.7. The general pattern of energy retained in fat and protein in lambs as affected by feed intake (shown as multiples of maintenance, M).

energy retained in protein. Fat gain is a function of the amount of energy available after maintenance costs and protein gain are accounted for; it therefore increases with feed intake in excess of maintenance. Rates of fat gain also increase with stage of maturity until approximately 70% maturity. As the limit of voluntary intake starts to decline at about this point, the difference between energy intake and maintenance energy costs plus the cost of protein accretion declines and, accordingly, the rate of fat accretion also declines.

Variation in growth rate due to variation in nutrient supply relative to potential requirements can cause variation in retail yield, fatness and possible eating quality of lambs. Management systems capable of attaining specific growth rates tailored for appropriate genotypes offer the best options to meet market specifications in terms of muscle development, fatness, including marbling, and consumer-assessed meat quality (Table 11.1).

To this point we have considered responses to energy-yielding nutrients without differentiating between nutrients. The supply of essential amino acids relative to total energy supply also influences the absolute and relative rate of protein and fat accretion in lambs. The clearest evidence of an effect on protein accretion has been obtained in milk-fed lambs (for an eloquent summary, see Black and Griffiths, 1975) and in ruminant lambs (Ørskov *et al.*, 1976). Briefly, response, measured as whole-body N retention, to amino acid supply at any fixed energy intake and weight can be described by a linear phase up to maximal protein gain (for that weight and energy intake), followed by no further response, as illustrated for $RE_{protein}$ in Fig. 11.7. Although this pattern of response to amino acid supply is readily observed in milk-fed lambs, where it is experimentally possible to provide amino acids independent of energy-yielding nutrients, it is much more difficult to demonstrate in ruminant lambs.

The ruminant pattern of digestion delivers microbial protein to the small intestine in proportion to the fermentable energy supply (see Annison *et al.*, Chapter 5, this volume). Accordingly, it is quite difficult to experimentally perturb the amino acid supply relative to the supply of

Table 11.1. Effect of growth rate on some important commercial attributes of lambs.

Lambs with faster growth when compared with slower-growing contemporaries of the same genotype and sex, at the same weight, are:

- Younger
- Fatter and have more intramuscular fat (marbling)
- Have smaller muscles

And, if they behave like cattle, it would be expected that faster-growing lambs would:

- Have lower ossification scores
- Have lower muscle compression – less connective-tissue toughness
- Have improved eating quality (as assessed by consumer panels)

energy-yielding nutrients in the ruminant lamb. If energy intake is sufficient to permit growth and the rumen is provided with sufficient nitrogenous substrate to maximize microbial protein production, then the response to additional amino acid supply is variable (Sainz *et al.*, 1994; Hegarty *et al.*, 1999). At MEI close to or below maintenance, where fat accretion is unlikely, an increase in postruminal amino acid supply has been shown to stimulate protein accretion (albeit to low levels) relative to fat accretion (Vipond *et al.*, 1989). However, even when substantial oversupply of amino acid is provided at low energy intake, the dominant fate of those amino acids is transamination, followed by conversion to energy-yielding substrates, including glucose (Oddy *et al.*, 1997).

In the free-ranging ruminant, supply of additional amino acid postruminally may lead to increased feed intake. If this occurs with low-quality (i.e. M/D < 8) roughages, feed intake will increase until rumen fill provides a ceiling on intake. Although there may be a small increase in body-protein deposition, most of the observed live-weight gain is rumen and intestine contents and associated increase in visceral weight (see Edwards *et al.*, 1989a, b). Intestinal tissues (portal-drained viscera) and liver have higher specific-energy expenditure (expressed as mol oxygen $(\text{kg}\cdot\text{min})^{-1}$) than peripheral tissues and skeletal muscle (Koong *et al.*, 1982). Accordingly, where the nutrient density of a feed is lower and internal organ weights are relatively greater, maintenance costs are higher and body gains are lower relative to animals consuming the same energy and amino acid supply in a more digestible feed.

Compensatory Growth

Most of the scientific literature on quantitative growth of animals is concerned with continuous growth. However, animals frequently undergo periods of nutrient restriction, followed by times of plenty. Growth is impaired during times of low feed quantity or quality, or both, and then improves when feed becomes abundant and of higher quality (realimentation). In some sheep-production systems, there are also significant effects of parasitic disease on lamb growth. Growth in the realimentation phase is often faster and more efficient than normal; this is called compensatory growth (Fig. 11.8). Animals undergoing compensatory growth may or may not recover the weight lost during the period of restriction. Where growth restriction occurs early in an animal's life or when it occurs for a prolonged period of time, animals may never achieve the same weight (Table 11.2) or body composition as unrestricted controls (Table 11.3). Growth restriction due to inadequate nutrition or disease is a regular occurrence in extensive situations, and compensatory growth is accepted as part of the production system. In many environments, producers depend upon compensatory growth to allow catch-up, and animals are generally not supplemented when feed supply restricts growth. Prediction of subsequent growth and body composition of lambs affected by previous growth retardation is a challenge to current feeding systems.

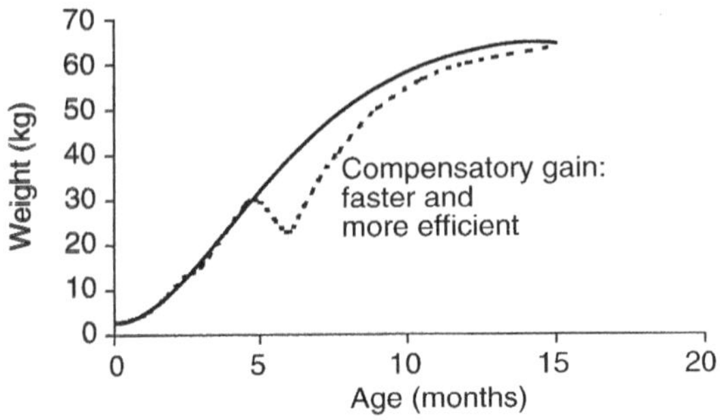

Fig. 11.8. An example of normal and compensatory gain in lambs.

Table 11.2. The effect of timing of nutritional setback relative to maturity on the degree of liveweight compensation in cattle (from R.M. Herd and V.H. Oddy, 1997, unpublished results).

Maturity at onset of restriction[a]	Compensation[b]
0.69	1.00
0.39	0.95
0.39	0.93
0.3	0.76

[a]Maturity = weight at onset of restriction/estimated mature weight (standard reference weight).
[b]Compensation = end weight of group of compensating animals/end weight of control group.

The composition of compensatory gain in lambs, at least in the period immediately after refeeding, contains more protein than in continuously grown lambs (Hegarty *et al.*, 1999). The rate of fat deposition may not differ in compensating and continuously grown lambs at similar energy intakes but, because protein gain is higher, the proportion of energy stored as protein is higher in the compensating lambs (Fig. 11.9). Because of their higher protein gain, and thus higher water retention, liveweight gain per unit energy available for production is higher in compensating lambs. The efficiency of energy retention is unchanged (Oddy, 1997) or may even be increased in compensating lambs (see Table 11.4).

Provision of additional dietary protein (as formaldehyde-treated casein) to compensating lambs did not increase feed intake, rate of liveweight gain or rate of protein deposition in the above studies. Neither compensating nor normally grown lambs showed significant responses to amino acid supply above that provided by microbial protein production from energy intake (Hegarty *et al.*, 1999). The data indicate that protein deposition in lambs, over the weight range studied, was more sensitive to energy than to amino acid supply. It is possible that in these studies amino

Table 11.3. Effect of growth impairment relative to maturity on subsequent growth and body composition and potential effects on composition of nutrient supply (from P.L. Greenwood and V.H. Oddy, 1999, unpublished lecture notes).

Growth check before 40% maturity	Growth check after 40% maturity
Reduce the long-term capacity to grow muscle and bone	Have little effect on the capacity to grow muscle and bone
During growth check body composition will shift to lower proportion of fatness	
On recovery predisposes to greater fatness due to:	On recovery will initially favour lean-tissue growth and lower proportion of fat deposition (compensatory growth)
Reduced capacity to grow lean tissues and impaired capacity to catch up	Enhanced lean-tissue growth but similar rates of fat deposition reduces proportion of fat in gain – capacity to catch up not impaired
Very high levels of feed intake per kg live weight upon resumption of improved nutrition may improve efficiency of feed utilization	Improved efficiency of feed utilization
Potentially high requirements for amino acids during early growth and recovery, which increases potential for nutritional imbalance in absorbed nutrients – principally too great a proportion of energy-yielding nutrients cf. amino acids	Relatively little effect on proportions of nutrients (amino acids cf. energy-yielding nutrients) for gain. May affect efficiency of nutrient utilization (see Table 11.4)

acid supply (from all sources – microbial and supplemented rumen-escape protein) was not limiting for protein deposition. What is remarkable is that rate of protein deposition in compensating lambs was almost double that of normally growing lambs at the same or lower predicted levels of amino acid availability. Perhaps, as Hodge (1974) observed in comparison of protein and fat deposition of non-ruminant lambs and piglets, protein deposition in lambs is indeed quite sensitive to energy supply, and efficiency of use of amino acids for body growth is limited by energy supply, even in older ruminant lambs.

Modelling Growth and Body Composition of Lambs

In order to make practical use of information on the effects of nutrition on the body composition of lambs, it must be integrated into a systematic framework. Computer simulations of sheep and lamb growth using empirical energy and protein feeding systems (e.g. Graham *et al.*, 1976) have evolved considerably since the early 1970s. Part of this process has been an increasing trend towards the incorporation of more mechanistic concepts, based on knowledge of the underlying biology, in the formulation of the equations used to represent animal function. This has been necessary because of the recognition of significant problems left unresolved by the

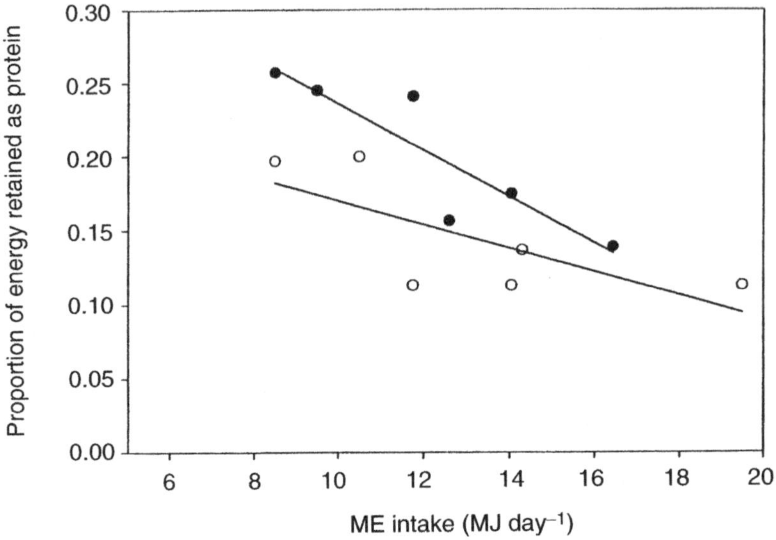

Fig. 11.9. The relationship between proportion of retained energy stored as protein and total metabolizable energy intake (MJ day^{-1}) in lambs with uninterrupted growth (open circles) and lambs exhibiting compensatory growth (closed circles). The values combine data from Hegarty *et al.* (1999) and from R.S. Hegarty, S.A. Neutze and V.H. Oddy (unpublished results).

Table 11.4. Effect on lambs[a] of previous nutrient restriction (Compensating)[b] compared to lack of restriction (Normal)[c] and the effect of diet[d] M/D (MJ kg^{-1}) on liveweight gain (LWG), protein gain and fat gain. Mean daily values are shown for ME intake and estimated ME available for production (ME_p), and the ratio of energy retained in protein to total energy retention after adjustment for ME_p per kg live weight$^{0.75}$ (ProtE/E). (From Hegarty *et al.*, 1999, and unpublished results by these authors.)

	ME intake (MJ day^{-1})	ME_p (MJ day^{-1})	LWG (g day^{-1})	Protein gain (g day^{-1})	Fat gain (g day^{-1})	ProtE/E
Regimen						
Compensating	12.9 ± 0.3	5.7 ± 0.2	219 ± 6	21.2 ± 0.7	65.4 ± 2.3	0.18 ± 0.01
Normal	14.8 ± 0.3	6.4 ± 0.2	154 ± 6	15.5 ± 0.7	62 ± 2.3	0.15 ± 0.01
M/D of diet						
7.7	10.0 ± 0.3	2.5 ± 0.2	149 ± 6	13.7 ± 0.8	31.3 ± 2.6	0.23 ± 0.02
9.2	13.4 ± 0.4	5.8 ± 0.3	174 ± 7	17.7 ± 0.9	61.6 ± 3.0	0.15 ± 0.01
10.9	18.0 ± 0.4	9.8 ± 0.3	237 ± 7	23.8 ± 0.9	98.1 ± 2.9	0.11 ± 0.02

[a]Lambs were second-cross Dorset Horn × (Merino × Border Leicester) desexed males, 20 weeks of age at the start.
[b]Compensating lambs weighed 27.7 ± 0.3 kg at the start and 47.5 ± 0.6 kg at the end of the 90-day feeding period.
[c]Normal lambs were 39.6 ± 0.3 kg at the start and 53.5 ± 0.6 kg at the end of the feeding period.
[d]The diets were pelleted and contained soluble protein in excess of that calculated to meet expected rumen microbial protein production, plus, on average, 45 g day^{-1} of formaldehyde-treated casein.

earlier models, which were very largely built on data from whole-animal studies. These problems include variance in apparent maintenance requirements, the effect of differences in the proportions of fat and protein on the efficiency of tissue accretion, the effects of age and previous plane of nutrition on current and future performance and the optimization of protein availability to producing animals.

Resolution of these problems will require greater use in our models of concepts derived from studies conducted at the tissue, cellular and subcellular levels. Significant progress towards this end has been achieved in recent years and it appears that a progressive increase in the mechanistic elements in the various feeding-system models will improve their accuracy of prediction and general applicability.

The components to be included and the principles upon which our current methods mechanistically model sheep growth were enunciated by Baldwin and Black (1979), as set out below.

1. The primary genetic determinant of organ size is the final number of cells, i.e. amount of DNA. It follows that a difference in organ size between species or between strains within a species is due largely to the amount of DNA observed in that organ in normally grown adults.
2. Each unit of DNA specifies, on a genetically defined basis for each tissue and each species, information required for the ultimate formation of a specific amount of cell material. Whether information specified by a unit of DNA leads to the formation of cell material depends on the nutritional and physiological status of the animal.
3. The specific activities, expressed as units per gram of tissue, of enzymes or groups of enzymes responsible for tissue growth and general metabolism vary as an exponential function of organ size.

In practice, the measurements required to implement models based on these principles cannot be made directly for groups of animals and for groups of feeds and it cannot be assumed that the nutrient supply from the digestion of a specific feed is the same across different animal genotypes. Accordingly, simpler dynamic approaches have been sought. For example, in the model developed by Oltjen *et al.* (1986a) for steers, body protein gain (ΔP) was represented as the difference between protein synthesis and degradation, with synthesis depending on the amount of DNA present at the time (see Equation (5) below). The daily increase (ΔD) in DNA is predicted as a function (Equation (4)) of the difference between the DNA mass at maturity (D_{max}) and the current DNA (D) and is modified by the level of nutrition. The nutritional factors (N_1 and N_2) that affect synthesis of protein and ΔD have a value of 1.0 if feed is offered *ad libitum*. At lower intakes, N_1 and N_2 are predicted from the ratio (R) of MEI to the ceiling intake (Equations (6) and (7)), based on data of Oltjen *et al.* (1986b). The rate constants (k_1, k_2 and k_3) are adjusted for mature body size, according to the scaling factor proposed by Taylor (1980) and k_2 can be modified if the rate of protein gain is increased by hormonal growth promotants.

$$\Delta D = k_1(D_{max} - D)N_1 \tag{4}$$

$$\Delta P = k_2D^{0.73}N_2 - k_3P^{0.73} \tag{5}$$

$$N_1 = -0.7 + 1.7R \tag{6}$$

$$N_2 = 0.83 + 0.2R/(0.15 + R) \tag{7}$$

Finally, daily gain (kg) in fat (ΔF) (energy content 39.27 MJ kg^{-1}) in the empty body is calculated in Equation (8) as the net energy, retained with an efficiency k_g, after the intake of ME (MJ) is used for maintenance (ME_m) and protein gain (23.18 MJ kg^{-1}).

$$\Delta F = ((MEI - ME_m)k_g - 23.18\Delta P)/39.27 \tag{8}$$

This model is equivalent to the NRC (1996) energy-utilization model, with mechanistic elements added to represent body composition. Since the model requires initial estimates of whole-body DNA, protein and fat, empirical relationships between these and animal weight, mature size and condition score are used to set starting values. The model accounts for variations attributable to initial body composition and mature size but does not always yield acceptable estimates of fat gain. This is not unexpected, as fat gain is predicted by difference and is therefore subject to errors in the estimates of maintenance and protein gain. Moreover, the model takes no account of the differences discussed earlier in the efficiency of retention of net energy as protein and fat.

To overcome these problems, an international team is currently collaborating in the design of a dynamic model of growth and body composition in the growing lamb (Soboleva *et al.*, 1999). In a particularly simple approach, two protein pools, viscera (V), with a fast turnover and a high rate of energy expenditure per kg, and muscle (M), with a slow turnover and a lower rate of energy expenditure, are represented in coupled differential equations. As with earlier models, fat deposition is determined by difference, after the prediction of visceral and muscle tissue gain. Upper bounds, V_{max} and M_{max}, are specified for viscera and muscle, respectively. For viscera, the upper bound is affected by current energy intake and previous nutrition and, while M_{max} is genetically determined, the possibility of reaching this level depends on current and previous nutrition. The model was developed using data for growth, body composition and heat production of ram lambs eating different amounts of feed (Ferrell *et al.*, 1986).

In the model, the energy retained as muscle and viscera is calculated as MEI less the total heat production for both maintenance and gain. The heat production for maintenance (H_m) is predicted from empty body weight (EBW) and MEI (Equation (9)) but is modified for changing level of intake according to Equation (10). This results in a lag in the change in maintenance requirements after intake changes from MEI_0 to MEI_t after time t (days) (Fig. 11.10). However, this model still assumes a constant efficiency of use of ME for gain, which we have already shown to be unlikely.

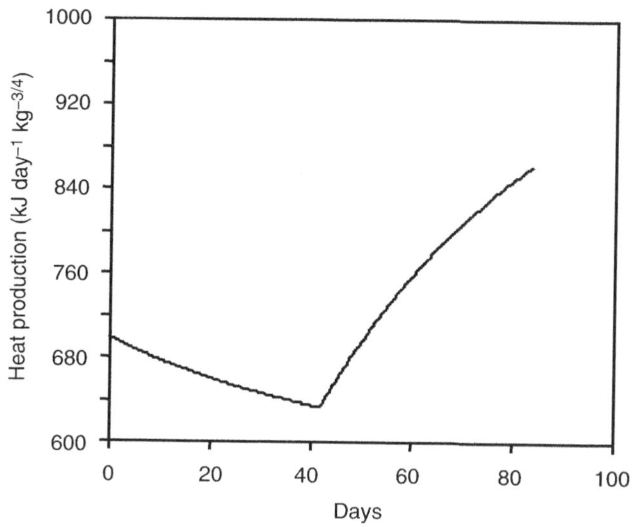

Fig. 11.10. Predicted pattern of change in heat production at maintenance in growing ram lambs eating less than maintenance energy intake for 40 days and then approximately twice maintenance thereafter. Values are simulated by the model of Soboleva *et al.* (1999) from data of Ferrell *et al.* (1986).

$$H_m = a_t \mathrm{EBW}^{0.75} + 0.09\mathrm{MEI} \tag{9}$$

$$a_t = a_0(1 + b(\mathrm{MEI}_t/\mathrm{MEI}_0 - 1)(1 - \exp(-t/\tau))) \tag{10}$$

where b and τ are constants and a_0 and a_t are the maintenance parameters at time 0 and t, respectively.

It is possible to reformulate the model to calculate heat production from protein metabolism so that the requirement for an independent estimate of maintenance and assumptions about a fixed efficiency of protein gain are removed. This approach was used by Knapp and Scharma (1996) to calculate heat production in various tissues of the pig. There are too few data to use this method directly with lambs; there are few experiments with adequate measurements of M and V, and their rates of accretion and heat production in response to nutrition. However, Ferrell *et al.* (1986) published data on 72 growing ram lambs that were used to estimate the relative contribution of M, V, dM/dt and dV/dt to heat production by multiple regression. The calculated regression coefficients for the four variables were, respectively, 1.017 (± 0.335), 10.54 (± 3.39), 61.1 (± 13.8) and 282.8 (± 91.6), with $r^2 = 0.987$.

It follows that heat production per kg V is much greater than for each kg M and is also much higher per unit gain of M or V than for the gross weights. This is consistent with direct observations of oxygen uptake per kg of viscera and muscle (Eisemann *et al.*, 1996). In the lamb growth model, V responds more than M to changing energy intake, with the result that maintenance requirement is a dynamic variable depending on nutritional history as well as current energy intake.

Comparative errors in estimating daily heat production from the model associated with Equations (9) and (10), compared with using the regression approach above, were, respectively, 0.133 and 0.105 MJ kg^{-1} $EBW^{0.75}$. This is a large improvement over the static maintenance functions used in traditional feeding systems, especially under variable nutritional conditions.

In summary, several dynamic, mechanistic models of animal growth are being developed for predictive purposes. As knowledge develops, these incorporate further levels of biological realism into existing empirical frameworks, with the intended, and usually achieved, result of improved applicability across a wider range of genotypes, physiological states, environmental conditions and dietary conditions.

Conclusion

Advances in the nutritional management of growing lambs for meat production will require a better understanding of the biology of growth and nutrient utilization. Meeting market specifications for weight, composition and quality involves achieving desired growth trajectories. Producers must optimize animal genotypes and their own feed resources in accordance with the demands of their markets. The number and complexity of these interactions is best accommodated using dynamic, mechanistic models that incorporate some degree of biological realism to aid decision making.

References

ARC (1980) *The Nutrient Requirements of Ruminant Livestock*. Commonwealth Agricultural Bureaux, Farnham Royal, UK, 351 pp.

Arthur, P.F., Archer, J.A.M., Herd, R.M. and Richardson, E.C. (1998) A review of variation in feed efficiency of beef cattle. In: *Proceedings of the 6th World Congress of Genetics Applied to Livestock Production* 25. University of New England, Armidale, pp. 85–88.

Baldwin, R.L. and Black, J.L. (1979) *Simulation of the Effects of Nutritional and Physiological Status on the Growth of Mammalian Tissues: Description and Evaluation of a Computer Program*. Technical Paper 6, Australian Animal Research Laboratories, Commonwealth Scientific and Industrial Research Organization, Melbourne, 35 pp.

Bernier, J.F., Calvert, C.C., Famula, T.R. and Baldwin, R.L. (1987) Energetic efficiency of protein and fat deposition in mice with a major gene for rapid postweaning gain. *Journal of Nutrition* 117, 539–548.

Black, J.L. (1983) Growth and development of lambs. In: Haresign, W. (ed.) *Sheep Production*. Butterworths, London, pp. 21–58.

Black, J.L. and Griffiths, D.A. (1975) Effects of liveweight and energy intake on nitrogen balance and total N requirement of lambs. *British Journal of Nutrition* 33, 399–413.

Blaxter, K.L. and Boyne, A.W. (1978) The estimation of the nutritive value of feeds as energy sources for ruminants and the derivation of feeding systems. *Journal of Agricultural Science, Cambridge* 90, 47–68.

Butterfield, R.M. (1988) *New Concepts of Sheep Growth.* Griffin Press, Netley, South Australia.

Buttery, P.J. and Annison, E.F. (1973) Considerations of the efficiency of the amino acid and protein metabolism in animals. In: Jones, J.G.W. (ed.) *The Biological Efficiency of Protein Production.* Cambridge University Press, Cambridge, pp. 141–172.

Corbett, J.L., Freer, M. and Graham, N.McC. (1987) A generalised equation to predict the varying maintenance metabolism of sheep and cattle. In: Moe, P.W., Tyrrell, H.F. and Reynolds, P.J (eds) *Energy Metabolism.* EAAP Publication No. 32, Rowman and Littlefield, Totowa, New Jersey, pp. 62–65.

Dawkins, R. (1983) *The Extended Phenotype.* Oxford University Press, Oxford.

Edwards, S.R., Neutze, S.A., Oddy, V.H., Warren, H.M. and Nandra, K.S. (1989a) Escape protein supplementation of lambs. I. Differential response in gastrointestinal tract and contents. *Proceedings of the Nutrition Society of Australia* 14, 137.

Edwards, S.R., Oddy, V.H., Neutze, S.A., Riley, K.D. and Jones, A.W. (1989b) Escape protein supplementation of lambs. II. Differential response in organ weight. *Proceedings of the Nutrition Society of Australia* 14, 138.

Eisemann, J.H., Huntington, G.B. and Catherman, D.R. (1996) Patterns of nutrient exchange and oxygen use among portal-drained viscera, liver and hindquarters of beef steers from 235 to 525 kg body weight. *Journal of Animal Science* 74, 1812–1831.

Ferrell, C.L., Koong, L.J. and Nienaber, J.A. (1986) Effect of previous nutrition on body composition and maintenance energy costs of growing lambs. *British Journal of Nutrition* 56, 595–605.

Goll, D.E., Thompson, V.F., Taylor, R.G. and Christiansen, J.A. (1992) Role of the calpain system in muscle growth. *Biochimie* 74, 225–237.

Graham, N.M.C., Black, J.L., Faichney, G.J. and Arnold, G.W. (1976) Simulation of growth and production in sheep – model 1. *Agricultural Systems* 1, 113–138.

Hegarty, R.S., Neutze, S.A. and Oddy, V.H. (1999) Effects of protein and energy supply on the growth and carcass composition of lambs from differing nutritional histories. *Journal of Agricultural Science, Cambridge* 132, 361–375.

Herd, R.M. (1992) Changing the size of beef cattle – implications for cow feed requirements. *Proceedings of the Australian Association of Animal Breeding and Genetics* 10, 334–337.

Herd, R.M., Oddy, V.H. and Lee, G.J. (1993) Effect of divergent selection for weaning weight on liveweight and wool growth responses to feed intake in Merino ewes. *Australian Journal of Experimental Agriculture* 33, 699–705.

Hodge, R.W. (1974) Efficiency of food conversion and body composition of the preruminant lamb and the young pig. *British Journal of Nutrition* 32, 113–126.

Kahn, L.P. (1996) Differences between Merino selection lines in microbial yield from the rumen and utilisation of protein for wool growth. PhD thesis, University of New England, Australia.

Kempster, A.J., Croston, D., Guy, D.R. and Jones, D.W. (1987) Growth and carcass characteristics of crossbred lambs by ten sire breeds, compared at the same estimated subcutaneous fat proportion. *Animal Production* 44, 39–49.

Kielanowski, J. (1965) Estimates of the energy cost of protein deposition in growing animals. In: Blaxter, K.L. (ed.) *Energy Metabolism.* Academic Press, London, pp. 13–20.

Knapp, P.W. and Scharma, J.W. (1996) Simulation of growth in pigs: approximation of protein turnover parameters. *Animal Science* 63, 533–547.

Koohmaraie, M., Shackleford, S.D., Wheeler, T.L., Lonergan, S.M. and Doumit, M.E. (1995) A muscle hypertrophy condition in lamb (callipyge): characterization of effects on muscle growth and meat quality traits. *Journal of Animal Science* 73, 3596–3607.

Koong, L.J., Ferrell, C.L. and Nienaber, J.A. (1982) Effects of plane of nutrition on organ size and fasting heat production in swine and sheep. In: *Energy Metabolism of Farm Animals*. EAAP Publication 29, Agriculture University, Ås, Norway, pp. 245–248.

Lines, E.W. and Pierce, A.W. (1931) *The Basal (Standard) Metabolism of the Australian Merino Sheep*. Bulletin No. 55, Council for Scientific and Industrial Research, Melbourne.

Lush, J.M., Gooden, J.M. and Annison, E.F. (1991) The uptake of nitrogenous compounds from the gut of sheep genetically different in wool production. *Proceedings of the Nutrition Society of Australia* 16, 144.

McDonagh, M.B., Fernandez, C. and Oddy, V.H. (1999) Hind-limb protein metabolism and calpain system activity influence post-mortem changes in meat quality of lamb. *Meat Science* 52, 9–18.

Nielsen, M.K. (1998) Genetic variation in feed energy utilisation in mice. In: *Proceedings of the 6th World Congress of Genetics Applied to Livestock Production* 26. University of New England, Armidale, pp. 89–96

NRC (1981) *Nutritional Energetics of Domestic Animals and Glossary of Energy Terms*. National Academy Press, Washington, DC.

NRC (1985) *Nutrient Requirements of Sheep*, 6th edn. National Academy Press, Washington, DC.

NRC (1996) *Nutritional Requirements of Beef Cattle*, 7th edn. National Research Council, Washington, DC, 242 pp.

Oddy, V.H. (1986) Protein metabolism in lambs. PhD thesis, University of Cambridge, Cambridge.

Oddy, V.H. (1993) Regulation of muscle protein metabolism in sheep and lambs: nutritional, endocrine and genetic aspects. *Australian Journal of Agricultural Research* 44, 901–913.

Oddy, V.H. (1997) Efficiency and compensatory growth. In: Hennessy, D.W., McLennan, S.R. and Oddy, V.H. (eds) *Growth and Development of Cattle: Proceedings of the Growth and Development Workshop*. The Cattle and Beef Industry Co-operative Research Centre, Armidale, Australia, pp. 29–32.

Oddy, V.H. (1999) Protein metabolism and nutrition in farm animals: an overview. In: Lobley, G.E., White, A. and MacRae, J.C. (eds) *Protein Metabolism and Nutrition, Proceedings of the VIIIth International Symposium on Protein Metabolism and Nutrition*. EAAP Publication No. 96, Wageningen Pers, The Netherlands, pp. 7–23.

Oddy, V.H., Warren, H.M., Ewoldt, C.L. and Riley, K.D. (1989) Pre-weaning growth and body composition of lambs genetically different in weight at weaning. *Proceedings of the Nutrition Society of Australia* 14, 139.

Oddy, V.H., Speck, P.A., Warren, H.M. and Wynn, P.C. (1995) Protein metabolism in lambs from lines divergently selected for weaning weight. *Journal of Agricultural Science, Cambridge* 124, 129–137.

Oddy, V.H., Edwards, S.R., Warren, H.M., Speck, P.A., Nicholls, P.J. and Neutze, S.A. (1997) Interrelationships between amino acid and glucose metabolism in lambs of different dietary history supplemented with rumen escape protein. *Journal of Agricultural Science, Cambridge* 128, 105–116.

Oltjen, J.W., Bywater, A.C., Baldwin, R.L. and Garrett, W.N. (1986a) Development of a dynamic model of beef cattle growth and composition. *Journal of Animal Science* 62, 86–97.

Oltjen, J.W., Bywater, A.C. and Baldwin, R.L. (1986b) Evaluation of a model of beef cattle growth and composition. *Journal of Animal Science* 62, 98–108.

Ørskov, E.R., McDonald, I., Grubb, D.A. and Pennie, K. (1976) The nutrition of the early weaned lamb IV. Effects on growth rate, food utilization and body composition of changing from a low to high protein diet. *Journal of Agricultural Science, Cambridge* 86, 411–423.

Owens, F.N., Gill, D.R., Secrist, D.S. and Coleman, S.W. (1995) Review of some aspects of growth and development of feedlot cattle. *Journal of Animal Science* 73, 3152–3172.

Pain, V.M. and Clemens, M.J. (1980) Mechanism and regulation of protein biosynthesis in eukaryotic cells. In: Buttery, P.J. and Lindsay, D.B. (eds) *Protein Deposition in Animals*. Butterworths, London, pp. 1–20.

Palsson, H. (1955) Conformation and body composition. In: Hammond, J. (ed.) *Progress in the Physiology of Farm Animals*, Vol. 2. Butterworths, London, pp. 430–542.

Palsson, H. and Verges, J.B. (1952) Effects of plane of nutrition on growth and the development of carcass quality in lambs. Part 1. The effects of high and low planes of nutrition at different ages. *Journal of Agricultural Science, Cambridge* 42, 1–92.

Rattray, P.V., Garrett, W.N. and Hinman, N. (1974) Energy cost of protein and fat deposition in sheep. *Journal of Animal Science* 33, 378–382.

Sainz, R.D. and Wolff, J.E. (1990) Development of a dynamic, mechanistic model of lamb metabolism and growth. *Animal Production* 51, 535–549.

Sainz, R.D., Wolff, J.E. and Upsdell, M.P. (1990) Effects of cimaterol on energy utilization for maintenance and for protein and fat depostion by wether and ewe lambs given chopped lucerne hay or lucerne–barley pellets. *Animal Production* 50, 129–139.

Sainz, R.D., Hosking, B.J., Hart, F.J. and Schricker, B.R. (1994) Exogenous growth hormone releasing factors and cottonseed meal improve growth performance and composition of gain in lambs fed lucerne chaff *ad libitum*. *Australian Journal of Agricultural Research* 45, 1111–1123.

SCA (1990) *Feeding Standards for Australian Livestock. Ruminants*. Standing Committee on Agriculture and CSIRO, Melbourne, 266 pp.

Soboleva, T.K., Oddy, V.H., Pleasants, A.B., Oltjen, J.W., Ball, A.J. and McCall, D.G. (1999) A dynamical model of body composition in sheep. *Proceedings of the New Zealand Society of Animal Production* 59, 275–278.

Taylor, StC.S. (1980) Genetic size scaling rules in animal growth. *Animal Production* 30, 160–165.

Thomson, B.C., Hosking, B., Sainz, R.D. and Oddy, V.H. (1997) The effect of nutritional status on protein degradation and components of the calpain system in skeletal muscle of weaned wether lambs. *Journal of Agricultural Science, Cambridge* 129, 471–477.

Tulloh, N.M., Brimblecombe, H. and Denniss, C. (1986) The effect of severe nutritional deprivation in early post-natal life: tissue and cellular responses during subsequent growth of lambs to the age of 4 months. *Journal of Agricultural Science, Cambridge* 106, 341–350.

Vernon, R.G. (1986) The growth and metabolism of adipocytes. In: Buttery, P.J., Haynes, N.B. and Lindsay, D.B. (eds) *Control and Manipulation of Animal Growth*. Butterworths, London, pp. 67–84.

Vipond, J.E., King, M.E., Orskov, E.R. and Wetherill, G.Z. (1989) Effects of fishmeal supplementation on performance of overfat lambs fed on barley straw to reduce carcass fatness. *Animal Production* 48, 131–138.

Waterlow, J.C., Garlick, P.J. and Millward, D.J. (1978) *Protein Turnover in Mammalian Tissues and in the Whole Body*. Elsevier North Holland, Amsterdam.

Webster, A.J.F. (1984) Energetics of maintenance and growth. In: Giradier, L. and Stock, J. (eds) *Mammalian Thermogenesis*. Chapman & Hall, London, pp. 178–207.

12 Nutrition of Sheep under Rangeland Conditions

P.J. O'Reagain[1] and N.P. McMeniman[2]

[1]*Queensland Beef Industry Institute, Department of Primary Industries, Charters Towers, Queensland, Australia;* [2]*School of Veterinary Science, University of Queensland, Brisbane, Queensland, Australia*

Introduction

Rangelands support a significant proportion of the world's sheep population and play a vital role in supporting low-cost, low-input, wool- and meat-production systems. The definition of what constitutes a rangeland is somewhat subjective, but for present purposes rangelands are broadly defined as any extensive, uncultivated and/or unfertilized area that supports production by large herbivores. This definition thus excludes deserts or forests and any cultivated or intensively managed pastures.

The world's rangelands are extremely diverse and may vary from semiarid shrublands, such as the chenopod shrublands of South Australia, to cool, temperate grasslands, such as those that occur in Mongolia, tropical savannahs, such as those that occur in Africa, or semiarid shrub steppe, such as those of Patagonia. Despite this diversity, most rangelands have a number of unifying characteristics that have important consequences for sheep nutrition and production in these environments and distinguish these systems from the more intensive systems based on cultivated pastures.

First, most rangelands are extensive and have limited infrastructure, such as fences and handling facilities. Further, carrying capacity and animal performance on most rangelands is relatively low when compared with that on cultivated pastures. This is due to basic biophysical constraints, such as rainfall and soil conditions, on productivity. Consequently, any management inputs, ranging from nutrient supplementation to land management, need to be cheap, easy to deliver and as simple as possible.

Secondly, all rangelands display marked spatial and temporal variability in both forage quality and supply. This variability occurs at a range of levels that vary from the plant part upwards to the plant, patch and landscape scales and over time-scales ranging from seasons to years. Although variability may also occur in cultivated pastures, it seldom, if ever, approaches the range and complexity commonly found in rangelands.

Thirdly, nearly all rangelands are characterized by the presence of poisonous or toxic plants. These may vary in toxicity from being lethal to causing subclinical depressions in animal performance. Plant toxicoses occasionally occur when animals consume cultivated pastures – for example, fescue toxicosis. However, with some exceptions, e.g. phalaris toxicity (see Waghorn *et al.*, Chapter 15, this volume), the toxic effects are usually a product of some other process, such as endophyte infection or nitrate accumulation, rather than plant toxicity *per se*.

Fourthly, in contrast to more intensive systems, drinking water is often poorly distributed in rangelands and may thus severely limit dry matter (DM) intake and hence animal production. Provision and distribution of water therefore often assume major importance for sheep production in rangeland environments.

Finally, resource management is of major significance in rangelands and has the potential to have major and sometimes irreversible impacts upon vegetation composition and structure and hence sheep nutrition. Although the productivity and composition of cultivated pastures also depend on management, a range of effective and economic interventions, such as reseeding and fertilization, are available that can largely ameliorate or remedy the consequences of poor management.

This chapter addresses these specific problems associated with the nutrition of sheep on rangelands and also the use of supplementary feeding to correct nutrient deficiencies for sheep grazing in these environments.

Variability in Feed Quality and Intake

Spatial variability in forage quality and supply

Plant level

On rangelands, sheep have access to a wide variety of plants, which may include some or all of the following: grasses, forbs (i.e. herbs other than grasses), shrubs and low-growing trees and even plant litter. These different classes vary widely in diet quality, both in nutrients and in their content of toxins and secondary chemicals, such as tannins (e.g. Cooper *et al.*, 1988).

Generally, forbs and shrub foliage are of higher digestibility and have higher levels of crude protein (CP) than grasses at similar stages of maturity (Table 12.1), probably due to higher levels of cell solubles and quicker access to this fraction by microbes. However, the extent of digestion of shrub material may be reduced through greater lignification. In forbs and shrubs, secondary chemicals, such as tannins, are also abundant and may suppress digestibility, even of higher-quality plant material (Holechek *et al.*, 1989).

Table 12.1. Examples of nitrogen concentration in the dry matter (N) and dry matter digestibility (DMD) of some common forage species in the wet and dry seasons on different rangelands (G, grass; S, shrub; F, forb).

	Species	Forage type	Composition	Wet season (%)	Dry season (%)
Australia					
Tropical savanna[a]	*Heteropogon*	G	N	2.1	0.6
	contortus	G	DMD	65	37
Mitchell grasslands[b]	*Astrebla* spp.	G	N	2.1	1.3
South Africa					
'Sour' grassland[c]	Mixed grasses	G	N	1.99	0.38
		G	DMD	69	40
Karoo shrubland[d]	*Stipagrostis obtusa*	G	N	1.68	0.52
	Pentzia incana	S	N	1.79	0.91
North America					
Temperate shrubland[e]	Mixed grasses	G	N	1.12	0.80
	Mixed shrubs	S	N	1.77	1.12
	Mixed grasses	G	DMD	53	42
	Mixed shrubs	S	DMD	55	41
Subtropical shrubland[f]	Mixed grasses	G	N	1.28	0.8
	Forbs	F	N	3.04	1.76
	Mixed grasses	G	DMD	44	31
	Forbs	F	DMD	59	53

[a]McIvor (1981); [b]Weston and Moir (1969); [c]O'Reagain *et al.* (1996); [d]Louw (1969); [e]Huston *et al.* (1981) and [f]Krysl *et al.* (1984), both cited in Holechek *et al.* (1989).

Even within a particular group of plants, such as grasses, individual plant species may vary widely in quality, mineral content, rate of ruminal degradation and secondary chemical content. Different species also vary widely in structural characteristics, such as leaf density, height, stemminess and thorniness, and hence in the rate at which animals can ingest them. For example, some grass species form a low-growing carpet of easily harvested leaf, while others may be tall and stemmy with leaves highly interspersed with stem and dead material. Even within species, there may be marked variability in plant structure and leaf quality, due to local differences in soil characteristics or differences in defoliation history between plants.

Sheep grazing on rangelands are highly selective and select strongly for some plant species while avoiding or rejecting others. Whereas sheep tend to be mixed feeders, consuming a range of grasses, forbs and browse, if available, the diets of cattle and goats tend to be dominated by grasses and browse, respectively.

For grasses, species acceptability appears to be determined by the interplay between leaf quality and the rate at which leaf can be harvested by the grazing animal. For example, sheep grazing the low-quality 'sour' grasslands in South Africa select short, non-stemmy species with high-quality leaves of low tensile strength. In contrast, tall, stemmy grass species with tough, low-quality leaves are avoided (O'Reagain, 1993). For forbs and shrubs, secondary chemicals are also likely to be important in species selection (Cooper *et al.*, 1988). Physical structures, such as thorns and spines, that reduce bite size and intake rates are also likely to be important and may strongly modify selection for forb and browse species. With sheep, as with other grazing and browsing ungulates, this selection appears to be based on the balance between nutrient content and the physical and metabolic costs of harvesting a particular plant species (O'Reagain, 2001).

On any rangeland, the different plant species encountered vary widely in their ability to support animal production, as would be expected from the large differences in ingestion rate and nutrient content recorded between species. Simulation of the potential animal production available from nine different African grasses indicated that a very large range in potential weight gains could be expected from different grasses (O'Reagain, 1996a). For example, while sheep in summer (the local growing season) could be expected to gain about 25 g day^{-1} grazing *Themeda triandra*, they would lose about 5 g day^{-1} grazing *Eragrostis plana*. Interestingly, the study also indicated that in winter none of the grass species compared were capable of providing maintenance energy or protein requirements for sheep, emphasizing the low quality of these grasslands.

Patch level

Most rangelands comprise a complex mosaic of patches that vary widely in sward structure or species composition, or both, and hence in the quality and availability of herbage to the grazing animal. In general, most patchiness arises from underlying variation in soil properties, such as fertility, texture or soil depth. This variability is compounded by various biotic processes, of which the most important is grazing. Selective grazing of certain areas, e.g. patches of high fertility, creates a mosaic of grazed and ungrazed patches of varying sizes. Once initiated, such patches are maintained by grazing, with preferred patches remaining short while avoided patches become rank and stemmy (Bakker *et al.*, 1983). Patches, varying in size from a few centimetres to many hectares in extent, may also arise due to urine deposition, fire, the presence of trees or the actions of other animals, such as termites or prairie dogs (Jaramillo and Detling, 1992).

Sheep on rangelands consistently select high-quality, productive patches but strongly avoid low-quality, unproductive patches. With increasing patch biomass, bite size and hence the instantaneous rate of DM intake (IIR) increase until an asymptote is reached, beyond which IIR can increase no further, due to the constraints set by the size of the animal's mouth (Fig. 12.1). For example, research conducted in South African

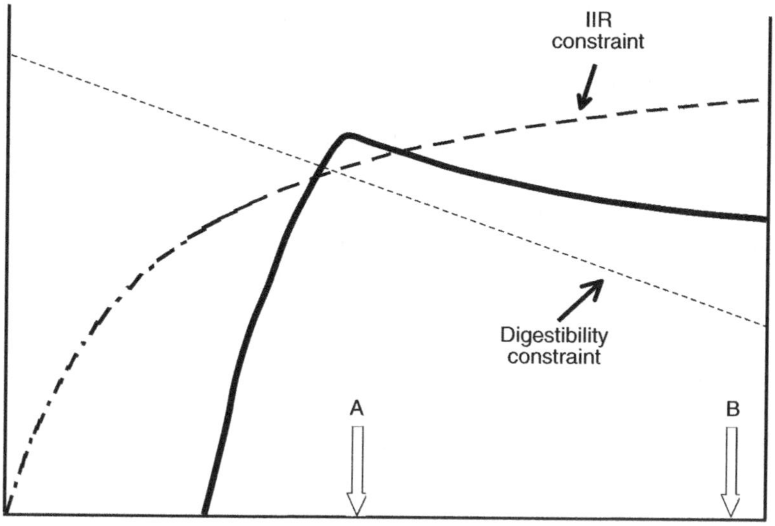

Fig. 12.1. Generalized depiction of the change in instantaneous intake rate (IIR) (dashed line), dietary *in vitro* digestibility (dotted line) and animal daily gain (solid line) with increasing sward height. A and B are the sward heights at which animal gain and IIR are maximized, respectively. (Adapted from O'Reagain, 1996a.)

grasslands indicates that sheep IIR increases with increasing patch height or biomass to reach an asymptote at a height of about 10 cm (O'Reagain, 1996b). However, on most pastures, herbage quality tends to decline with increasing biomass, resulting in a trade-off between IIR and the rate at which the material can be digested in the rumen. There should therefore be an optimum biomass or sward height on patches where the intake of digestible nutrients is maximized, given the opposing constraints of intake rate and herbage quality. Thus, on the 'sour' grasslands mentioned previously, simulation results suggest that sheep production should be maximized at sward heights considerably lower than the height at which IIR would be maximized (Fig. 12.1).

Landscape level

Most areas grazed by sheep in rangelands are extensive and may vary in size from a few hundred to many thousands of hectares. Spatial variability in feed quality and supply will thus also occur at the landscape level as well as at the plant and patch level. Landscapes are composed of landscape units, which may be defined as areas that differ in plant-species composition, soil fertility, depth, texture, rockiness or vegetation structure. As an example, a paddock may contain a combination of well-grassed, fertile alluvial plains, rocky slopes with low plant cover, ridge tops with shallow soil and mid-slopes of intermediate fertility and soil depth supporting open scrubland.

Superimposed over this landscape variability are other factors, such as the location of minerals and water, the location of shade and protection from the elements, barriers to movement, such as ravines or gullies, and predation refuges, such as thick undergrowth (Stuth, 1991). Provided water is available (see below) and barriers do not impede access by grazing animals, landscape selection is largely determined by the abundance of preferred plant species and the availability and quality of forage (Harrington, 1986). Animals thus appear to select landscape units that offer the greatest return per unit of foraging time invested.

Temporal variability in forage quality and supply

Short- to medium-term variability

As in more intensive pasture systems, sheep on rangelands frequently confront significant fluctuations in forage quality and supply, which may occur over time periods ranging from a few days to a few weeks. Such fluctuations may be natural and can result from normal biophysical processes, such as the changes in leaf nitrogen that may arise from short-term wetting and drying cycles in the soil (Heckathorn and DeLucia, 1994). However, the majority of changes that occur over this time-scale are animal-induced and simply result from the progressive depletion of the available forage through grazing.

In common with intensive pastures, grazing depletes overall forage availability resulting in a decline in bite size and bite quality. Sheep on rangelands commonly respond to such variability by simply shifting to other landscape units where forage is less restricted (Harrington, 1986). Where animals do not have access to other landscape units, either through fencing or because such units are already depleted, sheep may adopt a range of strategies, such as increasing biting rates or extending grazing time, in an attempt to maintain nutrient intakes (Roguet *et al.*, 1998).

However, in contrast to intensive pastures, the dominant effect of grazing in multispecies rangelands occurs at the plant rather than at the sward level. This results from the selective defoliation of the preferred plant species in the community and is manifested as a progressive change in the relative availability of different (ungrazed) species to the animal with time spent in a paddock.

The available evidence suggests that sheep follow a distinct three-phase pattern of species selection with time spent in a paddock (O'Reagain and Grau, 1995). Sheep first select the preferred plant species present and, to a limited extent, may also graze a few plants of intermediate acceptability in the paddock (Fig. 12.2). In the next phase, sheep graze the latter species in earnest and also regraze already defoliated plants of any preferred species present. In the third phase, sheep finally graze any species of low acceptability. This final phase is initiated only when the majority (> 80%) of all the plants of preferred and inter-

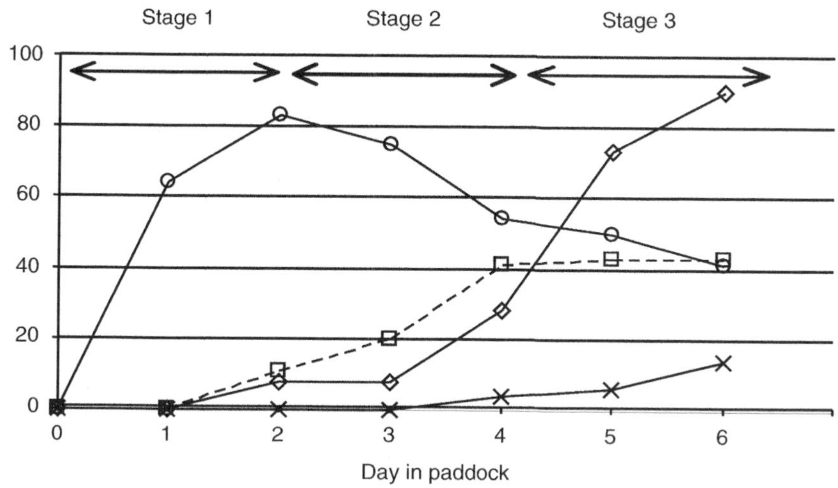

Fig. 12.2. Percentage of grass tillers of preferred species grazed either once (○) or twice (□), species of intermediate acceptability grazed once (◇) and avoided species grazed once (×), by sheep grazing a mesic grassland. (Adapted from O'Reagain and Grau, 1995.)

mediate acceptability have been grazed at least once. Evidence from other studies suggests that stocking density affects only the rate and not the sequence of selection (Stoltsz and Danckwerts, 1990). This sequence of species selection is likely to be considerably more complicated in larger rangeland paddocks with lower stocking densities or longer periods of stay in a paddock, or both. In certain situations, regrowth of the preferred species may occur following grazing. Under these conditions, animals may continually return to such regrowth without being forced to graze the intermediate or avoided species in the community.

At higher stocking densities or where regrowth is restricted, animal production is therefore likely to decline with time spent in a paddock as animals deplete the availability of better-quality species and are forced to consume lower-quality species in the community, depressing diet quality and hence nutrient intake. Simulation models of sheep grazing multispecies grassland strongly support this pattern but indicate that the rate and extent of the decline in animal production with time in a paddock is strongly dependent upon a number of factors (O'Reagain, 1996a). First, the inherent nutritive value of the plant species involved naturally determines both the upper and lower limits of the production that can be expected from a particular area. Secondly, the rate at which animal production will decline over a grazing period is directly determined by both the absolute and relative abundance of the different species in the rangeland. In practical terms, this means that animal production is likely to be maximized on rangelands with a high basal cover and a species composition dominated by high-quality, productive plant species.

Longer-term, intra-annual variability

Sheep on most, if not all, rangelands are confronted with major seasonal or intra-annual fluctuations in herbage quality and/or availability that occur over periods ranging from a few to many months. In some rangelands, these changes are largely associated with feed quality rather than feed availability. For example, in the high-rainfall 'sour' grasslands of southern Africa, the quality of winter forage may decline to such an extent that sheep lose significant amounts of body weight or may even starve to death, despite being surrounded by an apparent surfeit of feed. In other rangelands, shortages in both the quality and availability of feed may occur. Thus, in the semiarid shrub grasslands of East Africa, forage availability can decline by more than half and quality decline to submaintenance levels within 8 weeks of the end of the growing season (Schwartz, 1993).

Such intra-annual variability results from the coupling of plant growth and dormancy cycles to changes in temperature, light and soil-moisture availability in the environment. In most tropical rangelands, light and temperature are seldom limiting, so growth is largely a function of soil-moisture availability. In contrast, on temperate rangelands, temperature and, to some extent, day length are important determinants of productivity, and plant growth will not be initiated until certain threshold levels have been exceeded.

Whatever the relative importance of these factors for the rangeland environment, these seasonal fluctuations occur in four basic phases (Fig. 12.3). In phase 1, new leaf growth is initiated once both temperature and soil-moisture levels are adequate for plant growth. This leaf is usually of exceptionally high quality, partly due to its high content of non-structural carbohydrates and partly due to the ready availability of soil nitrogen at this stage. Many annual forbs or grasses may also germinate at this stage, further increasing forage quality. Herbage quality therefore increases rapidly to a peak, although availability may be restricted, due to the short and/or sparse nature of the growth characteristic of this phase. In phase 2, good growing conditions usually persist and herbage availability is usually high, due to the strong growth pulse initiated in the previous phase. Overall, forage quality is still high but starts to decline, due to increased leaf age, the depletion of plant-available nitrogen in the soil and a general decline in the leaf : stem ratio of the sward.

In phase 3, plant growth starts to decline or may cease altogether, due to the low availability of soil nitrogen and declining soil moisture and/or adverse changes in temperature. Most annual forbs or grasses set seed and die. Herbage quality declines rapidly, due to increased leaf senescence and the dilution of green leaf with increasing amounts of stem and dead material in the sward. In perennial grasses, this decline may be exacerbated by the translocation of nutrients and carbohydrates from leaves to crowns and roots in preparation for the approaching dormant season. In phase 4, growth ceases completely, due to adverse temperatures and/or restricted water availability. The availability of feed may consequently

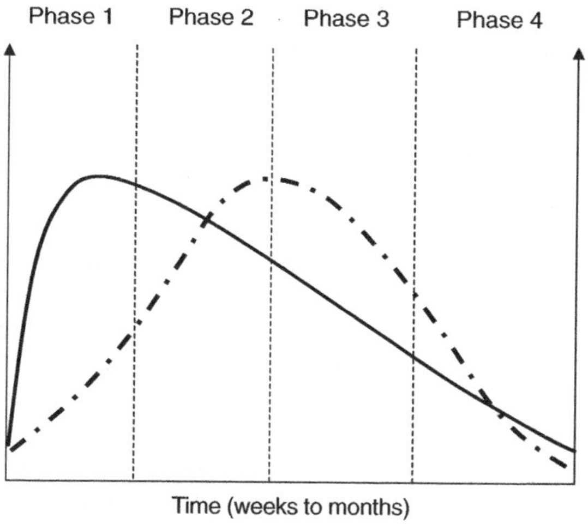

Fig. 12.3. Generalized depiction of the changes in forage quality (solid line) and availability (dashed line) encountered by sheep through the seasonal cycle on rangelands. Note that the overall changes in quality and availability, as well as phase length, are likely to vary significantly between different rangelands (see text for details).

decline, due to grazing and/or the weathering and loss of less-resistant leaf material from the pasture. Forage quality may similarly decline to a minimum, due to a lack of green leaf and the effects of adverse weather on standing herbage.

Although these basic phases are likely to hold for most situations, considerable variation in the shape, amplitude and periodicity of this basic curve may exist between different rangeland communities, according to the growing conditions that characterize a particular community. For example, rangelands with a very short growing season are likely to have a relatively longer phase 4 than those with a more extended season. Similarly, the amplitude of the curve is strongly dependent upon the biophysical characteristics of the community and will thus vary widely between different rangelands. Lastly, while these curves may be strongly cyclic and very predictable in rangelands that experience fairly regular, seasonal changes in growing conditions, e.g. some temperate systems, they are likely to be highly unpredictable in other systems where rainfall, for example, is aseasonal and has a high coefficient of variation.

Sheep, like all ungulates, have evolved a range of responses to cope with such seasonal variability and buffer the effects of such changes on nutrient intake (see O'Reagain and Schwartz, 1995). Animals may adjust foraging behaviour and increase grazing times in order to compensate for reduced availability (Allden and Whittaker, 1970) or may increase the time spent chewing and ruminating to improve the extent or rate of digestion of low-quality food. Increased particle retention time in the rumen, increased rumen capacity and improved urea recycling may also help sheep to cope with poor-quality forage (Lechner-Doll *et al.*, 1990).

However, possibly the most basic response for animals is to widen acceptance ranges and start utilizing plants, patches or different areas of the landscape that were previously avoided or only lightly utilized (O'Reagain, 2001). For example, in the mulga grasslands of Australia, the consumption of foliage from the leguminous shrub mulga (*Acacia aneura*) by sheep in the dry season allows them to maintain nitrogen intakes at a level considerably higher than that consumed by sheep with access to grass alone (McMeniman *et al.*, 1986a, b). Spatial variability at the plant, patch and landscape levels is thus a critical component of rangelands, in that it gives sheep the flexibility to buffer some of the temporal variability in nutrient supply that is characteristic of these environments (O'Reagain and Schwartz, 1995).

Despite a range of foraging and digestive strategies, sheep cannot eliminate but can only buffer the seasonal cycles in dietary quality and intake encountered on rangelands. Consequently, both wool and meat production tend to follow highly seasonal cycles in non-supplemented sheep, with maximum production in the early and mid-growing season, followed by low or zero production levels or even submaintenance levels in the dormant season (Lorimer, 1981).

Inter-seasonal variability

Most rangelands experience major inter-annual fluctuations in forage quality and supply, due to year-to-year variability in rainfall. In general, the coefficient of variation for rainfall is inversely correlated with mean annual precipitation (e.g. Tyson, 1986), so inter-annual variability tends to increase with decreasing rainfall. This can lead to huge inter-seasonal variability in arid and semiarid areas, with, for example, herbage production varying by up to four- to sixfold between years in some drier areas of Australia and Africa (e.g. Harrington, 1986; Freudenberger *et al.*, 1999). Such variability obviously has major consequences for nutrient intake and, hence, animal production. In dry years, liveweight gain, wool production and lambing percentages may be depressed (Freudenberger *et al.*, 1999), while, in extreme drought years, extensive animal mortality can occur unless there is substantial management intervention.

Paradoxically, while herbage availability is generally high in years with above-average rainfall, nutrient restrictions may still occur in such seasons, due to the low quality of the available feed. These so-called 'protein droughts' occur partly because of the dilution of the available nitrogen in the abundant plant material and partly because of the low leaf : stem ratios that commonly occur in such rank, overgrown swards. Animal production may thus show a quadratic relationship with rainfall, with production being maximized in years of intermediate precipitation (Fynn and O'Connor, 2000).

Although rainfall is the primary determinant of herbage production, management, particularly stocking rate, plays a crucial role in regulating the degree of variability encountered in herbage availability between years

(Danckwerts *et al.*, 1993). This occurs because of the strong interaction between grazing and rainfall in determining production and species composition in rangelands (Danckwerts *et al.*, 1993). In the short term, heavy stocking not only reduces feed availability through the direct effect of grazing; it also depresses plant vigour and rainfall effectivity, thus reducing overall herbage production. In the long term, heavy stocking invariably results in the replacement of perennial plant species with ephemeral or annual species, which produce little or no forage in dry or below-average rainfall years (Harrington, 1986; Freudenberger *et al.*, 1999). Consequently, sheep on heavily stocked properties are likely to encounter greater interannual variability in forage production and a greater number of feed deficits over the long term than sheep maintained at a moderate or light stocking rate (Dankwerts *et al.*, 1993).

Water Availability

Water is a critical nutrient, essential for animal life, irrespective of the production system involved. In more intensive, cultivated pasture systems, water is generally readily available and is unlikely to limit animal production. In contrast, water on rangelands is often scarce, poorly distributed and of low quality and therefore the provision of adequate drinking water assumes major significance in these environments.

The water requirement of sheep on rangelands is determined by a number of factors, including the physiological status of the animal, ambient temperature, water quality and the moisture and salt content of the feed on offer (e.g. Squires and Wilson, 1971; Squires, 1976, 1981). Sheep on fresh, green pasture can obtain a significant proportion of their water requirement from their feed and may only need to drink every few days (Lynch, 1974). In contrast, sheep grazing dry pasture have a greater water requirement and may need to drink once every 2 days or daily. Sheep grazing forage species such as saltbush (*Atriplex* spp.) with a high salt content are under particular stress and may even need to drink twice daily (Squires, 1981). For example, daily water intakes of wethers in Australia have been shown to vary from 0.6 to 3.1 l while on grassland, compared with 2.3 to 9.3 l while on saltbush (Squires, 1976).

Water quality is also an issue on some rangelands, with, for example, sheep having to contend with saline water in many paddocks in the Australian arid zone. Ironically, animals drinking saline water have to increase water intake in order to excrete the excess salt (Squires, 1981), further increasing their need to drink and the time and energy expended in walking to and from water.

Apart from its obvious role in basic physiological processes, water affects nutrient intake and hence animal production on rangelands in a number of different ways. Thus, where water is in short supply, DM intake is directly reduced, with obvious consequences for animal production. Further, in large paddocks where watering points are far apart, sheep may expend a significant proportion of time and energy in simply travelling between grazing areas and water, energy that would otherwise be available for growth and production. Research conducted in Australia indicates that animals may spend up to 40% of the day walking to water (Burnside *et al.*, 1990), which directly reduces the time available for grazing. Sheep on rangelands may walk between 4 and 17 km a day for water (Squires and Wilson, 1971), compared with 2–4 km for animals on cultivated pastures (Tribe, 1949).

In big paddocks, distance to water also directly affects the efficiency with which the surrounding country is utilized. Generally, there is a zone of intense utilization, termed the *piosphere*, immediately around the water point. Further out, utilization tends to decrease in direct proportion to distance from water. Depending upon the vegetation type, water quality, the physiological status of the animal and the frequency of drinking, most grazing is restricted to *c.* 3 km radius around water, although this distance may be substantially increased when feed is scarce (Squires, 1981). Accordingly, allowance needs to be made for distance from water for different land types in calculating the carrying capacity of a particular paddock. Paddocks with closely spaced watering points will thus have a relatively higher carrying capacity than equivalent-sized paddocks with widely spaced watering points.

In general, water points should be about 5–7 km apart for sheep in arid and semiarid areas (Squires, 1981; Burnside *et al.*, 1990), although this distance would be less in higher-rainfall areas where the overall carrying capacity was higher. This would allow access to about 4000 ha of surrounding pasture. To prevent excessive trampling and utilization of the surrounding pasture, water points should be established at a ratio of 1 water point to *c.* 500 sheep. However, this number would have to be reduced in times of seasonal stress to reduce the extent of landscape degradation. Considerable care needs to be taken in siting watering points to ensure that they are on non-erodable or depositional land types and that they also provide access to the more productive and favoured areas of the paddock (Burnside *et al.*, 1990).

Resource Management

Sustainable resource management is an essential and integral part of the management of both cultivated pasture and rangeland systems. This is especially so on rangelands, as these areas are generally far more fragile and less resilient to misuse than the better-watered and more fertile cultivated pastures. Rangelands are particularly vulnerable to poor management under sheep, as compared with cattle grazing (O'Reagain and Turner, 1992), due to the highly selective nature and short grazing habits of the former animals (O'Reagain and Grau, 1995).

In rangelands, poor resource management may precipitate vegetation change, with profound effects on the quality and availability of feed available to the grazing animal and hence on animal production. This generally arises through the replacement of the more palatable perennial plant species with annuals or unpalatable perennials, the loss of plant vigour and ground cover and an overall decline in resource productivity.

In brief, three basic rules need to be followed to achieve good resource management under sheep grazing (see also Harrington *et al.*, 1984; Stuth, 1991). First, stocking rate is the most important determinant of animal production and range condition (O'Reagain and Turner, 1992) and is probably the single most important variable under direct control of the manager (Danckwerts *et al.*, 1993). In general, stocking rates should be conservative and should not exceed the long-term carrying capacity of the land. Alternatively, in environments with a large inter-annual variation in rainfall and hence herbage production, flexible stocking rates may be employed, where animal numbers are varied according to forage availability (Holechek *et al.*, 1989). Whatever strategy is applied, stocking rates should be drastically reduced in drought years, in order to minimize animal loss and prevent overgrazing.

A second important rule is that different land types should be fenced to prevent selection and overutilization of the better areas in a paddock. Evidence from hill farms in Britain indicates that overuse of favoured land types by sheep occurs even at low stocking rates (Hunter, 1962), so that other management options, such as fencing, are necessary to prevent degradation of such sites. Fencing also allows different vegetation communities to be managed and stocked according to individual requirements and consequently prevents degradation of more sensitive areas. In some extensive situations, however, fencing of separate land types is impractical and uneconomic, due to the scale of operation involved and the relatively low levels of economic return possible from such areas. In such cases, animals can sometimes be moved around different areas by varying the placement of supplements, patch burning or even closing off different watering points at different times of the year.

Thirdly, it is important that all rangelands receive periodic resting or spelling, in order to allow vital plant processes, such as seed production or seedling recruitment, to proceed and so maintain a viable population of desirable plants. Spelling is also necessary for plants to maintain vigour under grazing and thus maintain productivity. Periodic spelling also allows the accumulation of a fodder reserve, which, in some situations, can smooth out the year-to-year variation in herbage availability and considerably reduce the risk of a feed deficit in years of below-average rainfall (Danckwerts *et al.*, 1993).

For sheep on rangelands, additional benefit may also be obtained by grazing them in conjunction with cattle, at a replacement ratio of about six to ten sheep to one cattle unit. This not only reduces the detrimental effect of sheep by evening out the grazing, but may also increase sheep production through cattle-induced grazing facilitation (O'Reagain and Turner, 1992). However, this is not an option on all rangelands and, in some situations, may be precluded by economics or the vegetation under consideration.

In conclusion, good resource management is an essential part of managing rangelands and ensuring an adequate supply of nutrients to grazing sheep. In general, this can be achieved by following the three basic rules of maintaining the correct stocking rate, separating land types and regular spelling. In some situations, the application of fire may also be necessary. Although more intensive grazing systems, such as cell grazing, are sometimes claimed to give superior animal production and result in better range condition, the evidence in support of such systems is equivocal and largely anecdotal (O'Reagain and Turner, 1992).

Supplementation under Rangeland Conditions

Pastures grown in response to seasonal rainfall deteriorate in nutritive value once vegetative growth stops (Fig. 12.3). Therefore, in areas with summer rainfall, any unconsumed pastures present in a sward from mid- to late winter through to the following summer rains will be dry and of low nutritive value. The extent to which the nitrogen content of Mitchell grass (*Astrebla* spp.) falls as it dries out is shown in Table 12.1. Similarly, in winter-rainfall regions, pasture quality and possibly quantity will be low from midsummer until the following autumn rains begin. For sheep consuming these dry pastures, the first limiting nutrient is usually rumen-degradable protein (RDP), especially in summer-rainfall regions (see McMeniman *et al.*, 1986b). Once RDP deficiencies are corrected, energy and then, possibly, undegraded dietary protein (UDP) usually become the next limiting nutrients (see Coleman and Henry, Chapter 1, this volume). Under the extensive grazing conditions common in rangelands, supplementation programmes to overcome these seasonal nutrient deficiencies usually need to be low in cost and targeted at reproducing or young growing sheep.

RDP supplements

In summer-rainfall rangelands regions, spring lambing is the preferred management option. As a result, autumn-joined ewes that are in the later stages of pregnancy or are lactating frequently graze RDP-deficient pastures. Under these conditions, it has been shown that an RDP supplement in the form of urea is both cheap and effective. In sheep-grazing systems, 8 g urea per head per day can improve ewe survival rates, lamb birth weights, milk production by ewes and, as a consequence, lamb growth rates and survival (Stephenson *et al.*, 1981). Urea supplementation of non-reproducing sheep that are consuming similar pastures has also been shown to reduce or prevent liveweight loss. When urea is being used, it is advisable to also provide a sulphur source, so that the N : S ratio in the supplement is between 10 : 1 and 13 : 1, in order that the requirements of the rumen microorganisms be met. Ammonium sulphate has been found to be a suitable sulphur source.

When the only water available to grazing sheep is in troughs, an effective method of providing urea is to dissolve it in the drinking water, ensuring that all sheep receive the urea supplement. Reliable commercial devices that deliver predetermined amounts of urea into water lines and troughs are now available. Urea can also be provided as a dry lick by mixing it with salt and feeding it out in troughs. A feeding regimen that has been recommended is to give sheep free access to salt for 2 weeks to satisfy any 'salt hunger' they may have and then to add urea to the salt in the ratio of one part urea to four parts salt. After a further 4 weeks, the urea-to-salt ratio is increased to 1 : 3 and 5% ammonium sulphate is added to the mix. Adult sheep should consume 24–30 g of this mix per day. Troughs should have drain holes to prevent accumulation of rainwater, which might dissolve high concentrations of urea. Alternatively, troughs can be covered to prevent rain from wetting the mix (see Miller, 1998).

Producers and advisers have formulated numerous 'home-made' blocks containing urea and an example would be the mix shown in Table 12.2 (Miller, 1998). The ingredients are mixed with a cement mixer before being poured into containers and allowed to set over a number of days. An adult sheep would need to consume approximately 50 g of this block per day to receive the required 7–8 g urea per day. Disadvantages of making blocks on the property include timely supply of ingredients and the time and effort involved in the mixing. A number of proprietary blocks containing urea are available but they have varying compositions. For example some are based on molasses, others have high concentrations of salt and most contain added minerals and/or vitamins. It is usually more convenient to purchase rather than produce blocks on farm, but purchased blocks will usually be more expensive than farm-produced blocks. Care should be taken when feeding proprietary blocks to ensure that they do not contain nutrients that could be toxic to the sheep. For example, some blocks with high inclusion rates of copper are designed for use in copper-deficient areas, but, if they are fed to sheep in areas that are not copper-deficient, copper toxicity could result.

Table 12.2. Toorak urea block (from Miller, 1998).

Ingredients	Order of mixing	Units of mix (%) Starter mix	Units of mix (%) Final mix
Hot water	1	10	10
Molasses	2	20	20
Urea	3	5	15
Salt	4	15	10
Bran	5	15	10
Ammonium sulphate	6	5	5
Bentonite	7	30	30
Total nitrogen (% of mix)			8.4
Crude protein equivalent (%)			52.5

A further method of supplementing sheep with urea is to dissolve it in a molasses–water mix and give sheep access to the mixture by means of a roller drum floating on top of the urea/molasses mixture. Molasses contains approximately 7 g sulphur kg^{-1} DM, so there is no need for additional sulphur in a urea and molasses mix. Sheep must not have direct access to the mixture or they will drink it and suffer from urea poisoning. The sheep must also be adapted to the urea, and a suggested adaptation procedure is shown in Table 12.3 (Miller, 1998). The on-farm use of a urea/molasses supplement similar to that shown in Table 12.3 requires provision of molasses storage facilities, mixing equipment and suitable troughs to feed out the mixture. In some regions of Australia and other countries, commercially produced mixes of urea and molasses can be purchased for direct delivery to supplementation points on a property. However, expense would probably preclude this approach in the more extensive rangelands regions.

The phosphorus concentrations in dry pastures, especially subtropical or tropical pastures, can be below theoretical requirements, even for non-reproducing sheep. However, except in the case of mulga (see below), no positive response to phosphorus supplementation of sheep on theoretically phosphorus-deficient pastures has been recorded (Entwistle, 1972), even though cattle grazing the same pasture types do respond. The reasons for the lack of response by sheep are not clear but have been ascribed to the fact that sheep select a diet with a higher nutrient content than do cattle and that sheep have a smaller skeletal mass. Notwithstanding this, many advisers recommend that, when sheep grazing dry pastures are supplemented with an RDP source, they should also be provided with a phosphorus supplement.

UDP supplements

Weaners, ewes in late pregnancy and lactating ewes may have protein requirements in excess of that provided by microbial protein (ARC, 1980). Therefore, if these animals are grazing dry pastures with low protein concentrations, they may respond to UDP as well as RDP supplementation. Protein supplementation is usually expensive, so careful consideration should be given to the cost : benefit ratio of a supplementation programme before it is implemented. Several experiments have shown that supple-

Table 12.3. Programme for introducing urea roller-drum mix (from Miller, 1998).

Ingredients	Starter mix: days 1–3	Introduction: days 4–7	Build-up: days 8–14	Final mix: day 14 onwards
Water (l)	100	100	125	150
Molasses (l)	100	100	100	50
Urea (kg)	0	5	10	20
% urea	–	2	3.6	8.5

mentation of ewes during the last trimester of pregnancy and during lactation with protein sources such as cottonseed meal, copra meal, whole cottonseeds and lupins can increase the birth weight of lambs, milk production of ewes and growth rate and survival of lambs (McMeniman *et al.*, 1982; Bird *et al.*, 1990; Cajas and Hinch, 1998). However, the responses obtained to protein supplementation may not be entirely due to their UDP content. Proteins also provide RDP that may be more slowly released in the rumen than RDP from urea and so be used more efficiently by the rumen microbes. Proteins are also a source of digestible organic matter (OM), which would provide metabolizable energy (ME) and promote synthesis of additional microbial protein. The recommended level of protein supplementation for late-pregnant and lactating sheep is 50 and 75 g per head per day, respectively. Whole cottonseeds and lupins can be fed on the ground, while meals should be fed out in troughs. It may be necessary to entice sheep to accept some protein sources by mixing them with small quantities of molasses or salt until the required level of intake is reached.

Energy supplements

Energy supplements are not usually an option in extensive grazing, due to the high cost. The usual procedure is to utilize standing dry paddock feed as efficiently as possible, with strategic use of urea or protein supplements, which usually stimulate intake of dry roughage and hence improve the ME intake by animals. The necessity to use energy supplements to maintain live weight or support pregnancy and lactation usually indicates the beginning of drought conditions, and it is not the intention to discuss drought feeding in this section. Strategic energy supplementation of sheep in more intensive regions, particularly in the winter-rainfall areas, is discussed by Dove (Chapter 6, this volume).

If the decision is made to provide an energy supplement, then molasses has been shown to be useful in extensive grazing conditions. Molasses contains approximately 11 MJ ME kg^{-1} DM. Molasses plus either 3% urea (M3U) or 8% urea (M8U) have been successfully used for sheep, with the mixture provided *ad libitum* in open troughs. Three per cent urea provides the RDP required by rumen microbes to digest the OM in molasses, but it has been found, especially with cattle, that overconsumption of M3U can occur, with the inherent danger of molasses toxicity. Increasing the urea concentration to 8% makes the mixture somewhat unpalatable and restricts intake. With both M3U and M8U, the urea must be thoroughly and evenly dissolved into the molasses to prevent potential urea toxicity. Liveweight maintenance of dry sheep would be all that could be expected with a dry grass diet supplemented with urea and molasses. If a higher level of response was required – for example, growth of weaners or maintenance of pregnant or lactating ewes – then up to 10% protein meal (for example, cottonseed meal) could be mixed into molasses (see Wythes and Ernst, 1984).

Hay supplements

Pasture hay in large bales is made in some extensive areas following periods of good pasture growth. This hay can be fed back to sheep when standing dry pastures become scarce. However, the protein content and digestibility of some pasture hays are low, especially if they have been harvested after pastures have flowered (Stephenson *et al.*, 1986). It is possible to improve the RDP content of such hay by injecting a solution of urea and molasses into the bales 3–4 days before they are fed out (Stephenson *et al.*, 1984; see also Annison *et al.*, Chapter 5, this volume). A suggested solution is 20 kg urea, 50 kg molasses and 4 kg ammonium sulphate dissolved in 70 l water. This solution is injected into the bales under pressure at the rate of 100 l per t of hay (Miller, 1998).

Forage supplements

Mulga (*A. aneura*) is a tree legume that is distributed over a wide area of semiarid and arid Australia (see Plate 12.1). Mulga leaves are readily eaten by sheep, constituting up to 10% of the diet in normal seasons and up to

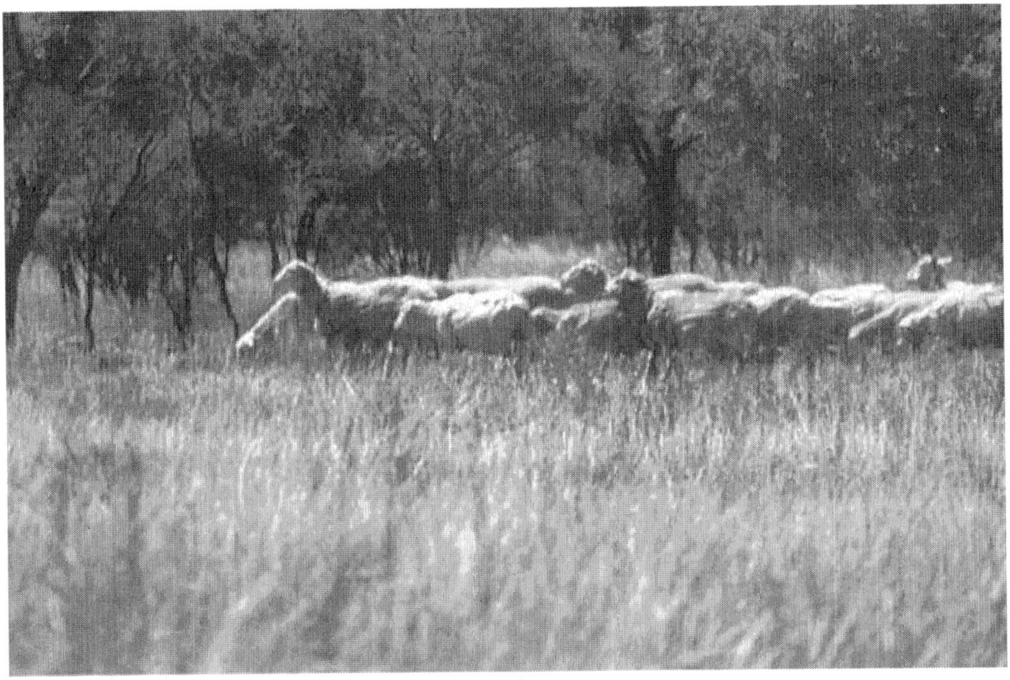

Plate 12.1. Merino wethers near Louth, New South Wales, Australia, grazing in rangeland dominated by mulga trees (*Acacia aneura*) and the native perennial grasses woollybutt (*Eragrostis eriopoda*), bandicoot grass (*Monachather paradoxa*) and mulga grass (*Thyridolepis mitchelliana*). (Photo courtesy of K.C. Hodgkinson, CSIRO Sustainable Ecosystems, Canberra, Australia.)

100% of the diet when fed under drought conditions. Sheep offered a diet containing only mulga maintain or slowly lose live weight. Although mulga has a DM digestibility (DMD) of 50% and a CP content of 10–14%, the digestibility of the protein is low (35–40%), because high concentrations of condensed tannins bind the protein during rumen digestion. The low protein digestibility results in mulga-fed sheep being sulphur- and sometimes RDP-deficient. Mulga also has a low phosphorus concentration, but sheep do not respond to phosphorus supplementation unless the first limiting nutrients, sulphur and possibly RDP, are provided (McMeniman, 1976). Goodchild and McMeniman (1994) found that supplementing a low-quality forage diet with mulga at up to 42% of the diet resulted in a progressive reduction in the intake of the low-quality roughage but an increase in overall digestible OM intake.

The digestibility of mulga protein can be improved by dosing sheep daily with the polymer polyethylene glycol (8 g per head), which displaces tannins from tannin–protein complexes in the gut. However, because of the cost of the chemical and labour, this is not an economical approach (Pritchard *et al.*, 1988).

A dry lick containing (per head per day) RDP (6–12 g), sulphur (1–1.5 g), phosphorus (1–2 g) and sodium (1–2 g) is recommended for dry sheep consuming diets of dry grass and mulga. Pregnant or lactating sheep consuming similar diets would require protein supplementation as well (Miller, 1998).

Saltbushes (*Atriplex* spp.) and bluebushes (*Kochia* spp.) dominate a large area of the Australian semiarid and arid rangelands. These species contain relatively high levels of CP (approximately 18%), which are maintained during periods when native pastures are dry. Although this suggests a role for these plants as supplements for grazing sheep, published reports indicate that the performance of sheep consuming diets containing these shrubs and dry pasture was little better than that of sheep consuming dry pasture alone (Leigh *et al.*, 1970; Warren *et al.*, 1990). The shrubs do, however, have a place as a drought reserve.

Tagasaste (*Chamaecytisus palmensis*) is a leguminous perennial shrub that grows in winter-rainfall areas with well-drained soils. Tagasaste leaves have a reasonable nutritive value (15–18% CP and an *in vitro* digestibility of 68–70%) and could be expected to have a place as a supplement to dry summer pastures (see Norton *et al.*, 1996).

References

Allden, W.G. and Whittaker, I.A.M. (1970) The determinants of herbage intake by grazing sheep: the inter-relationship of factors influencing herbage intake and availability. *Australian Journal of Agricultural Research* 21, 755–766.

ARC (1980) *The Nutrient Requirements of Ruminant Livestock*. Commonwealth Agricultural Bureaux, Farnham Royal, UK, 351 pp.

Bakker, J.P., De Leeuw, J. and Van Wieren, S.E. (1983) Micro-patterns in grassland created and sustained by sheep grazing. *Vegetatio* 55, 153–161.

Bird, A.R., Rignet, S.J., Stephenson, R.G.A. and O'Sullivan, B.M. (1990) Copra meal supplementation of lambing ewes in north west Queensland. *Proceedings of the Australian Society of Animal Production* 18, 456.

Burnside, D., Williams, A. and Curry, P. (1990) *Spacing Water Points in the Southern Pastoral Areas of Western Australia*. Bulletin No. 4162, Western Australian Department of Agriculture, Perth, 10 pp.

Cajas, S. and Hinch, G.N. (1998) Lupin supplementation of Merino ewes grazing native pastures in New England: effects on birth weight and maternal behaviour. *Proceedings of the Australian Society of Animal Production* 22, 286.

Cooper, S.M., Owen-Smith, N. and Bryant, J.P. (1988) Foliage acceptability to browsing ruminants in relation to seasonal changes in the leaf chemistry of woody plants in a South African savanna. *Oecologia* 75, 336–342.

Danckwerts, J.E., O'Reagain, P.J. and O'Connor, T.G. (1993) Range management in a changing environment: a southern African perspective. *Australian Rangeland Journal* 15, 133–144.

Entwistle, K.W. (1972) Performance of Merino ewes grazing Mitchell grass pastures when supplemented with nitrogen, phosphorus and vitamins A, D, E. *Proceedings of the Australian Society of Animal Production* 9, 235–240.

Freudenberger, D., Wilson, A. and Palmer, R. (1999) The effects of perennial grasses, stocking rate and rainfall on sheep production in a semi-arid woodland of eastern Australia. *Rangelands Journal* 21, 199–219.

Fynn, R.W.S. and O'Connor, T.G. (2000) Effect of stocking rate and rainfall on rangeland dynamics and cattle performance in a semi-arid savanna, South Africa. *Journal of Applied Ecology* 37, 491–507.

Goodchild, A.V. and McMeniman, N.P. (1994) Intake and digestibility of low quality roughages when supplemented with leguminous browse. *Journal of Agricultural Science, Cambridge* 122, 151–160.

Harrington, G.N. (1986) Herbivore diet in a semi-arid *Eucalyptus populnea* woodland. 1. Merino sheep. *Australian Journal of Experimental Agriculture* 26, 413–421.

Harrington, G.N., Wilson, A.D. and Young, M.D. (1984) *Management of Australia's Rangelands*. CSIRO, Australia, 354 pp.

Heckathorn, S.A. and DeLucia, E.H. (1994) Drought induced nitrogen retranslocation in perennial C4 grasses of tall-grass prairie. *Ecology* 75, 1877–1886.

Holechek, J.L., Pieper, R.D. and Herbel, C.H. (1989) *Range Management: Principles and Practices*. Prentice Hall, Englewood Cliffs, New Jersey, 501 pp.

Hunter, K.F. (1962) Hill sheep and their pasture: a study of sheep-grazing in south-east Scotland. *Journal of Ecology* 50, 651–680.

Jaramillo, V.J. and Detling, J.K. (1992) Small-scale patch heterogeneity in a semi-arid North American grassland. II. Cattle grazing of simulated urine patches. *Journal of Applied Ecology* 29, 9–13.

Lechner-Doll, M., Rutagwenda, T., Schwartz, H.J., Schultka, W. and Engelhardt, W.V. (1990) Seasonal changes in ingesta mean retention time and forestomach volume in indigenous grazing camels, cattle, sheep and goats in a thornbush savanna pasture. *Journal of Agricultural Science, Cambridge* 115, 409–420.

Leigh, J.H., Wilson, A.D. and Williams, O.B. (1970) An assessment of the value of three chenopodiaceous shrubs for wool production of sheep grazing semi-arid pastures. In: Norman, M.J.T. (ed.) *Proceedings of the 11th International Grasslands Congress*. University of Queensland, Brisbane, pp. 55–59.

Lorimer, M.S. (1981) Forage selection studies 2. Diet quality, liveweight change and wool production of sheep grazing *Astrebla* spp. pastures in north-west Queensland. *Tropical Grasslands* 15, 183–192.

Louw, G.N. (1969) The nutritive value of natural grazings in South Africa. *Proceedings of the South African Society of Animal Production* 8, 57–61.
Lynch, J.J. (1974) Behaviour of sheep and cattle in the more arid areas of Australia. In: Wilson, A.D. (ed.) *Studies in the Australian Arid Zone II. Animal Production*. CSIRO, Melbourne, pp. 37–49.
McIvor, J.G. (1981) Seasonal changes in the growth, dry matter distribution and herbage quality of three native grasses in northern Queensland. *Australian Journal of Experimental Agriculture and Animal Husbandry* 21, 600–609.
McMeniman, N.P. (1976) Studies on the supplementary feeding of sheep fed mulga (*Acacia aneura*). 3. The provision of phosphorus, molasses and urea supplements under pen conditions. *Australian Journal of Experimental Agriculture and Animal Husbandry* 16, 819–822.
McMeniman, N.P., O'Dempsey, N., Niven, D.R., Jordan, D. and O'Brien, J. (1982) The effect of cottonseed meal and urea supplementation on the reproductive performance of ewes in central and south west Queensland. *Proceedings of the Australian Society of Animal Production* 14, 447–450.
McMeniman, N.P., Beale, I.F. and Murphy, G.M. (1986a) Nutritional evaluation of south-west Queensland pastures. I. The botanical and nutrient content of diets selected by sheep grazing on Mitchell grass and mulga grassland associations. *Australian Journal of Agricultural Research* 37, 289–302.
McMeniman, N.P., Beale, I.F. and Murphy, G.M. (1986b) Nutritional evaluation of south-west Queensland pastures. II. The intake and digestion of organic matter and nitrogen by sheep grazing on Mitchell grass and mulga grassland associations. *Australian Journal of Agricultural Research* 37, 303–314.
Miller, D. (1998) *Livestock Nutrition in Western Queensland*. Information Series Q198040, Queensland Department of Primary Industries, Brisbane.
Norton, B.W., Gutteridge, R.C., Johnson, P.W., Beale, I.F., Oldham, C.M. and McNeill, D.M. (1996) Beyond the herb layer – shrubs and trees as drought reserves. In: Rowe, J. and Cossins, N. (eds) *A User's Guide to Drought Feeding Alternatives*. University of New England, Armidale, Australia, pp. 99–109.
O'Reagain, P.J. (1993) Plant structure and acceptability of different grasses to sheep. *Journal of Rangeland Management* 46, 232–236.
O'Reagain, P.J. (1996a) Predicting animal production on sourveld 1. A species based approach. *African Journal of Range and Forage Science* 13, 113–123.
O'Reagain, P.J. (1996b) Predicting animal production on sourveld 2. A sward based approach. *African Journal of Range and Forage Science* 13, 124–130.
O'Reagain, P.J. (2001) Foraging strategies on rangelands: effects of intake and animal performance. In: Gomide, J.A., Mattos, W.R.S. and da Silva, S.C. (eds) *Proceedings of the XIX International Grassland Congress*. Brazilian Society of Animal Production, São Paulo, pp. 277–284.
O'Reagain, P.J. and Grau, E.R. (1995) Sequence of species selection by cattle and sheep grazing South African sourveld. *Journal of Rangeland Management* 48, 314–321.
O'Reagain, P.J. and Schwartz, H.J. (1995) Dietary selection and foraging strategies of animals on rangelands. Coping with spatial and temporal variability. In: Journet, M., Grenet, E., Farce, M.-H., Theriez, M. and Demarquilly, C. (eds) *Proceedings IV International Symposium on the Nutrition of Herbivores*. INRA, Paris, pp. 407–423.
O'Reagain, P.J. and Turner, J.R. (1992) An evaluation of the empirical basis for grazing management recommendations for rangeland in southern Africa. *Journal of the Grassland Society of Southern Africa* 9, 38–49.

O'Reagain, P.J., Goetsch, B.C. and Owen-Smith, R.N. (1996) Effect of species composition and sward structure on the ingestive behaviour of cattle and sheep grazing South African sourveld. *Journal of Agricultural Science, Cambridge* 127, 271–280.

Pritchard, D.A., Stocks, D.C., O'Sullivan, B.M., Martin, P.R., Hurwood, I.S. and O'Rourke, P.K. (1988) The effect of polyethylene glycol on wool growth and liveweight of sheep consuming a mulga (*Acacia aneura*) diet. *Proceedings of the Australian Society of Animal Production* 17, 290–293.

Roguet, C., Prache, S. and Petit, M. (1998) Feeding station behaviour of ewes in response to forage availability and sward phenological stage. *Applied Animal Behaviour Science* 56, 187–201.

Schwartz, H.J. (1993) The use of marginal areas for animal production. *Animal Research and Development* 38, 100–110.

Squires, V.R. (1976) Walking, watering and grazing behaviour of Merino sheep on two semi-arid rangelands in south-west New South Wales. *Australian Rangeland Journal* 1, 13–23.

Squires, V. (1981) *Livestock Management in the Arid Zone*. Inkata Press, Melbourne.

Squires, V.R. and Wilson, A.D. (1971) Distance between food and water supply and its effects on drinking frequency, and food and water intake of Merino and Border Leicester sheep. *Australian Journal of Agricultural Research* 22, 283–290.

Stephenson, R.G.A., Edwards, J.C. and Hopkins, P.S. (1981) The use of urea to improve milk yields and lamb survival of Merinos in a dry tropical environment. *Australian Journal of Agricultural Research* 32, 497–509.

Stephenson, R.G.A., Pritchard, D.A. and Connell, J.A. (1984) Evaluation of treatments for fortifying round bales of barley stubble using a spear technique. *Proceedings of the Australian Society of Animal Production* 15, 604–607.

Stephenson, R.G.A., Martin, P., Pritchard, D.A., Cobon, D.H. and O'Sullivan, M. (1986) The value of native pasture hay in western Queensland. *Proceedings of the Australian Society of Animal Production* 16, 363–366.

Stoltsz, C.W. and Danckwerts, J.E. (1990) Grass species selection patterns on rotationally-grazed Döhne sourveld during autumn and early winter. *Journal of the Grassland Society of Southern Africa* 7, 92–96.

Stuth, J.W. (1991) Foraging behaviour. In: Heitschmidt, R.K. and Stuth, J.W. (eds) *Grazing Management: an Ecological Perspective*. Timber Press, Portland, Oregon, pp. 65–83.

Tribe, D.E. (1949) Some seasonal observations on the grazing habits of sheep. *Empire Journal of Experimental Agriculture* 17, 105–115.

Tyson, P.D. (1986) *Climatic Change and Variability in Southern Africa*. Oxford University Press, Cape Town, 214 pp.

Warren, B.E., Bunny, C.J. and Bryant, E.R. (1990) A preliminary examination of the nutritive value of four saltbush (*Atriplex*) species. *Proceedings of the Australian Society of Animal Production* 18, 424–427.

Weston, E.J. and Moir, K.W. (1969) Grazing preferences of sheep and nutritive value of plant components in a mitchell grass association in north-western Queensland. *Queensland Journal of Agricultural and Animal Science* 26, 639–650.

Wythes, J.R. and Ernst, A.J. (1984) Molasses as a drought feed. *Proceedings of the Australian Society of Animal Production* 15, 213–226.

13 Trace-element and Vitamin Nutrition of Grazing Sheep

J. LEE,[1] S.O. KNOWLES[1] AND G.J. JUDSON[2]

[1]*AgResearch Limited, Grasslands Research Centre, Palmerston North, New Zealand;* [2]*South Australian Research and Development Institute, Glenside, South Australia, Australia*

Introduction

Trace elements and vitamins, here defined collectively as micronutrients, occur in living tissues at low concentrations and are the reaction catalysts of biological systems. Their presence is essential in maintaining normal cellular metabolism in animals. Together with adequate supplies of energy and protein, they are required for optimal health of the well-fed sheep. Hence the study of micronutrients has immense practical importance, as inadequate or excessive supply of any one trace element or vitamin can impair the health and productivity of the animal. This chapter examines the essentiality of micronutrients in sheep metabolism and nutrition. Principles underpinning recommendations for optimal supply are discussed, along with dietary factors that affect availability, transport, absorption and utilization – factors that will vary for each micronutrient. Furthermore, function may be influenced by interactions with other nutrients, which may be additive, synergistic or antagonistic. In this chapter, we shall discuss the utilization of copper (Cu), selenium (Se) and vitamin B_{12} as 'case-studies' of those principles – many of which are applicable to other micronutrients. Supplementation strategies are briefly summarized and also the effect of micronutrients on end-product quality.

Function

Essentiality

All elements must be obtained from diet, whether required at trace, micro- or macroconcentrations. As many as 19 elements are metabolically essential and, for sheep at pasture, deficiencies and excesses of many, but not all, have been reported. Only a handful of elements are commonly responsible for nutritional problems that affect growth, milk production or fertility performance of sheep. The seven of practical significance (in approximate order of importance) are Se, cobalt (Co) (as vitamin B_{12}), Cu (and its antagonist molybdenum (Mo)), iodine (I), zinc (Zn), iron (Fe) and manganese (Mn). Macroelements (calcium, chlorine, potassium, magnesium, sodium, phosphorus and sulphur) are discussed elsewhere in this text and will only be mentioned in this chapter where they are of special significance to the behaviour of micronutrients. The reader is directed to the major work of Underwood and Suttle (1999) on the essentiality of trace elements for an element-by-element coverage. Similarly, McDowell (2000a) is recommended as an introduction to the function and metabolism of vitamins.

Vitamins are supplied through diet, synthesized by the animal or produced via microbial activity in the rumen. Given adequate protein, energy and precursors, normal rumen function will produce sufficient B-group vitamins and vitamin K to meet animal needs. Vitamin C is synthesized endogenously from glucose and galactose, while vitamin D is produced in the skin through the interaction of ultra-violet (UV) radiation and precursor sterols. Only vitamin A, its precursor β-carotene and vitamin E are diet-dependent and are therefore of general practical significance. Of the B vitamins, the supply of vitamin B_{12} and, to a lesser extent, thiamine is of interest. Sporadic outbreaks of thiamine deficiency in sheep at pasture are thought to be due to a marked increase in thiaminase activity in the rumen (McDonald, 1982); thiaminase may be present in ingested plants, such as ferns, but more often arises from microbial activity in the rumen. Although vitamin B_{12} is produced by microbial activity, its synthesis depends on sufficient Co in the diet. The preruminant lamb relies on vitamin B_{12} from milk or from fetal reserves.

Micronutrients of practical significance, plus several others typically present in pasture but with no known therapeutic or physiological roles, are identified, along with their major metabolic roles, in Table 13.1. Other elements (e.g. arsenic (As), cadmium (Cd) and nickel (Ni), considered to be 'newer' trace elements) may in fact also be essential, but their functions are as yet undefined.

Toxic risks

All essential micronutrients have a therapeutic range that covers the amount necessary to meet the animal's minimal requirements, but which is less than a toxic overdose. Chronic toxic accumulation of micronutrients rarely occurs in grazing sheep; exceptions include Cu, which readily accumulates in the liver, and fluorine (F) from excessive fertilizer application, artesian water for stock use or volcanic activity (Cronin *et al.*, 2000). Although high concentrations of some trace elements and heavy metals, notably Cu, As, Cd, mercury (Hg) and lead (Pb), can affect marketability of sheep products, they usually have little impact on sheep health. Producers will come under increasing pressure to meet market specifications for residues of these elements.

Table 13.1. Examples of trace-element and vitamin function and essentiality in sheep.

Micronutrient	Chemical form and mechanism	Example enzymes and cofactors	Metabolic functions	Disease consequences of deficiency
Copper	Chemical coordination[a] bonds forming Cu–O and Cu–S centres (electron transfer)	Ferroxidase (ceruloplasmin), cytochrome c oxidase, lysyl oxidase, CuZn superoxide dismutase	Iron transport and storage, mitochondrial respiration, collagen/elastin cross-linking, cellular antioxidant	Enzootic ataxia (sway-back), non-Fe-responsive anaemia, arterial aneurysms
Iron	Coordination bonds forming porphyrin ring or Fe–S cluster (oxygen transport or electron transfer)	Ferrochetalase substrate, cytochromes, aconitase	Haem formation and oxygen transport, redox centres and cellular respiration, carbohydrate utilization	Fe-responsive anaemia, fatigue, anorexia
Iodine	Covalently bound as T_4 and T_3[b]	Iodinase substrate	T_4 and T_3 thyroid hormones regulating cell growth and metabolic rates	Goitre, low birth weight, neonatal mortality
Manganese	Coordination bonds forming mononuclear centre (cyclic oxidoreduction)	Mn superoxide dismutase, pyruvate carboxylase, arginase	Mitochondrial antioxidant, glucose utilization, bone-matrix development	Skeletal and cartilage malformation
Molybdenum	Coordination bonds forming molybdopterin cofactor (oxygen transfer)	Xanthine oxidases, sulphite oxidases	Purine nucleotide metabolism, sulphite metabolism	Copper toxicity from high-copper diets
Selenium	Covalently bound as selenocysteine (an ionizable selenol reaction centre)	Glutathione peroxidases, thioredoxin reductase, iodothyronine deiodinase	Intra- and extracellular antioxidants, thyroxine metabolism	Cardiomyopathy, white-muscle disease, reduced fertility, poor growth
Zinc	Flexible coordination bonds (maintaining protein spatial and configurational relationships)	Many metalloenzymes, zinc-finger motif[c] for DNA binding	Structural, non-catalytic, cell signalling	Wool deterioration, slow wound healing, reduced appetite, delayed puberty
Cobalt (vitamin B_{12})	Coordination bonds in a porphyrin-like corrin ring[d] (methyl transfer)	Cyanocobalamin cofactors	Gluconeogenesis (propionate metabolism) and methionine synthesis (methionine synthase)	Poor growth, reduced wool, watery eyes, phalaris toxicity staggers, anaemia
Vitamin A	Retinol and retinal dehydrogenases		Many functions including maintenance of epithelial cells, vision, gene regulation, immune-cell function	Inability to produce rhodopsin, keratinization of mucous membranes, depressed immune function Night blindness, ill thrift, scouring, infertility, disorganized bone growth, increased susceptibility to disease

Continued

Table 13.1. *Continued.*

Micronutrient	Chemical form and mechanism	Example enzymes and cofactors	Metabolic functions	Disease consequences of deficiency
Vitamin E	Biologically most active form is *RRR*-α-tocopherol. Non-specific chain-breaking antioxidant		Protects PUFA in membrane and plasma phospholipids, as α-tocopherol is located in unsaturated subcellular fractions of cell membranes[e]	Peroxidation of membrane lipids affects cell function, diffuse dark red or greyish-white areas in muscle, white-muscle disease (nutritional myopathy)
Vitamin B_1	Coenzyme for all enzymatic decarboxylations of α-keto acids		Metabolism of carbohydrate via citric acid and pentose phosphate cycles Role in nervous tissue	Increase in blood lactate and pyruvate, cerebral cortical necrosis, reduced growth rate, ill thrift, polioencephalomalacia
Vitamin D	Irradiation of sterols with UV light to form precursor of hormone 1,25-dihydroxycholecalciferol (active form of vitamin D)[f]		Maintenance of plasma Ca and P concentrations required for normal mineralization	Failure of bone mineralization, ill thrift, hypocalcaemia, rickets

[a]Coordination compounds or complexes, in which a central atom or ion chemically unites or binds with one or more ligands, are of particular importance in the chemistry of the transition elements (e.g. Co, Cu, Fe, Mn, Mo, Zn).
[b]Thyroxine (L-3,5,3′,5′-tetraiodothyronine or T_4) and tri-iodothyronine (L-3,5,3′-tri-iodothyronine or T_3).
[c]DNA-binding domain in which eight cysteine residues provide binding sites for two Zn^{2+} ions; important in gene regulation.
[d]Coenzyme B_{12}, the cofactor form of vitamin B_{12}, consists of Co (as Co^{3+}) coordinatively bound to four nitrogen atoms in a corrin ring system (chemically related to the porphyrin ring system of haem proteins).
[e]The mechanism by which peroxidation of membrane lipids leads to cellular damage is not clear.
[f]Action of 1,25-dihydroxy-D_3 is mediated by the nuclear vit. D receptor, a phosphoprotein that binds the hormone and regulates expression of genes. Vit. D receptors are found in various organs, including the parathyroid gland, skin, immune system, pancreas and ovary.
PUFA, polyunsaturated fatty acids.

Identification of needs

Early studies (in a number of countries) identified those micronutrient deficiencies that had a major impact on animal productivity (Underwood, 1977). This work quickly led to recognition of trace elements as necessary for successful farming of sheep and other livestock, but accurate benchmarking of requirements for improved productivity and the development of strategies to ensure adequacy under a range of environmental conditions is ongoing (SCA, 1990). Severe deficiencies are clinically recognizable and hence treated through supplementation (Grace, 1983a; SCA, 1990; Grace and Clark, 1991; Masters and White, 1996; Underwood and Suttle, 1999). Identifying the more common and widespread marginal deficiencies is often problematic, as marginal deficiencies are frequently exacerbated by interactions among micronutrients or are confounded by variations in protein and energy supply (Underwood and Suttle, 1999). Benchmarks for the vitamins are not so well defined, particularly for the B vitamins and vitamins D and K, because of the difficulty of accounting for endogenous and intestinal synthesis of these vitamins. Establishing vitamin E requirements is difficult because they depend on dietary levels of polyunsaturated fatty acids, antioxidants, sulphur amino acids and Se. Similarly, for sheep at pasture, vitamin A requirements are met from carotenes, with β-carotene having the highest provitamin A activity. Data on the bioavailability of β-carotene are limited and it probably varies with pasture and with the quantity of carotenoids ingested. Further, carotenoids have been shown to have biological actions independent of vitamin A. Recent evidence indicates a beneficial role for supplemental vitamin E and carotene above physiological levels for enhanced immunocompetence and for vitamin E for the preservation of meat products (McDowell, 2000b). Minimum levels of vitamin E and carotene to produce these desired effects have not been established.

Consequences of deficiency

Underwood and Suttle (1999) have described a model of the physiological events occurring during dietary insufficiency of a micronutrient, which spells out the progression of depletion, deficiency, dysfunction and disease. Chronic marginal dietary deficiency, which gradually reduces tissue storage pools, ultimately leads to dysfunction, and each micronutrient has a characteristic response. Figure 13.1 presents a diagram of this model generalized for micronutrients pertinent to sheep nutrition. The early stage of micronutrient deficiency, frequently exacerbated by complex interactions, is one of the most challenging themes of micronutrient science. An understanding at the molecular level of the biological behaviour of each micronutrient is a prerequisite for practical solutions to identifying and ameliorating the causes of marginal deficiencies common in sheep husbandry.

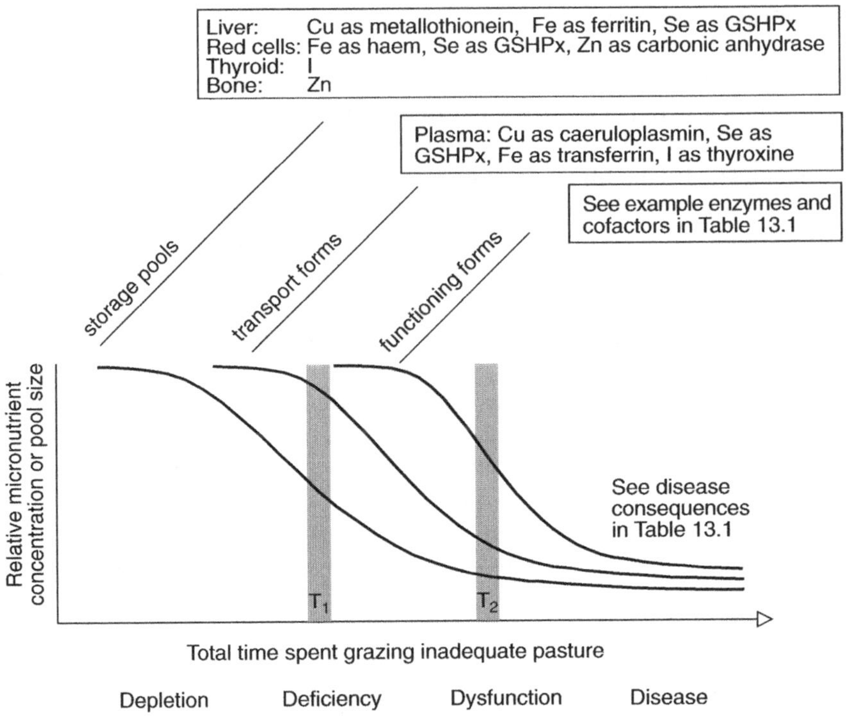

Fig. 13.1. Physiological events occurring during insufficiency of a micronutrient (adapted from Underwood and Suttle, 1999). The consequences of feeding inadequate micronutrient supply are a function of time. Short durations (grey bar T_1) may markedly deplete measured concentrations of the storage form of a nutrient, but have little or no effect on the pool sizes of transport and functional forms. Longer durations (grey bar T_2) can lead to drastically reduced transport pool size, which limits incorporation into functional forms, thus causing reduced or failed function. If unchecked, disease and death will follow.

Requirements and Availability

Intake and diet

Adequate dietary intake of each micronutrient is essential for optimum wool, meat and milk production from sheep. An understanding of the micronutrient requirements of sheep is desirable in order for producers and nutritional advisers to predict the likelihood or risk of deficiency and to develop appropriate supplementation strategies. Published tables of dietary recommendations for sheep essential micronutrients vary in the range of values given (ARC, 1980; NRC, 1985; SCA, 1990). Although some of the variation reflects the methodology employed to derive optimum intakes (Grace and Clark, 1991), the main differences arise from the inclusion of a variable safety margin over and above the minimum requirement (White, 1996). In practice, the recommended requirement of a trace nutrient will often include the safety margin to account for variations in intake, productivity and availability of the nutrient over a broad range of conditions. Desirably, the recommended requirement will meet the need for functions, such as the immune system, that may have a higher requirement than those traits (growth rate, reproduction) that are normally measured when determining minimum requirements of the animal.

In general, there is no recommended dietary requirement for the water-soluble vitamins in sheep with a functioning rumen. Endogenous synthesis of ascorbic acid is usually sufficient to meet the vitamin C requirements of sheep and their requirements for vitamin K and the B vitamins are usually met from microbial synthesis. Suckled lambs meet their needs for the water-soluble vitamins from tissue stores but primarily from milk. However, deficiencies of a number of these vitamins have been reported and, for sheep at pasture, deficiencies of vitamin B_{12} and occasionally thiamine are of concern. The minimum daily vitamin B_{12} requirement of sheep is about 0.3 μg kg^{-1} body weight (Marston, 1970).

It is difficult to assess nutrient intake from pasture analysis because of selective grazing, adventitious intake of soil and interaction of ingested nutrients; hence regular monitoring of a productivity trait and/or testing blood or tissues for an indication of nutrient status is desirable. In intensive sheep-production systems, supplementary-feeding options are more readily available. For further reading on micronutrient recommendations for sheep, the reader is directed to publications by Grace and Clark (1991), Masters and White (1996) and Underwood and Suttle (1999).

Figure 13.2 draws on data from all these sources to compare generally accepted 'standard' reference ranges (low–high) for sheep dietary requirements of key micronutrients with concentrations often found in grazed pastures (Ballet *et al.*, 2000; MacPherson, 2000). Globally, forage samples vary widely in range and quantity of micronutrient provided and in factors affecting their utilization. For instance, vitamin E concentrations in dry summer and autumn pastures in southern Australia may be as low as 1–3 mg kg^{-1} dry matter (DM). Seleniferous areas throughout the world support plants that accumulate high concentrations of Se, which may be toxic to grazing animals. Sheep grazing pastures growing on peat soils are frequently at risk of Cu deficiency, as plant uptake of Cu is restricted, while Mo uptake is high.

Absorption

Micronutrient absorption, together with transport, storage and excretion, are components of the dynamic system, which, across a range of 'normal' dietary intakes and conditions, will result in homoeostasis (Buckley, 2000). Estimation of dietary requirements depends on knowledge of the absorption coefficient of the micronutrient and on various production parameters for growth (including that for wool), pregnancy and lactation. Estimates of trace-element requirements for sheep (e.g. ARC, 1980) have often been based on the factorial model, the principles of which have been discussed

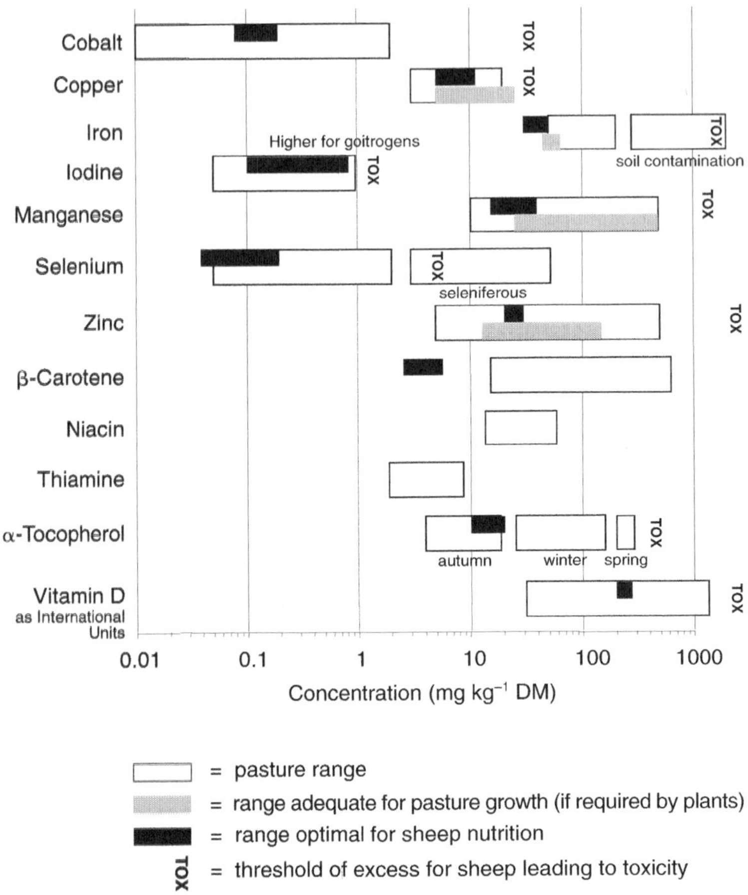

Fig. 13.2. Optimum ranges for some micronutrients to meet sheep requirements relative to typical ranges found in grazed pastures. Not all micronutrients necessary for sheep nutrition are required for pasture growth.

by Grace and Clark (1991) and its strengths and limitations by Underwood and Suttle (1999). The model uses data from nutritional balances, whole-animal compositional analyses and radioisotope-tracer studies. The latter serve to quantify the fraction of a trace element that is consumed, absorbed, retained by tissue pools or excreted.

Newer approaches, based on the use of stable isotope tracers and advanced measurement technologies, are now available, which will enable better estimates of these parameters (Buckley, 1991; Knowles *et al.*, 2000). Typical absorption coefficients for a range of trace elements and vitamin B_{12} in sheep are summarized in Table 13.2. The feature of this table is the variation in absorption for many micronutrients. This variation is partly a function of animal need, age and physiological state, but environmental and dietary factors also contribute. For several of the essential transition metals (e.g. Cu, Fe), absorption may be very low, partly as a result of low solubility

Table 13.2. Absorption, distribution and excretion of key trace elements by grass-fed sheep.

Micro-nutrient[a]	Absorption coefficient[b]	Absorption site	Whole body distribution[c]	Major excretion route	Conditions and features
Copper	0.01–0.13	Small intestine	0.8 ± 0.3[d] (0.08–150)	Bile, faeces	Binds to metallothionein in the gut mucosa Some breeds very susceptible to high accumulation in liver
Iodine	> 0.9	Rumen, small intestine	– (1200–2000)[e]	Urine	Endogenous loss from abomasum, with resorption from small intestine Eighty per cent of whole-body I found in thyroid
Iron	0.05–0.6	Duodenum	45 ± 2 (1–850)	Faeces	Absorption varies according to need and dietary intake, but is typically low in grazing sheep and high in milk-fed lambs Red cells contain 40% of whole-body Fe
Manganese	Not defined but < 0.05	Small and large intestine	0.5 ± 0.03 (0.02–4.3)	Faeces	Requirements higher for testicular growth in sheep (Masters *et al.*, 1988)
Molybdenum	–	–	0.028 ± 0.005[f] (0.005–1.5)	Urine, faeces	High absorption is curtailed by presence of Cu and S, when excretion via faeces predominates Highest concentrations in liver
Selenium	0.3–0.6	Small intestine (anterior)	0.03 ± 0.008 (0.02–0.35)	Urine, faeces, exhalation	Incorporated into rumen microbial fraction Readily resorbed from bile
Zinc	0.2–0.75	Abomasum, small intestine	26 ± 1.6 (0.7–100)	Pancreatic secretions, faeces	Absorption varies according to need and dietary intake, declining as intake exceeds requirement Absorption by ruminants high, as rumen degrades potentially chelating plant phytates
Cobalt (vitamin B_{12})	0.03–0.05	Small intestine	– (0.06–1.4)[g]	Bile, faeces	Absorption varies according to need and dietary intake Significant resorption from bile About 13% of Co is converted to vitamin B_{12}

[a]Other vitamins not listed do not have a readily definable absorption coefficient.
[b]Absorption coefficient = [dietary intake – (faecal output – endogenous loss)] / dietary intake (see Underwood and Suttle, 1999). Ranges depend on animal and environment conditions.
[c]Concentrations (mg $kg^{-1} \pm$ SD fresh tissue) in an entire sheep, and (range) among sheep organs (Grace, 1983b; Grace and Lee, 1990).
[d]Fleece-free empty body minus liver (Grace, 1983b).
[e]Thyroid only (Underwood and Suttle, 1999).
[f]Grace and Martinson (1985), J. Lee and S.O. Knowles (unpublished data).
[g]Vitamin B_{12} in liver.

in the anaerobic environment of the rumen. Sheep are particularly vulnerable to both Cu deficiency and toxicity – deficiency as a result of digestive processes in the rumen forming poorly absorbed Cu sulphides (exacerbated by interactions with Mo – see below) or toxicity from excessive Cu accumulation in the liver. A balance of dietary intake and Cu excretion in bile maintains Cu homoeostasis in animals.

By way of example, a generalized factorial model for the metabolism of Cu for a 50 kg Romney ewe at maintenance is illustrated in Fig. 13.3. The model depicts the movement of pasture Cu through the body. Irretrievable loss occurs via the fetus and milk outputs of the pregnant and lactating ewe, respectively, and also via wool, although this is comparatively small. In this model, total daily output by excretion or secretion of Cu is about 1 mg day^{-1} (endogenous loss + milk (or fetus) + urine + wool) for the lactating or pregnant ewe. For simplicity, steady state has been imposed on the tissue compartments, as the animal is neither gaining nor losing weight and the transfer of Cu between pools follows first-order kinetics. In reality, both compartment sizes and fluxes will be continuously changing over time. Movement of Cu from the liver into the blood pool is assumed to be similar to that from biliary excretion (Buckley, 1991), although in the sheep the movement of Cu from the liver into plasma may be greater than that leaving via bile. Total salivary output is about 0.2 mg day^{-1} and, together with output in pancreatic

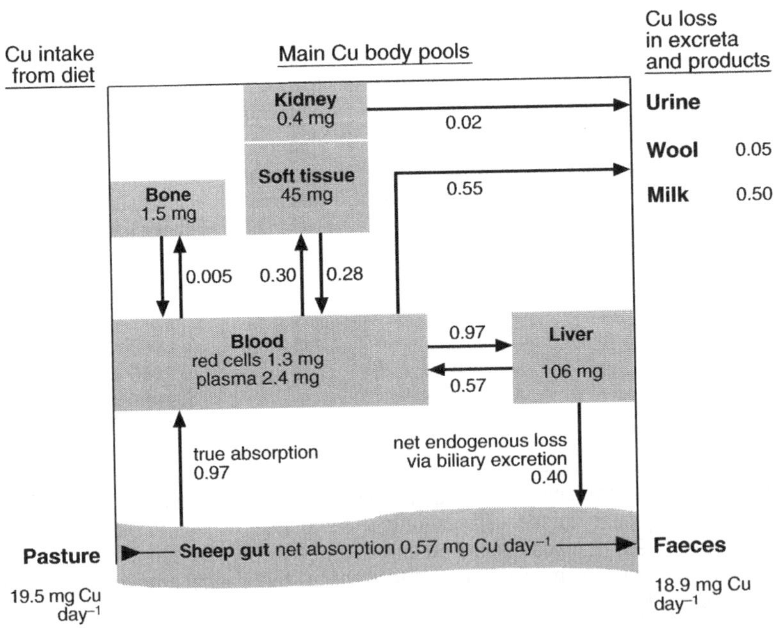

Fig. 13.3. An example of a factorial model, in this case for Cu absorption and utilization, showing whole-body distribution and movement of Cu between pools in a mature lactating ewe (pool sizes, mg; fluxes, as mg day^{-1}).

juice (0.06 mg Cu day^{-1}) and bile (0.3 mg Cu day^{-1}) (Grace and Gooden, 1980), combined secretions exceed endogenous loss, with no allowance made for erosion of intestinal cells. The extent to which Cu in some of these secretions is resorbed is not known, although resorption of Cu in bile is thought to be low. Urinary Cu output for sheep (as in cattle (Buckley, 1991)) is generally less than 2% of the daily flux leaving the liver. Few tracer studies have been conducted to measure endogenous loss in sheep or cattle, so there is uncertainty on the magnitude of this loss from the body. In the present model, Cu requirements are met, and therefore any decrease in the absorption coefficient and/or dietary intake will require mobilization of Cu from the liver to meet the Cu demands of the tissues. This must be sustained until further absorption of Cu. In the sections below, we summarize some of the factors and interactions that affect Cu absorption.

Factors Affecting Bioavailability

The regulation of micronutrients in sheep metabolism involves factors that affect availability, absorption, transport and utilization. The fate of soluble micronutrients in the rumen depends on flow between pools, sorption with digesta (feed particles), uptake by microorganisms and membrane transport. The highly anaerobic rumen environment dictates the chemical speciation or form of trace elements entering the intestines. Chemical equilibrium is further modified through progressive changes in pH and chemical composition. For instance, insoluble sulphides account for most of the Cu, Fe and Zn present in the solid fractions of the rumen contents.

Feed components and soil ingestion

Forages vary widely in micronutrient content, as a consequence of species, stage of maturity, soil type, seasonal and temporal climatic factors and soil fertility or fertilizer applications (Ballet *et al.*, 2000; MacPherson, 2000). Changes in pasture quality – energy and protein digestibility – along with pasture contamination and faecal and soil ingestion complicate the estimation of apparent absorption and digestibility of trace elements by grazing sheep and thus may confound micronutrient requirements. High-protein pasture is known to reduce Cu absorption. Vegetative growth stages may have lower concentrations of elements that are not essential to plant growth (e.g. Co, Se) through growth dilution. On unimproved pastures and rangelands, 'accumulator' plants and browsed leaves of trees and shrubs that contain high concentrations of some elements can affect trace-element supply.

Carotenoids are the most diverse and widespread group of pigments found in plants and microorganisms, but are not synthesized by animals. Less than 10% of the carotenoids can be metabolized to retinol and function as vitamin A precursors in mammals, with β-carotene the most active of these. The degree of green colour in forages is a credible index of its carotene content, and good pasture will provide a liberal supply of carotene. The type of pasture, whether it is grass or legume, is of minor importance, but plants at maturity can have substantially less carotene than the growing plant, since the carotene is readily destroyed by oxidation.

Plant tocopherols are present in lipid-containing fractions of green leaves and seeds. Of the four isomers with vitamin E activity, α-tocopherol is the most biologically active. Although green forages are generally a good source of vitamin E, there is wide variation in pasture concentrations. Stability of tocopherol is poor and substantial losses of vitamin E activity can occur with maturity and drying of pasture. Vitamin D_2 (ergocalciferol) is the major naturally occurring form of this vitamin in plants; it is formed by natural irradiation of sterols with UV light. Plants are generally a poor source of this vitamin, but sun-dried herbage contains more vitamin D than does fresh herbage when compared on a dry-matter basis. Glucosinolates in brassica plants produce goitrogenic effects in sheep and these are exacerbated when dietary I is low (see Waghorn *et al.*, Chapter 15, this volume).

Soil intake affects the absorption and storage of trace elements in ruminants (Grace *et al.*, 1996). Grazing sheep inevitably ingest some soil, and the amount varies between 2 and 25% of DM intake, with ingestion high for sheep on very short pastures or during a wet winter. Soil may contribute up to 20% of the total dietary intake for some trace elements, notably Co, Fe, Mn and I, which are more concentrated in soil than in herbage. Other than providing a source of Co for rumen synthesis of B_{12}, soil ingestion does not contribute significantly to the intake of vitamins.

Rumen microflora

The availability and metabolic utilization of micronutrients depends on their passage through the rumen, as interactions with the microbial pool may affect their subsequent release and transformation. The rumen microflora of sheep has first call on ingested micronutrients but, for the most part, microbial growth and synthesis are not limited by supply of essential trace elements in normal grazing situations. Rumen microbes respond rapidly and efficiently to changes in dietary Co to synthesize vitamin B_{12} (cobalamin), although efficiency of conversion decreases as dietary Co increases. One form of cobalamin (methylcobalamin) is required by microbes for methane, acetate and methionine synthesis, and deficiency leads to succinate accumulation in rumen liquor as a result of inhibition of propionate metabolism (for review, see Underwood and Suttle, 1999). It appears that some species of rumen microorganisms (propionate-producing bacteria) are cobalamin-dependent, with *in vitro* studies using Co-deficient substrates demonstrating shifts in microbial populations of some cultures (McDonald and Suttle, 1986).

Molybdenum affects sulphide production in the rumen, and a very high concentration of dietary Mo (50 mg kg^{-1} DM) may inhibit the number of sulphide-producing bacteria in the rumen of sheep. Supplements of Se have been shown to increase hepatic retention of Cu in sheep (Millar *et al.*, 1988), and Cu and Se together increased Se concentrations in liver to a greater extent than Se supplementation alone (Hartman and van Ryssen, 1997).

It appears that significant quantities of α-tocopherol and β-carotene are subjected to microbial metabolism in the rumen. Both micronutrients appear to have beneficial effects on the growth of rumen microbes and fibre digestion (Hino *et al.*, 1993).

Micronutrient interactions

Micronutrient absorption, availability and utilization are sensitive to inorganic and organic interactions among dietary components. The sparing of Se by vitamin E is a rare example of synergistic interaction, but more commonly the interactions are antagonistic, with marginal deficiencies of trace elements frequently exacerbated. The utilization of dietary Cu is sensitive to inhibition by co-consumed antagonists (notably Fe, Mo and S), and provides a good example of how dietary factors affect trace-element bioavailability, absorption and accumulation (see Fig. 13.4). The effect of increasing pasture Mo concentration, in the presence of dietary S, on absorption and storage of Cu by grazing sheep remains an important problem, as Mo concentrations as low as 1 mg Mo kg^{-1} DM in pasture have a significant impact on Cu absorption in sheep (Knowles *et al.*, 2000). The formation in the rumen of poorly absorbed Cu–thiomolybdate complexes results in an induced Cu deficiency or low Cu status, which in turn is linked with bone and nervous disorders, poor liveweight gain and impaired reproductive performance (Mason, 1981; Gooneratne *et al.*, 1989). Interestingly, this interaction is used beneficially in treating chronic Cu poisoning in sheep (van Ryssen, 1994).

Predictive regression equations derived from pasture concentrations of Cu, Mo and S and from Cu concentrations in liver show pasture Mo as the main factor linked to Cu deficiency (Suttle, 1996; Underwood and Suttle, 1999; Knowles *et al.*, 2000), but Cu absorption is also impaired through interactions with Fe and Zn (Fig. 13.5). Increasing dietary Fe intake of lambs reduces Cu concentration in the liver (Wang and Masters, 1990), perhaps via the formation of insoluble mixed Fe and Cu sulphides in the gastrointestinal tract. The form of Fe may be important, as intake of Fe oxides from soil ingestion does not affect either Fe or Cu concentrations in the liver (Grace *et al.*, 1996). Excess dietary Zn reduces absorption of Cu and decreases Cu concentrations in plasma and liver. This effect is related to the extent of metallothionein (MT) protein expression, initial Cu pool size in the liver, duration of the Zn dose, level of DM intake and age of animal (Lee *et al.*, 1994). High dietary Zn increases the output of Cd in faeces

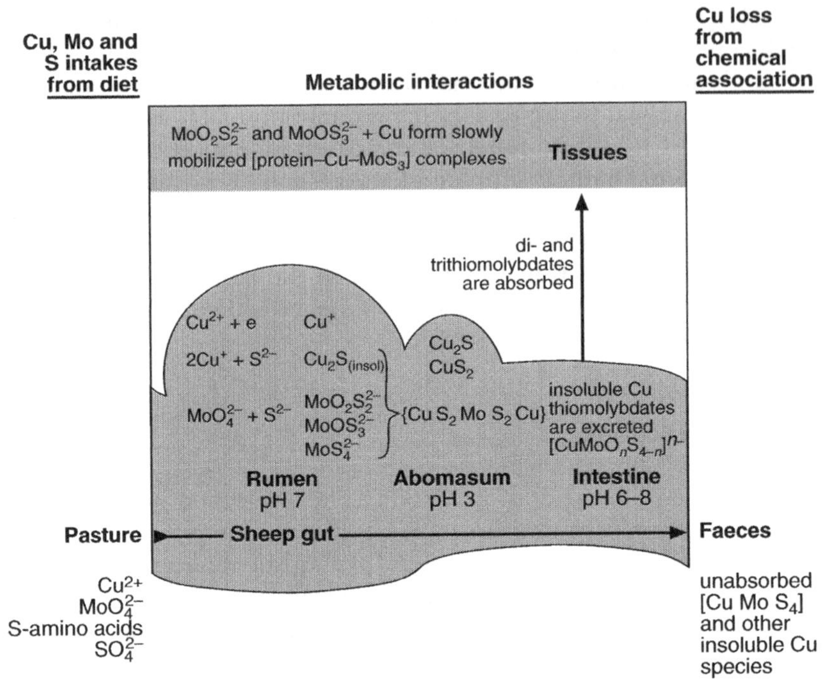

Fig. 13.4. The biochemical association of dietary Mo with Cu in the presence of S at rumen and abomasum pH results in the formation of unabsorbable Cu-tetrathiomolybdates and other insoluble Cu species.

and reduces Cd absorption in sheep (Lee *et al.*, 1996a), but accretion of Cd in the kidneys with time occurs through its association with MT. Zinc induces MT synthesis, which improves the ability of the kidney to sequester Cd (Lee *et al.*, 1994).

Adequate amounts of both I and Se are required for optimal thyroid metabolism. Thyroxine (T_4) is the major hormone produced by the thyroid, but 5′-monodeiodination of T_4 is necessary to create the biologically active form, tri-iodothyronine (T_3). Two deiodinase enzymes (ID1 and ID2), both selenoenzymes, are responsible for the conversion of T_4 to T_3. ID1 in liver and kidney is the major source of plasma T_3, whereas ID2 is a major source of intracellular T_3 in the central nervous system and brown adipose tissue. The effects of Se deficiency on thyroid-hormone metabolism are mediated through changes in deiodinase activities, particularly ID1 activity, and Se deficiency has been shown to compound the harmful effects of I deficiency (Arthur and Beckett, 1994). Selenium supplementation may also ameliorate I deficiency via a compensatory deiodinase response in the thyroid gland and an increased activity of cytosolic glutathione peroxidase (cGSHPx) activity to protect the thyrocyte against toxic effects of hydrogen peroxide. The latter is needed for the oxidation of I before iodination of tyrosine residues in the *de novo* synthesis of T_4 (Zagrodzki *et al.*, 1998).

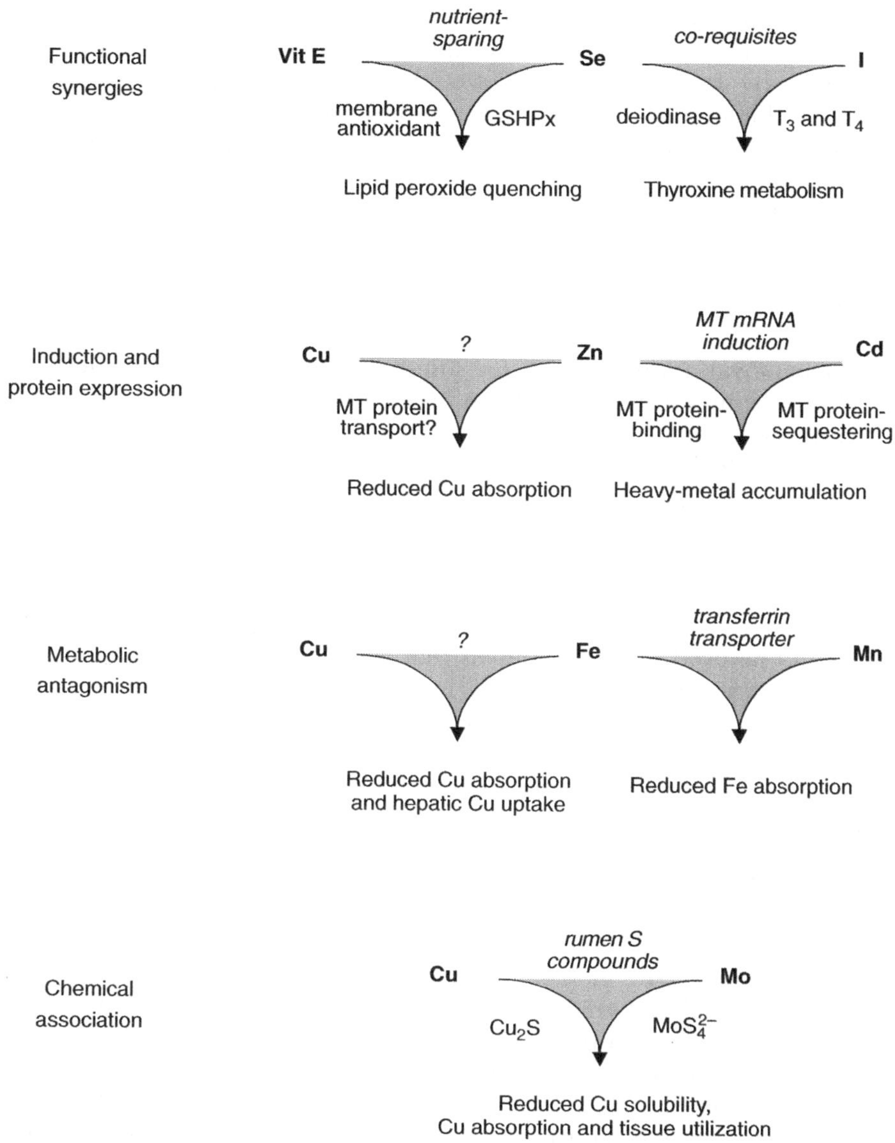

Fig. 13.5. Multiple interactions among elements may be synergistic or antagonistic, with mutual interactions not always of equal strength. A complex three-way interaction among Cu, Zn and Cd is mediated by metallothionein (MT).

Supplements of Se and vitamin E in excess of dietary requirements have complementary functions in reducing the severity and duration of diseases. For instance, both micronutrients appear to have discrete and interactive effects on the immune system (Finch and Turner, 1996). Also, both vitamin E and Se as GSHPx are potent antioxidants. Vitamin E protects tissue membranes by blocking the formation of hydroperoxides from polyunsaturated fatty acids, whereas GSHPx protects cell components against a range of oxidants, including superoxide, hydrogen peroxide and hydroxyl radicals. These micronutrients work together to protect cells from biological damage that can lead to cardiac and skeletal muscle myopathies (white-muscle disease). Unfortunately, this apparent reciprocal sparing effect is not without limits; in severe deficiencies of either nutrient, the other will not prevent oxidative myopathy.

Breed effects

Genetic variation accounts for some differences in trace-element metabolism within and between sheep breeds (Suttle, 1996). Judson *et al.* (1994) reported genetic heritability estimates and phenotypic correlations for several elements in liver from Merino sheep, with high heritability for liver Cu, Se and Zn. Phenotypic differences in liver concentrations of Cu and Mo and in erythrocyte Cu/Zn superoxide dismutase activity have been observed between flocks of Romney sheep (Knowles *et al.*, 1998). Susceptibility to Cu toxicity varies within and between breeds of sheep (Wiener *et al.*, 1985), and Wiener and others suggest that genetic selection could be used to select animals that would be better suited to specific Cu intakes. Recent developments in genetic techniques and bioinformatics will allow important micronutrient traits to be mapped, with the identification of quantitative trait loci ultimately enabling marker-assisted selection for animals better able to meet requirements.

Physiological state

An animal's requirement for micronutrients varies during its lifetime, due to changes in the metabolic demands of individual tissues brought on by physiological and environmental stressors. For instance, additional inputs are required to support pregnancy and lactation over and above requirements for maintenance and growth (Grace, 1983a; Masters and White, 1996). This additive effect necessitates increased dietary intake, changes to homoeostatic mechanisms (such as increased absorption or reduced excretion) or the mobilization of trace elements from maternal pools (such as Zn from bone or Cu, Se and vitamin B_{12} from liver). Less clear are the adaptations needed to meet conditions of stress involving infection with parasites, bacteria or viruses, or diseases caused by toxins from plants and fungi. Interesting and important future work on this theme will include evaluation of micronutrient roles in maintaining a fully competent immune system.

Efficiency of absorption changes with age and this affects the nominal requirement of many micronutrients. The largest differences are observed for the preruminant lamb. Provision for the neonate is made through reserves built up in the fetal liver during the latter stages of gestation, when an adequate supply of micronutrients is critical. Although the concentrations of many trace elements in milk are quite low (and, for Cu, Fe and Zn, not responsive to supplementation), the suckling lamb is able to absorb more than 70% of that ingested. For Cu, this compares with less than 10% in the weaned lamb. The growing lamb is more susceptible to vitamin B_{12} deficiency than mature animals (Grace, 1983a).

Iodine deficiency in sheep is indicated by an enlarged thyroid (goitre) and, in newborn lambs, low serum T_4 concentrations, with the latter declining with age (Andrewartha *et al.*, 1980). Iodine supplementation and cold temperatures may raise serum T_4 concentrations in sheep. Variation in T_4 concentrations may also occur because Se inadequacy decreases the conversion of T_4 to T_3 and this can result in significant depression of plasma T_3 and an increase in T_4, even in ewes and lambs consuming adequate I (Donald *et al.*, 1994).

Parasite, toxins and immune interactions

Nematode infections, endemic to all pasture systems grazed by sheep, will increase the dietary requirement for many micronutrients. Larval infection can induce Cu deficiency in sheep on normally sufficient pastures, with a combination of reduced absorption and increased endogenous loss decreasing the effective supply of Cu to metabolic processes (Judson *et al.*, 1985; Suttle, 1996). Anthelmintics can increase the concentration of Cu in plasma of sheep, which indicates that even a low worm burden impairs Cu metabolism (Suttle, 1996). Oral treatment of young sheep with Cu needles has been shown to reduce parasite burdens of *Haemonchus contortus* and *Ostertagia circumcinca*, but not the intestinal parasite *Trichostrongylus colubriformis* (Bang *et al.*, 1990).

Macrominerals and trace elements, in particular Cu, Co, Mo, Se and Zn, can influence host–parasite relationships (Suttle and Jones, 1989). Sheep that are naturally low in Cu or have been selected for low plasma Cu are more susceptible to bacterial infections (Suttle and Jones, 1989). Dietary Mo at relatively high intakes reduces faecal egg counts and total worm burden in sheep (McClure *et al.*, 1999), while abomasal parasitism in lambs has been shown to influence the Cu/Mo/S antagonism and lower Cu status (Ortolani *et al.*, 1993). Observations of high worm burdens, elevated worm-egg outputs, reduced prepatent periods and increased mortality have been reported in Co-deficient lambs (Ferguson *et al.*, 1989). Selenium deficiency can have a profound effect not only on the immune system of the animal but also on the virulence of the invading organism (Beck and Matthews, 2000). However, there is no evidence that Se status has any influence on parasite infestation; Se-deficient sheep experimentally given *H. contortus* showed the same infestation establishment, abomasal worm burden and inflammatory response in the abomasum as Se-supplemented sheep (Jelinek *et al.*, 1988).

There is increasing evidence that trace elements influence the pathophysiology arising from the ingestion of toxins. Sheep of low Co status appear more susceptible to annual ryegrass toxicity, possibly because of the increased risk from liver damage (Davies *et al.*, 1995). Lupinosis, a mycotoxicosis caused by the fungus *Phomopsis leptostromiformis* in grazing sheep, leads to liver damage associated with increased concentrations of Cu and Se and decreased concentrations of Zn and Fe in liver. The accumulation of Cu and reduction in Zn in liver was shown to be a consequence and not a cause of liver damage. Lupinosis may therefore lead to secondary Zn deficiency (White *et al.*, 1994). Novel interactions involving phomopsin, vitamin E and Se as selenomethionine are proposed as being involved in lupinosis-associated myopathy, a muscle disease observed in weaner sheep grazing phomopsis-infected lupin (Smith and Allen, 1997).

Plants belonging to the *Heliotropium*, *Echium* and *Senecio* genera contain pyrrolizidine alkaloids. As with lupinosis, the liver is the main target organ for the toxin, and affected sheep may show elevated concentrations of Cu and reduced concentrations of Zn in the liver (Seaman, 1987) (see Waghorn *et al.*, Chapter 15, this volume).

Intervention for Health and Quality

Supplementation

A regional or district history of disorders among grazing animals attributable to trace element or vitamin deficiencies is typically the first impetus to provide micronutrient supplements. Evidence that perceived deficiencies are affecting health and productivity of the animal should be obtained from diagnostic tests (see above) and/or dose–response trials before implementing a potentially costly supplementation programme.

Various methods are available for supplying micronutrients to the grazing animal (Judson, 1996; Lee *et al.*, 1999; McDowell, 2000a). Table 13.3 lists supplements suitable for seasonal or long-term dietary inadequacies. Delivering the supplement as a drench is not normally recommended because of the limited effectiveness of this method and the requirement for frequent or repeated doses because of rapid passage time through the rumen. An exception is in the treatment of thiamine deficiency in sheep at pasture, where a single oral dose of thiamine was regarded as the most appropriate means of suppressing intestinal thiaminase activity (Thomas, 1986). Selenium drenches for sheep can be effective for up to 2 months (Judson, 1996).

Successful use of long-term treatments has not been without problems, as experienced with the intraruminal pellets of Se and Co. The short effective life of the pellet in releasing Se was attributed to the use of small, rather than large, particles of elemental Se as the active constituent, and in releasing Co to possible subtle differences in the Co oxide used in the

Table 13.3. Examples of trace-element and vitamin supplement strategies for sheep (see also Judson (1996) and Lee *et al.* (1999)).

Micronutrient	Chemical form	Presentation	Dosage	Efficacy	Comments and references
Copper	Copper in organic complexes	Injectable s.c. or i.m.	0.5–1 mg Cu kg^{-1} to all ages	> 6 months	Cu complexes of glycinate, EDTA, methionate or heptonate differ in their Cu release rate and in severity of injection-site reaction
Copper	Copper oxide	Oral needle or particles	1.25 g to lambs, 2.5 g to sheep	6–9 months	Cu oxide is inert in the rumen but soluble in acid environment of the abomasum. Slow trickle of particles from the rumen to abomasum reduces the risk of Cu toxicity. Effectiveness might be reduced if given to sheep with scours
Selenium	Barium selenate in oil carrier	Injectable s.c. or i.m. at anterior neck	1 mg Se kg^{-1} to all ages	> 1 year	Slow dissolution of barium selenate at injection site allows sustained release. Se depot persists at injection site and must be discarded at slaughter
Selenium	5% elemental Se in Fe matrix	Oral rumen pellet	10 g pellet to weaned sheep	> 1 year	Pellet retained in rumen. Alternatively, an oral drench of selenate at 0.1 mg Se kg^{-1} given before weaning has 2–3-month efficacy.
Cobalt (vitamin B_{12})	Microencapsulated B_{12} in oil carrier	Injectable s.c.	0.25 mg kg^{-1} to lambs or ewes	8 months	Microspheres of lactide–glycolide polymer slowly release micro-encapsulated vitamin B_{12} (Grace and Lewis, 1998). Urinary loss of the vitamin is thus reduced compared with aqueous carrier preparations, which offer only 1–2 months' efficacy (based on MMA levels in prime lambs)
Cobalt (vitamin B_{12})	30% cobaltic oxide in Fe matrix	Oral rumen pellet	10 g pellet to weaned lambs or sheep	> 1 year	Pellet retained in rumen for long-term protection against Co deficiency. The abrasive action of a co-administered grub screw may assist in the release of Co from the pellet and prevent salt deposition
Iodine	26% I_2 in oil	Injectable i.m.	390 mg I to ewes	8–12 months	Administer premating for maximum efficacy. Prevents goitre in lambs when ewes graze low-I pasture or brassica crops
α-Tocopherol (vitamin E)	Aqueous emulsion of α-tocopherol acetate	Oral drench or injectable s.c.	2 g to weaners	2–3 months	Injection is more effective than oral route for raising liver vitamin E reserves
Multi (Co, Cu, Se, Zn)	Elements in soluble PO_4 glass matrix	Oral rumen pellet	16 g pellet to lambs, 33 g pellet to sheep	6–8 months	Pellet retained in rumen, where the phosphate glass readily dissolves to release elements. Not affected by salt deposition and hence suitable for suckling animals (Mackenzie *et al.*, 2000)
Multi (Co, Cu, I, Mn, Se, Zn, vit. A, vit. D, vit. E)	Nutrients compressed and coated for controlled release	Oral rumen pellet	30 g pellet to weaners	> 4 months	Nutrients are compressed into a cylindrical pellet and coated, apart from the flat end, with a resin. Pellet is retained in rumen and release of ingredients occurs from the exposed end of the mix. For seasonal coverage of trace element and vitamins. May be unsuitable for lambs on Cu-adequate pasture (Hemingway *et al.*, 1997)

s.c., subcutaneously; i.m., intramuscularly; EDTA, ethylenediamine tetra-acetic acid; MMA, methylmalonic acid.

pellet. Recent developments in intraruminal devices include multi-element glass boluses and polymer-coated boluses containing trace elements and fat-soluble vitamins, as well as those of variable geometry that are able to provide a constant or variable supply of micronutrients over extended periods (Judson, 1996). A number of these devices permit the use of organic forms of the trace elements, which may increase the availability of the element, although initial findings regarding the use of these complexes have not been encouraging (Lee *et al.*, 1999).

Recent developments in the subcutaneous or intramuscular injection of micronutrients include long-acting barium selenate and vitamin B_{12} supplements (Table 13.3) (see Plate 13.1). These remedies provide a depot of the active constituent at the injection site and ideally should cause little tissue reaction and no residue of carrier after exhaustion of the active constituent. Supplements supplied as both licks and blocks or via drinking-water often have limited success because of unregulated intake. The option of soil or plant treatments should not be overlooked, since such applications may also produce a response in pasture production. The synthesis of α-tocopherol and β-carotene in plants usually results in levels of these vitamins in green pasture well in excess of the apparent dietary requirement by sheep.

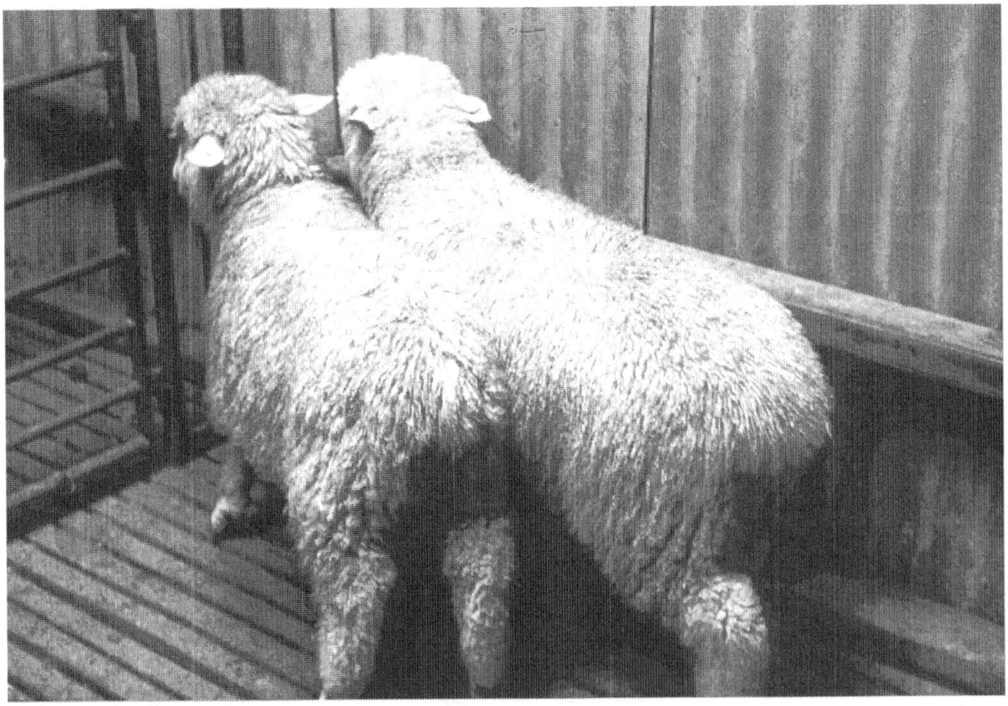

Plate 13.1. Housed cross-bred lambs showing the results of different nutritional histories with respect to vitamin B_{12}. At 6 weeks of age, the lambs were the same weight; the lamb on the right was given an injection of vitamin B_{12}. As a result, it was heavier than its age-mate when this photo was taken 20 weeks later.

Micronutrients and product quality

Dietary intake of micronutrients by sheep can enhance the quality characteristics of meat, offal and wool, but, conversely, excessive intakes may be unhealthy for the consumer (Howell, 1996). The nutritional ideal would have meat and milk contain those trace elements that are beneficial to human health (i.e. Fe, Se and Zn in meat products and Fe, I and Se in milk) at concentrations sufficient to meet human recommended dietary requirements, while deleterious elements, such as Cd in kidney and liver, do not accumulate above regulatory maximum residue limits.

Meat products are a significant source of dietary micronutrients for humans, including vitamin B_{12} and other B-group vitamins, Fe, Zn and potentially Se. Supplements given for animal-health reasons can increase trace-element concentrations in tissues, notably in the liver, but the changes in muscle tend to be small and well within accepted safety standards (Masters *et al.*, 1992). Bioavailability of Fe in sheep diets has been manipulated, using metal-chelating agents, to reduce muscle Fe and thus improve colour. However, Fe supplied at three times the normal intake for sheep grazing ryegrass/white clover pasture did not affect meat Fe, but markedly reduced the concentration of Cu in both liver and carcass (Grace and Lee, 1990). Manipulation of dietary Fe in order to effect changes to either meat colour or Fe concentration should be accompanied by monitoring of the Cu status of the animal because of the potential for Fe to reduce Cu status.

Pharmacological doses of Zn oxide given as a drench for the prevention of facial eczema (see Waghorn *et al.*, Chapter 15, this volume) increased Zn concentrations in muscle of sheep (Lee *et al.*, 1994). A combination of breed and diet can result in differences between concentrations of Fe and Zn in lamb from different countries (Lin *et al.*, 1988). Selenium concentration in muscle reflects Se dietary intake, and supplementation to sheep may be a method for raising Se intake of humans. Supplementation with either inorganic Se (selenite or selenate) or selenomethionine increases muscle Se concentration, but the organic form is more effective because of direct incorporation of selenomethionine into proteins in place of methionine (Knowles *et al.*, 1999).

High concentrations of some trace elements and heavy metals in animal products frequently occur when sheep graze pastures that have accumulated contaminants from fertilizer. Elements such as As, Cd, F, Hg and Pb accumulate in fertilized soils. Absorption and accumulation of Cd in sheep kidney and liver is age-dependent and can be predicted from knowledge of pasture Cd concentrations and phosphate-fertilizer history (Loganathan *et al.*, 1999). Cadmium concentrations in muscle are low compared with those in liver and kidney, and remain low regardless of the Cd intake and age of the animal (Lee *et al.*, 1996b).

Wool accumulates trace elements during its growth, and this may reflect the trace-element status of the sheep at the time of wool-fibre development. However, little is known about the factors that influence the trace-element composition of wool (Lee *et al.*, 1999). Copper, Se and Zn have been implicated as influencing wool properties (Purser, 1978), while breed, diet and season may also change wool trace-element content. The role of trace elements in wool growth is discussed more fully by Hynd and Masters (Chapter 8, this volume).

Conclusion

The micronutrient deficiencies most commonly encountered in the field are of a marginal nature, often with non-specific ill thrift as the only sign of a disorder. Therefore, tests of blood and tissue are relied on to identify which micronutrient might be limiting productivity. For many of the micronutrients, biochemical changes in blood precede dysfunction, so monitoring of these changes provides early warning. Although some production responses are unambiguous, the complex interrelationships between micronutrients, immune function and disease are only beginning to be unravelled.

In spite of a proliferation of tabled values, the concept of requirements or dietary allowances remains poorly defined for micronutrients. For practical purposes, however, intakes should permit best productivity and health (including immune competency) and provide for adequate body reserves of the micronutrient over a range of environmental conditions. Improving productivity through 'smarter' nutritional application brings with it increased demands for micronutrients. Considerable progress has been made in methods of supplying additional micronutrients to the grazing animal, particularly with the development of sustained-release devices that reside in the rumen or implants that are subcutaneous. There is an increasing trend for commercial suppliers to incorporate micronutrients in products such as anthelmintic drenches and vaccines.

Research continues to discover new roles and describe novel involvement of micronutrients in structural and catalytic functions within the cell and in gene expression in particular. Such progress improves our understanding of tissue requirements and permits more sophisticated manipulation of the micronutrient content of wool and meat to meet future specifications for these products.

References

Andrewartha, K.A., Caple, I.W., Davies, W.D. and McDonald, J.W. (1980) Observations on serum thyroxine concentrations in lambs and ewes to assess iodine nutrition. *Australian Veterinary Journal* 56, 18–21.

ARC (Agricultural Research Council) (1980) *The Nutrient Requirements of Ruminant Livestock*. Commonwealth Agricultural Bureaux, Farnham Royal, UK, 351 pp.

Arthur, J.R. and Beckett, G.T. (1994) Roles of selenium in Type I iodothyronine 5′-deiodinase and in thyroid hormone and iodine metabolism. In: Burk, R.F. (ed.) *Selenium and Biology and Human Health*. Springer-Verlag, New York, pp. 93–115.

Ballet, N., Robert, J.C. and Williams, P.E.V. (2000) Vitamins in forages. In: Givens, D.J., Owen, E., Axford, R.F.E. and Omed, H.M. (eds) *Forage Evaluation in Ruminant Nutrition*. CAB International, Wallingford, UK, pp. 399–431.

Bang, K.S., Familton, A.S. and Sykes, A.R. (1990) Effect of ostertagiasis on copper status in sheep: a study involving use of copper oxide wire particles. *Research in Veterinary Science* 49, 306–314.

Beck, M.A. and Matthews, C.C. (2000) Micronutrients and host resistance to viral infection. *Proceedings of the Nutrition Society* 59, 581–585.

Buckley, W.T. (1991) A kinetic model of copper metabolism in lactating dairy cows. *Canadian Journal of Animal Science* 71, 155–166.

Buckley, W.T. (2000) Trace element dynamics. In: D'Mello, J.P.F. (ed.) *Farm Animal Metabolism and Nutrition*. CAB International, Wallingford, UK, pp. 161–182.

Cronin, S.J., Manoharan, V., Hedley, M.J. and Loganathan, P. (2000) Fluoride: a review of its fate, bioavailability, and risks of fluorosis in grazed-pasture systems in New Zealand. *New Zealand Journal of Agricultural Research* 43, 295–321.

Davies, S.C., White, C.L. and Williams, I.H. (1995) Increased tolerance to annual ryegrass toxicity in sheep given a supplement of cobalt. *Australian Veterinary Journal* 72, 221–224.

Donald, G.E., Langlands, J.P., Bowles, J.E. and Smith, A.J. (1994) Sub-clinical selenium insufficiency 6. Thermoregulatory ability of perinatant lambs born to ewes supplemented with selenium and iodine. *Australian Journal of Experimental Agriculture* 34, 19–34.

Ferguson, E.G.W., Mitchell, G.B.B. and MacPherson, A. (1989) Cobalt deficiency and *Ostertagia circumcincta* infection in lambs. *Veterinary Record* 124, 1–20.

Finch, J.M. and Turner, R.J. (1996) Effects of selenium and vitamin E on the immune response of domestic animals. *Research in Veterinary Science* 60, 97–106.

Gooneratne, S.R., Buckley, W.T. and Christensen, D.A. (1989) Review of copper deficiency and metabolism in ruminants. *Canadian Journal of Animal Science* 69, 819–845.

Grace, N.D. (1983a) *The Mineral Requirements of Grazing Ruminants*. Occasional Publication No. 9, New Zealand Society of Animal Production, Palmerston North, 150 pp.

Grace, N.D. (1983b) Amounts and distribution of mineral elements associated with fleece-free empty body weight gains in the grazing sheep. *New Zealand Journal of Agricultural Research* 26, 59–70.

Grace, N.D. and Clark, R.G. (1991) Trace element requirements, diagnosis and prevention of deficiencies in sheep and cattle. In: Tsuda, T., Sasaki, Y. and Kawashima, R. (eds) *Physiological Aspects of Digestion and Metabolism in Ruminants. Proceedings of the Seventh International Symposium on Ruminant Physiology*. Academic Press, Tokyo, pp. 321–346.

Grace, N.D. and Gooden, J.M. (1980) Effect of increasing intakes of Zn, Cu, and Mn on their secretion via bile and pancreatic juice and their excretion in faeces and urine in sheep fed lucerne pellets. *New Zealand Journal of Agricultural Research* 23, 293–298.

Grace, N.D. and Lee, J. (1990) Effect of Co, Cu, Fe, Mn, Mo, Se and Zn supplementation on the elemental content of soft tissues and bone in sheep grazing ryegrass/white clover pasture. *New Zealand Journal of Agricultural Research* 33, 635–647.

Grace, N.D. and Lewis, D.H. (1998) An evaluation of an injectable micro-encapsulated vitamin B_{12} to increase and maintain serum and liver vitamin B_{12} concentrations in lambs. *New Zealand Veterinary Journal* 47, 4–7.

Grace, N.D. and Martinson, P.L. (1985) The distribution of Mo between the liver and other organs and tissues of sheep grazing a ryegrass white clover pasture. In: Mills, C.F., Bremner, I. and Chester, J.K. (eds) *Trace Elements in Man and Animals – 5: Proceedings of the Fifth International Symposium on Trace Elements in Man and Animals.* Commonwealth Agricultural Bureaux, Farnham Royal, UK, pp. 534–536.

Grace, N.D., Rounce, J.R. and Lee, J. (1996) Effect of soil ingestion on the storage of Se, vitamin B_{12}, Cu, Cd, Fe, Mn and Zn in the liver of sheep fed lucerne pellets. *New Zealand Journal of Agricultural Research* 39, 325–331.

Hartman, F. and van Ryssen, J.B.J. (1997) Metabolism of selenium and copper in sheep with and without sodium bicarbonate supplementation. *Journal of Agricultural Science* 128, 357–364.

Hemingway, R.G., Parkins, J.J. and Ritchie, N.S. (1997) Sustained-release boluses to supply trace elements and vitamins to calves. *Veterinary Journal* 153, 221–224.

Hino, T., Andoh, N. and Ohgi, H. (1993) Effects of β-carotene and α-tocopherol on rumen bacteria in the utilization of long-chain fatty acids and cellulose. *Journal of Dairy Science* 76, 600–605.

Howell, J. (1996) Toxicities and excessive intakes of minerals. In: Masters, D.G. and White, C.L. (eds) *Detection and Treatment of Mineral Nutrition Problems in Grazing Sheep.* Monograph No. 37, ACIAR, Canberra, pp. 95–117.

Jelinek, P.D., Ellis, T., Wroth, R.H., Sutherland, S.S., Masters, H.G. and Petterson, D.S. (1988) The effect of selenium supplementation on immunity and establishment of an experimental *Haemonchus contortus* infection, in weaner Merino sheep fed a low selenium diet. *Australian Veterinary Journal* 65, 214–217.

Judson, G.J. (1996) Trace element supplements for sheep at pasture. In: Masters, D.G. and White, C.L. (eds) *Detection and Treatment of Mineral Nutrition Problems in Grazing Sheep.* Monograph No. 37, ACIAR, Canberra, pp. 57–80.

Judson, G.J., Brown, T.H., Beveridge, I. and Ford, G.E. (1985) Effect of anthelmintic treatment and stocking rate on trace element and vitamin B_{12} status of young sheep. In: Mills, C.F., Bremner, I. and Chester, J.K. (eds) *Trace Elements in Man and Animals – 5. Proceedings of the Fifth International Symposium on Trace Elements in Man and Animals.* Commonwealth Agricultural Bureaux, Farnham Royal, UK, pp. 549–551.

Judson, G.J., Walkley, J.R.W., James, P.J., Klenmann, D.O. and Ponzoni, R.W. (1994) Genetic variation in trace element status of Merino sheep. *Animal Production in Australia* 20, 438.

Knowles, S.O., Rounce, J.R., Grace, N.D. and Lee, J. (1998) Variation in copper metabolism between two flocks of Romney sheep in response to increasing dietary copper. *Proceedings of the New Zealand Society of Animal Production* 58, 195–198.

Knowles, S.O., Grace, N.D., Wurms, K. and Lee, J. (1999) Significance of amount and form of dietary selenium on blood, milk, and casein selenium concentrations in grazing cows. *Journal of Dairy Science* 82, 429–437.

Knowles, S.O., Grace, N.D., Rounce, J.R., Litherland, A.J., West, D.M. and Lee, J. (2000) Dietary Mo as an antagonist to Cu absorption: stable isotope (^{65}Cu) measurements in grazing sheep. In: Rousel, A.M., Anderson, R.A. and Favier, A.E. (eds) *Trace Elements in Man and Animals – TEMA – 10. Proceedings of the 10th International Symposium on Trace Elements in Man and Animals, Evian, France.* Kluwer Academic, Plenum, New York, pp. 717–721.

Lee, J., Treloar, B.P. and Grace, N.D. (1994) Metallothionein and trace element metabolism in sheep tissues in response to high and sustained zinc dosages. II. Expression of metallothionein mRNA. *Australian Journal of Agricultural Research* 45, 321–332.

Lee, J., Rounce, J.R., Grace, N.D. and Gregoire, D.C. (1996a) Effect of dietary zinc on absorption and tissue accumulation of cadmium in Romney sheep. In: Fischer, P.W.F., l'Abbe, M.R., Cockell, K.A. and Gibson, R.S. (eds) *Trace Elements in Man and Animals – TEMA – 9. Proceedings of the 9th International Symposium on Trace Elements in Man and Animals, Banff, Canada*. NRC Research Press, Ottawa, pp. 199–200.

Lee, J., Rounce, J.R., Mackay, A.D. and Grace, N.D. (1996b) Accumulation of cadmium with time in Romney sheep grazing ryegrass–white clover pasture: effect of cadmium from pasture and soil intake. *Australian Journal of Agricultural Research* 47, 877–894.

Lee, J., Masters, D.G., White, C.L., Grace, N.D. and Judson, G.J. (1999) Current issues in trace element nutrition of grazing livestock in Australia and New Zealand. *Australian Journal of Agricultural Research* 50, 1341–1364.

Lin, K.C., Cross, H.R., Johnson, H.K., Breidenstein, B.C., Randecker, V. and Field, R.A. (1988) Mineral composition of lamb carcasses from the United States and New Zealand. *Meat Science* 24, 47–59.

Loganathan, P., Louie, K., Lee, J., Hedley, M.J., Roberts, A.H.C. and Longhurst, R.D. (1999) A model to predict kidney and liver cadmium concentrations in grazing animals. *New Zealand Journal of Agricultural Research* 42, 423–432.

Mackenzie, A.M., Kendell, N.R., Illingworth, D.V., Jackson, D.W., Gill, I.M. and Telfer, S.B. (2000) The effect of copper, cobalt and selenium bolus on sheep from three upland Scottish farms. In: Rousel, A.M., Anderson, R.A. and Favier, A.E. (eds) *Trace Elements in Man and Animals – TEMA – 10. Proceedings of the 10th International Symposium on Trace Elements in Man and Animals, Evian, France*. Kluwer Academic, Plenum, New York, pp. 749–752.

MacPherson, A. (2000) Trace mineral status of forages. In: Givens, D.J., Owen, E., Axford, R.F.E. and Omed, H.M. (eds) *Forage Evaluation in Ruminant Nutrition*. CAB International, Wallingford, UK, pp. 345–371.

Marston, H.R. (1970) The requirement of sheep for cobalt or for vitamin B_{12}. *British Journal of Nutrition* 24, 615–633.

Mason, J. (1981) Molybdenum–copper antagonism in ruminants: a review of the biochemical basis. *Irish Veterinary Journal* 35, 221–229.

Masters, D.G. and White, C.L. (1996) *Detection and Treatment of Mineral Nutrition Problems in Grazing Sheep*. Monograph No. 37, ACIAR, Canberra, 117 pp.

Masters, D.G., Paynter, D.I., Briegel, J., Baker, S.K. and Purser, D.B. (1988) Influence of manganese intake on body, wool, and testicular growth of young rams and on the concentration of manganese and the activity of manganese enzymes in tissues. *Australian Journal of Agricultural Research* 39, 517–524.

Masters, D.G., White, C.L., Peter, D.W., Purser, D.B., Roe, S.P. and Barnes, M.J. (1992) A multi-element supplement for grazing sheep. 2. Accumulation of trace elements in sheep fed different levels of supplement. *Australian Journal of Agricultural Research* 43, 809–817.

McClure, S.J., McClure, T. J. and Emery, D.L. (1999) The effect of molybdenum on primary infection and subsequent challenge by the nematode parasite *Trichostrongylus colubriformis* in weaned Merino lambs. *Research in Veterinary Science* 67, 17–22.

McDonald, J.W. (1982) Mortality and ill thrift associated with thiamine deficiency in lambs. *Australian Veterinary Journal* 58, 212–213.

McDonald, P. and Suttle, N.F. (1986) Abomasal fermentation in continuous cultures or rumen micro-organisms given cobalt-deficient hay or barley as the food substrate. *British Journal of Nutrition* 56, 369–378.

McDowell, L.R. (2000a) *Vitamins in Animal and Human Nutrition.* Iowa State University Press, Ames, Iowa, 793 pp.

McDowell, L.R. (2000b) Re-evaluation of the metabolic essentiality of the vitamins: review. *Asian–Australian Journal of Animal Science* 13, 115–125.

Millar, K.R., Meads, W.J., Albyt, A.T., Sheppard, A.D. and Scahill, B.G. (1988) The effect of copper on the response of lambs to selenium supplementation when grazing a selenium deficient pasture. *New Zealand Veterinary Journal* 36, 59–62.

NRC (National Research Council) (1985) *Nutrient Requirements of Sheep,* 6th edn. National Academy Press, Washington, DC, 99 pp.

Ortolani, E., Knox, D., Jackson, F., Coop, R. and Suttle, N.F. (1993) Abomasal parasitism lowers liver Cu status and influences the Cu × Mo × S antagonism in lambs. In: Anke, M., Meissner, D. and Mills, C.F. (eds) *Trace Elements in Man and Animals – 8. Proceedings of the Eighth International Symposium on Trace Elements in Man and Animals.* Verlag Media Touristik, Gersdorf, Germany, pp. 331–332.

Purser, D.B. (1978) Effect of minerals upon wool growth. In: Black, J.L. and Reis, P.J. (eds) *Physiological and Environmental Limitations of Wool Growth.* University of New England Publishing Unit, Armidale, Australia, pp. 243–255.

SCA (Standing Committee on Agriculture) (1990) *Feeding Standards for Australian Livestock. Ruminants.* CSIRO Publications, Melbourne, 266 pp.

Seaman, J.T. (1987) Pyrrolizidine alkaloid poisoning of sheep in New South Wales. *Australian Veterinary Journal* 64, 164–167.

Smith, G.M. and Allen, J.G. (1997) Effectiveness of α-tocopherol and selenium supplements in preventing lupinosis-associated myopathy in sheep. *Australian Veterinary Journal* 75, 341–348.

Suttle, N.F. (1996) Non-dietary influences on the mineral requirements of sheep. In: Masters, D.G. and White, C.L. (eds) *Detection and Treatment of Mineral Nutrition Problems in Grazing Sheep.* Monograph No. 37, ACIAR, Canberra, pp. 31–44.

Suttle, N.F. and Jones, D.G. (1989) Recent developments in trace element metabolism and function: trace elements, disease resistance and immune responsiveness in ruminants. *Journal of Nutrition* 119, 1055–1061.

Thomas, K.W. (1986) Oral treatment of polioencephalomalacia and subclinical thiamine deficiency with thiamine propyl disulphide and thiamine hydrochloride. *Journal of Veterinary Pharmacology and Therapeutics* 9, 402–411.

Underwood, E.J. (1977) *Trace Elements in Human and Animal Nutrition,* 4th edn. Academic Press, London, 545 pp.

Underwood, E.J. and Suttle, N.F. (1999) *The Mineral Nutrition of Livestock,* 3rd edn. CAB International, Wallingford, UK, 614 pp.

van Ryssen, J.B.J. (1994) The effectiveness of using supplementary zinc and molybdenum to reduce the copper content in the liver of hypercuprotic sheep. *Journal of the South African Veterinary Association* 65, 59–63.

Wang, Z.S. and Masters, D.G. (1990) Effects of supplementary iron on tissue trace elements and plasma folate and vitamin B_{12} in young sheep. *Proceedings of the Nutrition Society of Australia* 15, 142.

White, C.L. (1996) Understanding the mineral requirements of sheep. In: Masters, D.G. and White, C.L. (eds) *Detection and Treatment of Mineral Nutrition Problems in Grazing Sheep.* Monograph No. 37, ACIAR, Canberra, pp. 15–29.

White, C.L., Masters, D.G., Paynter, D.I., Howell, J.McC., Roe, S.P., Barnes, M.J. and Allen, J.G. (1994) The effects of supplementary copper and a mineral mix on the development of lupinosis in sheep. *Australian Journal of Agricultural Research* 45, 279–291.

Wiener, G., Woolliams, J.A., Suttle, N.F. and Jones, D. (1985) Genetic selection for Cu status in the sheep and its consequences for performance. In: Mills, C.F., Bremner, I. and Chester, J.K. (eds) *Trace Elements in Man and Animals – 5. Proceedings of the Fifth International Symposium on Trace Elements in Man and Animals*. Commonwealth Agricltural Bureaux, Farnham Royal, UK, pp. 193–196.

Zagrodzki, P., Nicol, F., McCoy, M.A., Smyth, J.A., Kennedy, D.G., Beckett, G.J. and Arthur, J.R. (1998) Iodine deficiency in cattle: compensatory changes in thyroidal selenoenzymes. *Research in Veterinary Science* 64, 209–211.

14 Interactions between Gastrointestinal Parasites and Nutrients

R.L. Coop[1] and A.R. Sykes[2]

[1]*Moredun Research Institute, Pentlands Science Park, Edinburgh, UK;* [2]*Animal and Food Sciences Division, Lincoln University, Canterbury, New Zealand*

Introduction

Grazing sheep are invariably infected with a range of nematode species, which are the most important parasites of the gastrointestinal (GI) tract (Table 14.1) and which frequently lead to significant impairment of productivity (Sykes, 1994). Control of GI nematodes in ruminants is currently achieved through prophylactic or therapeutic use of anthelmintics, combined, where farm practice allows, with grazing-management strategies that are aimed at reducing contact between the host and the infective stages of the parasite on pasture. The continued use of suppressive anthelmintic strategies is unsustainable, as nematode resistance to the three main classes of broad-spectrum anthelmintics is now widespread in small ruminants throughout many areas of the world (Waller, 1997). In many parts of the southern hemisphere, anthelmintic resistance is one of the main threats to sustainable livestock production. The ability of nematodes to rapidly develop resistance to new drug families and formulations is of paramount importance, as it is unlikely that many new drugs with novel modes of action will be licensed for future veterinary use in small ruminants, due to the high cost of development for a limited market. A further issue arising from extensive use of anthelmintics is the increasing public awareness of potential drug residues in meat and milk products and also concern about the possible ecotoxicological effects of excretion of certain anthelmintics on the environment, especially beneficial microfauna. These issues have led to a drive to find alternative sustainable control strategies for helminth infections, which are less reliant on chemotherapy (Waller, 1999). One approach has been to investigate the role of dietary supplementation in enhancing the resistance and resilience of livestock that are susceptible to GI parasitism.

Table 14.1. Common gastrointestinal helminths of sheep.

Abomasum	*Teladorsagia* (*Ostertagia*) *circumcincta*[a]
	Teladorsagia (*Ostertagia*) *trifurcata*
	Trichostrongylus axei
	Haemonchus contortus[a]
Small intestine	*Trichostrongylus vitrinus*[a]
	Trichostrongylus colubriformis[a]
	Nematodirus battus[a]
	Nematodirus filicollis
	Nematodirus spathiger
	Cooperia curticei
	Strongyloides papillosus
	Bunostomum trigonocephalum
	Moniezia expansa
Large intestine	*Chabertia ovina*
	Oesophagostomum venulosum
	Oesophagostomum columbianum[a]
	Trichuris ovis

[a]Frequently associated with outbreaks of parasitic gastroenteritis.

In this context of parasite control involving reduced anthelmintic input, greater emphasis is being placed on recognition of sources of contamination (eggs passed in faeces) and their availability to susceptible livestock. The latter is the young naïve lamb, whose protection has traditionally been provided by direct anthelmintic therapy. Increasingly, it is being recognized that reduction in anthelmintic usage will be more readily achieved by limitation of exposure rather than chemical treatment in the face of challenge. This approach recognizes increasingly that the characteristic breakdown in established immunity, characteristic of mammals in the periparturient period, could be a major source of early-season infection to the lamb. Recent work suggests a nutritional involvement in this breakdown, which may be mitigated by supplementation (Donaldson *et al.*, 1998).

In this chapter, parasite/nutrition interactions will be considered from two aspects: first, the impact of infection on the host's metabolic processes and, secondly, the influence of the nutritional status of the host on its ability to resist or tolerate a parasitic challenge.

Effects of Gastrointestinal Nematodes on Host Metabolism

The consequence of parasitic infection on ruminant metabolism has been the subject of several recent reviews (MacRae, 1993; Coop and Holmes, 1996; van Houtert and Sykes, 1996). Gastrointestinal nematodes impair animal productivity primarily through reductions in voluntary feed intake and/or reductions in the efficiency of food utilization, particularly the inefficient use of absorbed nutrients. The magnitude of either effect will be influenced by the extent of larval challenge, the number and species of nematodes, the host's previous experience of parasites and its age and breed. For example, a consistent feature of infection of sheep or cattle with the abomasal nematode (*Teladorsagia/Ostertagia*) is a marked depression of appetite, whereas comparable infection with intestinal *Trichostrongylus* spp. mainly results in impaired ability to use absorbed nutrients for normal body growth.

Malabsorption of nutrients was originally suggested to account for reduced productivity of parasitized ruminants, but recent evidence, cited by van Houtert and Sykes (1996), would support the view that, in many subclinical GI nematode infections, there is only a transient effect or no effect on apparent digestibility of crude protein (CP) or energy. Where radiolabelled tracers have been used to measure 'true' digestibility of protein in sheep, it has been demonstrated that infection with GI nematodes did not significantly affect digestion and absorption of protein during the phase of infection where extensive damage to the GI tract would be expected (Poppi *et al.*, 1986; Bown *et al.*, 1991a).

Effects on feed intake

A common feature of many parasitic infections is a depression in voluntary feed intake, with reductions of 10–30% commonly observed in subclinical infections. Food intake generally recovers once animals have developed immunity to nematodes and presumably are harbouring low worm populations. The degree of inappetence has been shown to be influenced by the intake of dietary protein or phosphorus (P) or both. The magnitude of the reduction in feed intake is less when it is expressed per unit of body weight. Despite the importance of induced inappetence, the mechanisms involved are little understood (Symons, 1985; Kyriazakis *et al.*, 1998).

Studies with cattle infected with the abomasal nematode *Ostertagia ostertagi* have shown direct associations between increased concentrations of the GI hormone gastrin and impaired feed intake (Fox, 1997) and it was suggested that the mode of action might be via alterations in reticulorumen motility and digesta flow. There is evidence that GI nematode infection in sheep can alter the rate of digesta transit (Gregory *et al.*, 1985). Other studies have investigated the possible influence of parasitic infection on central satiety signals and related hormones. Although peripheral activity of the GI peptide cholecystokinin (CCK) appears to have no direct influence on short-term appetite regulation in parasitized sheep (Dynes *et al.*, 1990), recent experiments, in which CCK receptor antagonists were administered either systemically or centrally to sheep infected with *Trichostrongylus colubriformis*, have suggested a role of central brain CCK receptors in the regulation of feed intake (Dynes *et al.*, 1998). These experiments provided evidence that central satiety signals might be involved in the depression of feed intake that accompanies many parasite infections. Parallel studies, in rats infected with the intestinal nematode *Nippostrongylus brasiliensis*, have suggested that changes in hypothalamic neuropeptide gene expression are associated with the reduction in appetite that accompanies infection (Horbury *et al.*, 1995). These data suggest that there may be other suppressive neuroendocrine interactions that can modify the feeding stimulus; signals from adipose tissue could also be involved. An interesting observation is that, if the parasite burden is removed with an anthelmintic drug, then feed intake is rapidly restored to a similar level to that in comparable non-infected sheep (Kyriazakis *et al.*, 1996), despite the fact that the damaged intestinal mucosa has not yet recovered morphologically. These data have led to speculation that GI nematodes might secrete cytokine-like substances that can influence the host's appetite-control mechanisms.

There is a need for further research to clarify the role of hypothalamic neuropeptides and hormones and also the possible influence of cytokines, which are known to influence food intake, in the induction of inappetence by GI nematode infections. Although inappetence undoubtedly contributes to reduced productivity in many parasitic infections, it is not the sole cause. Comparisons of the performance of parasitized sheep with that of uninfected controls offered the same amount of feed (pair-fed animals) have shown that GI nematode infection also depresses the efficiency of feed utilization (Coop and Holmes, 1996; van Houtert and Sykes, 1996).

Effects on efficiency of feed utilization

Protein

A feature of many of these nematode infections is an increased loss of endogenous protein into the GI tract, which is partly attributable to increased leakage of plasma protein or whole blood or both and partly due to increased secretion of mucoproteins and increased sloughing of epithelial cells into the tract as a result of increased turnover of the GI mucosa. Plasma-protein losses are frequently increased four- to fivefold by GI parasitism and, in those infections which cause haemorrhage, the additional loss of erythrocytes can be considerable. The nitrogen (N) balance of sheep parasitized with intestinal nematodes can be 3–5 g day^{-1} less than in uninfected pair-fed control animals. Whether or not the majority of the protein passing into the lumen of the GI tract is reabsorbed depends, to some extent, on whether the lesions are in the anterior or distal tract and whether there is sufficient compensatory absorptive capacity.

In parasitic infections of the abomasum, most of the endogenous protein losses will be reabsorbed in the small intestine (Rowe *et al.*, 1988). Any losses not reabsorbed in the proximal intestine are likely to be degraded in distal regions of the tract, will be absorbed as ammonia to be excreted as urea and will be unavailable for productive processes. Using cannulated animals and/or infusion of radiolabelled tracers, it has been estimated that the amount of non-reabsorbable endogenous N leaving the terminal ileum of sheep parasitized with GI nematodes can be as high as 4–5 g day^{-1} (Poppi *et al.*, 1986; Bown *et al.*, 1991a). Even when the majority of the endogenous protein is reabsorbed as amino acid, experiments with pair-fed animals have shown that there is poor protein deposition in the body, probably because energy is directed to protein synthesis for the preferential repair of GI tissue and to maintain homoeostasis and replacement of endogenous secretions. Recently, the increased protein turnover of the parasitized ovine GI tract has been quantified, using trans-organ catheterization and mass isotope tracer kinetics, with leucine as the marker amino acid (Yu *et al.*, 2000). These authors showed that sequestration of amino acid by the total GI tract from arterial pools was increased by 24% and also that the GI-tract oxidative losses of leucine were increased by 22–41% in sheep infected subclinically with *T. colubriformis*. A reduction in the availability of absorbed amino acids for metabolism in peripheral tissues is in agreement with the observation of reduced rates of protein synthesis in wool and muscle of sheep infected with *T. colubriformis* (Jones and Symons, 1982) and also with recent data (Bermingham *et al.*, 2000), which showed that experimental *T. colubriformis* infection reduced liveweight gain of sheep but had no effect on the whole-body irreversible loss rate of valine or cysteine, implying repartitioning of amino acid utilization between tissues. Scarce resources, such as essential amino acids, are diverted from productive processes (growth and reproductive effort) into those areas which are essential to maintain homoeostasis, such as repair of the GI tract, maintenance of blood proteins and components of the immune response and mucus production (Fig. 14.1). These effects will be exacerbated in those infections where the overall nutrient availability is further limited by reductions in voluntary feed intake.

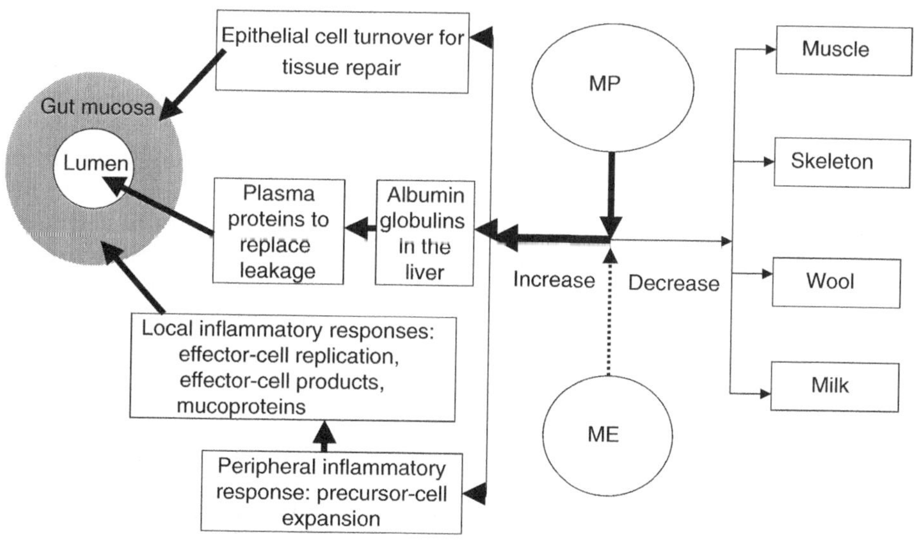

Fig. 14.1. Effects of gastrointestinal nematode infection on protein metabolism in sheep. The net effects are that amino acids from metabolizable protein (MP) are diverted from production (skeleton, muscle, wool and milk) to maintain integrity of the GI tract and to mount an effective local immune response. There is a concomitant diversion of metabolizable energy (ME) to the maintenance of the gut.

The overall conclusion must be that parasitism reduces the supply of metabolizable protein (MP) while increasing demand – an induced protein deficiency.

Energy

Gastrointestinal parasitism has a major effect on the energy metabolism of the host, largely through reductions in feed intake. This is especially the case in the young naïve lamb (MacRae *et al.*, 1982) but also in the mature ewe during lactation following the breakdown of immunity around parturition (Leyva *et al.*, 1982), as discussed earlier. Early experiments that compared energy deposition in the carcass of sheep infected with *Teladorsagia circumcincta* or *Trichostrongylus colubriformis* with that in pair-fed controls, showed significant additional effects on energy metabolism – namely, reduced energy deposition in the body relative to gross energy intake. This could be due to either reduced digestibility of energy or reduction in efficiency of use of digested energy. The majority of experiments have shown no change or an extremely small (1 or 2 percentage units) reduction in feed-energy digestion (Sykes and Coop, 1976, 1977), though MacRae *et al.* (1982) did observe a larger reduction. Precise attribution of the cause of reduced efficiency of energy use may therefore be equivocal. However, increased protein endogenous losses (see above) must lead to increased protein synthesis by GI tissue for which there is direct evidence (Jones and Symons, 1982; Yu *et al.*, 2000). This, together with the fact that GI tissue accounts for 30–40% of energy expenditure in the uninfected animal (see Corbett and Ball, Chapter 7, this volume), must lead to the conclusion that absorbed energy is diverted to maintenance of the alimentary tract and its immune function and away from productive functions. Efficiency of use of metabolizable energy (ME) for growth or other productive functions must, by definition, be reduced. The extent of such changes in energy partitioning may well vary with the site of infection. Whereas reduction in feed intake seems to be the major cause of reduced energy deposition in infections of the abomasum, reduction in efficiency of use of digested energy seems to be more important in infections of the small intestine (Sykes, 1994). This is demonstrated graphically in Fig. 14.2. The whole subject of the nutrient requirement of the digestive tract, especially in response to pathogens, merits further investigation.

Minerals

For the effects of parasitism on mineral metabolism, most information is available for calcium (Ca) and P, as GI nematode infection has a marked effect on skeletal growth and mineralization of bones (Sykes *et al.*, 1975, 1977). The effects are influenced by the location of the parasite within the GI tract and the extent of the lesions. With intestinal nematode infection (*Trichostrongylus* spp.), which causes extensive villous atrophy in the ante-

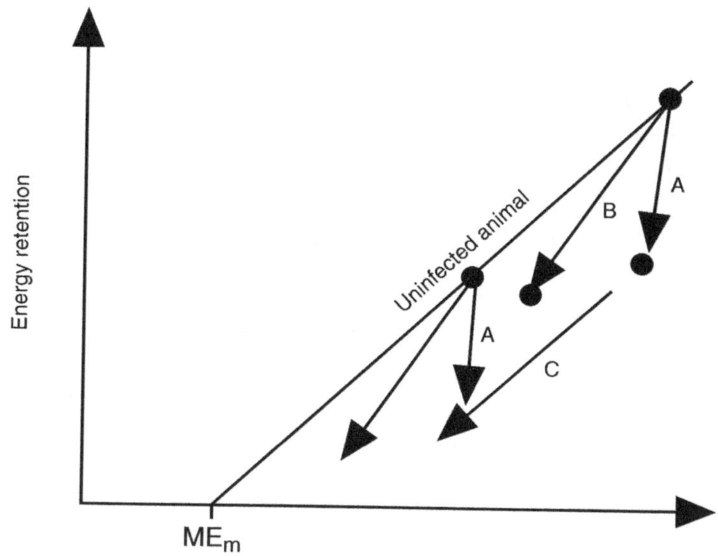

Fig. 14.2. Change in efficiency of use of metabolizable energy (ME) as a result of infection with parasites. This can occur as a result of reduction of feed intake (C), reduction in efficiency of use of energy for bodyweight gain (A) or a combination of the two (B). Abomasal infections with *T. circumcincta* tend to be due to changes dominated by route C and those in the intestine with *T. colubriformis* by route A, particularly in the initial stages of infection. ME_m, maintenance ME.

rior small intestine (Plate 14.1), absorption and retention of P can be markedly reduced (Poppi *et al.*, 1985; Bown *et al.*, 1989), leading to lowered plasma P concentrations and depressed secretion of P in the saliva (Coop and Field, 1983). There is also evidence for increased endogenous loss of Ca (Wilson and Field, 1983), but the overall effects of intestinal parasitism on Ca absorption are less clear, as Ca homoeostasis is regulated through Ca absorption in ruminants, rather than by renal clearance as in non-ruminants. These disturbances in P metabolism and, by association, Ca can lead to severe osteomalacia and osteoporosis in parasitized sheep.

Absorption of Ca and P is unaffected by nematode infections of the abomasum (Wilson and Field, 1983) and the reduced growth of the skeleton observed in these infections is considered to result from disturbances in protein, rather than mineral, metabolism. There is little information available for interactions between GI nematode infection and other macrominerals. Bown *et al.* (1989) reported that absorption of magnesium was unaffected in parasitized sheep. One study has shown that the elevation of abomasal pH, typical of infections in that organ, can lead to reduction in the availability of copper (Cu) from therapeutic Cu oxide wire particles (Bang *et al.*, 1990b). Otherwise, the information regarding trace-element metabolism is sparse and, in some cases, equivocal and will be considered below in relation to its influence on the resistance and resilience of sheep to parasitism.

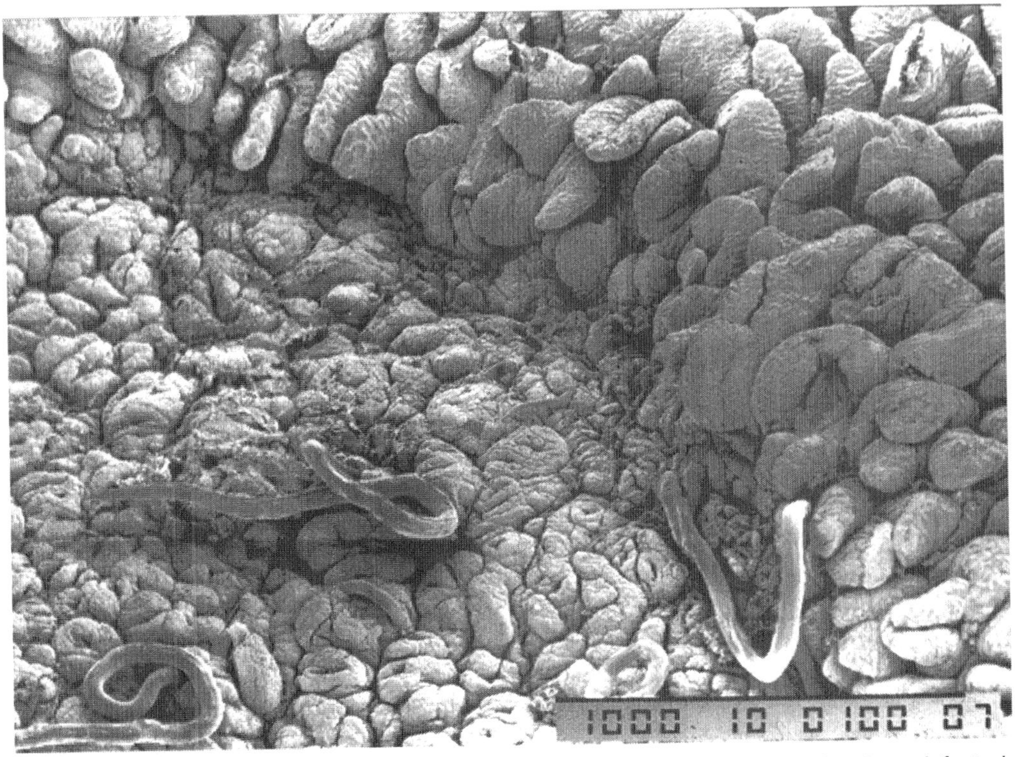

Plate 14.1. Scanning electron micrograph of the lining of the small intestine of a sheep infected with *Trichostrongylus* spp. nematodes. The area colonized by the worms shows marked villous atrophy compared with the normal villi in the surrounding area. (Photo reproduced from Henderson (1990), *The Veterinary Book for Farmers*, Farming Press, Ipswich, UK.)

Effect of Nutrition on the Resistance and Resilience of the Host to Parasitism

Two terms have been used to describe the response of the host to parasitic infection. Resistance has been used to define the ability of the host to limit larval establishment and the longevity or fecundity (egg-laying capacity) of adult worms since, in the main, resistance has been judged by the host's ability to limit faecal egg count. Resilience has been used to describe the ability of an animal to function or maintain normal productivity in the face of larval challenge or nematode egg count in faeces. Almost inevitably these two terms are inseparable as, for example, increased resistance to a larval intake will result in a reduced faecal egg count and any improvement in performance, as a consequence, will be attributed to resilience unless there is frequent sampling of the host population to assess worm burden. Even then, we are not in a position to correct or adjust resilience for observed changes in resistance. Moreover, it has become increasingly clear that both are significantly affected by the protein nutrition of the host, possibly reflecting the considerable change in protein metabolism induced in the host by infection, as described above.

Resistance

Following continuous exposure to GI nematodes, sheep gradually acquire a degree of immunity that will protect them from subsequent challenge infections. However, expression of an adequate immune response is only partial in animals under about 6 months of age, so young growing lambs are susceptible to GI nematode infections. Many factors, such as age, sex, breed, productive state and nutritional status of the host, influence this expression of immunity to a nematode infection.

The detailed mechanisms involved are not fully understood (Balic *et al.*, 2000). However, although a general peripheral eosinophilia and humoral immune response can be observed, it is becoming clear, not unexpectedly, that a cell-mediated immune response at the parasite–mucosal interface is important. Following infection, a rapid influx of eosinophils is observed within the mucosal lamina propria and, during the development of immunity, the numbers of mucosal mast cells increase dramatically. These latter cells contain numerous highly potent biological mediators, including histamine, leukotrienes and proteases, and these are secreted following the cross-linking of surface immunoglobulin E (IgE) by worm allergens. Whether these mast-cell products affect worms directly or indirectly remains unclear. Nevertheless, there is increasing evidence that the immune response is directed via the T-helper 2 (Th2) cell system and involves local IgA and IgE responses and recruitment of mucosal mast cells and their secretory products.

At issue still is the extent to which variation in immune responses occurs through variation in the competition for nutrients between the productive requirements and the requirements of the immune system of the animal. For example, the demand for MP, compared with ME is at its highest in the young growing animal and will be greater in the male than the female because of the greater growth potential of male livestock. This is normally provided for in the high protein-to-energy ratio in milk and the fact that milk protein passes directly to the abomasum via the reticular groove. Demand for MP relative to ME declines rapidly as the young lamb grows, and only when the lamb achieves a weight of about 30–35 kg does it receive an optimum protein : energy ratio from pasture alone. The breakdown of established immunity in the ewe in the peripartum period is associated with a rapid increase in demand for protein relative to energy at levels only seen in the young lamb and which are not attainable from pasture alone (Robinson, 1990).

Evidence in the literature supports the view that protein supplementation has little or no effect on the 'innate' ability of young growing livestock to prevent the early establishment of a parasite infection (Coop and Holmes, 1996; van Houtert and Sykes, 1996). The major effect of protein appears to be on the speed or degree to which the animal can 'acquire' or express immunity against a parasitic challenge. The MP supply can influence the extent of expression of immunity to GI nematodes in ruminants (van Houtert and Sykes, 1996), which is manifest as reduced establishment or inhibited development of incoming larvae and reduced survival and/or lowered fecundity of an established parasite population. Studies using 'trickle' infections of *Haemonchus contortus* (Abbott *et al.*, 1988) showed that faecal egg output of an established infection could be reduced by approximately 30% when sheep were fed a high-protein diet (169 g CP kg^{-1} dry matter (DM)) in comparison with animals offered a low-protein ration (88 g CP kg^{-1} DM). Approximately three times as many worms were recovered at necropsy from the sheep that were offered the low-protein ration.

Experimental studies with *T. colubriformis* infection in growing sheep have demonstrated that provision of additional protein, either as a direct infusion into the abomasum (Bown *et al.*, 1991b; Coop *et al.*, 1995) or fed as a dietary supplement (Kambara *et al.*, 1993; van Houtert *et al.*, 1995a; Datta *et al.*, 1998), can lower the fecundity and/or increase the rate of expulsion of parasites from the host. The decrease in faecal nematode egg count or in the apparent rate of worm expulsion appears to be influenced by the level of protein supplementation offered (van Houtert *et al.*, 1995a; Datta *et al.*, 1998). There is evidence that these effects of supplementation on the expression of resistance are greatest in the young animal, which has the greatest demand for a high protein : energy ratio (Kambara *et al.*, 1993). Recently, it has been demonstrated that intake of digestible energy can also increase resistance of growing sheep to *T. colubriformis* infection (Kahn *et al.*, 2000).

The results from studies in which grazing animals have been given a protein supplement have been more variable (van Houtert *et al.*, 1995b, 1996). Some have shown reductions in faecal nematode egg output but no effect of additional protein on worm populations at slaughter. Recently, the long-term benefits of providing short-term (9 weeks) protein supplementation to sheep have been investigated (Datta *et al.*, 1999). Following their turnout on to infected pasture, higher liveweight gain, wool production and lower worm egg counts were recorded in sheep previously supplemented than in unsupplemented animals. These beneficial effects of short-term protein supplementation persisted for at least 16 months.

It is well established that the immune status of ewes may be relaxed to varying degrees during the periparturient period. This periparturient relaxation of immunity (PPRI) is particularly evident for abomasal nematode infections. The timing of PPRI is variable, but, in general, the immune status of the ewe is lowered from about 2–3 weeks before and up to 6–8 weeks after parturition (McAnulty *et al.*, 2001). Outside this period the ewe is fairly refractory to GI nematode infection. The causes of PPRI are still subject to debate, but there is supporting evidence that it may have a nutritional basis. Termination in late pregnancy or removal of lambs at birth or during lactation will restore the normal immune expression of the ewe to nematode infection. In addition, the relaxation of immunity is influenced by nutritional demand, being greater in ewes carrying or rearing twin lambs compared with singles. Most of the studies of this breakdown of immunity have focused on nutrition/parasite interactions involving the abomasal nematode *T. (Ostertagia) circumcincta*, as this is the predominant parasite contributing to PPRI in ewes in temperate areas. Recent investigations (Donaldson *et al.*, 1998, 2001) have experimented with ewes infected concurrently with *T. cir-*

cumcincta and *T. colubriformis*. The results indicate that supplementation with protein in late pregnancy or early lactation or both can reduce the faecal nematode egg output and, in some cases, also reduce the worm populations. Similarly, in ewes bearing or rearing twins, Houdijk *et al.* (2000) showed that an increased intake of MP during pregnancy and lactation improved resistance and resilience to experimental infections with *T. circumcincta*.

A pivotal experiment undertaken by Donaldson *et al.* (1998) demonstrated that protein supply appears to be more important than energy supply in these host/parasite interactions in the ewe, a finding similar to that reported for young growing animals (Bown *et al.*, 1991b). These data and those from recent experiments (Houdijk *et al.*, 2001a, b) support the view that an increase in MP supply or a reduction in MP demand will partially ameliorate PPRI to *T. circumcincta* during periods when there is a scarcity of MP. Interestingly, the studies also suggest that the effect of supplementation may be more beneficial in more fecund sheep, further strengthening the argument that competitive demand for nutrients may be the cause of PPRI in ewes. It is also known that genetic selection for enhanced resistance in sheep can reduce the extent of PPRI, and the interactions between nutrition and genotype in breeding ewes merit further research (Kahn *et al.*, 1999).

Coop and Kyriazakis (1999) have developed a framework to consider this partitioning of nutrients between somatic tissue and the immune system during different phases of the growth cycle. This argues from available information in the literature that the poor growth of lambs during early infection occurs because acquisition of immunity is more important for survival and would have priority over gain in body protein and hence the high susceptibility to infection. The partitioning framework suggests that responses of the immune system to protein supplementation would be small during this early acquisition phase but would be more apparent later in a parasitic infection, when the host is expressing a degree of immunity. In contrast, in the reproductive female, it appears that immunity is foregone in the interests of production. In the case of the latter, however, it appears that intakes of protein more than 30% greater than the conventional requirement may enable maintenance of immunity (Donaldson *et al.*, 2001). There is general recognition that the milk-fed ruminant is well protected against infection, though whether this is a direct effect of the abundant protein supply or protection from the need to graze and therefore from exposure to infective larvae has not been tested.

Investigation of the mechanisms by which nutrition influences the specific immune responses has only just started. This reflects, in part, the recent recognition of the importance of nutrition, but also the rudimentary status of our understanding of the precise immune response. There is currently an accumulation of evidence to show that supplementation with rumen-undegradable protein can increase the numbers of immune-system effector cells in the intestinal mucosa (eosinophils and mucosal mast cells (MMC)) or peripheral blood (eosinophils), or both, of young lambs exposed to nematode larvae (Kambara *et al.*, 1993; Coop *et al.*, 1995; van Houtert *et al.*, 1995a; Datta *et al.*, 1998) and in ewes around parturition (Houdijk *et al.*, 2000).

In some cases, these increases in cellular responses are associated with increased resistance to nematode infection. Changes in the humoral responses following protein supplementation in sheep with intestinal nematode infections are more variable (Kambara *et al.*, 1993). It is likely that some components of the host's immune response may have a disproportionate demand for specific amino acids. For example, leukotrienes, which are involved in cell-signalling, are rich in cysteine. Similarly, the increased mucus production that frequently accompanies GI parasitism will have a high requirement for proline, threonine and serine (MacRae, 1993). Interestingly, Coop *et al.* (1997) showed enhanced resilience to infection and increased numbers of intestinal MMC and mast-cell protease in sheep that were 'trickle'-infected with *T. colubriformis* larvae and which received an additional supplementation of 'protected' methionine.

Although the focus has centred on protein metabolism because of the large nutritional changes induced in the host, there may well be other similarly specific nutrient or environmental demands in the GI mucosa. The changes in resistance to larval establishment and worm fecundity shown in response to changes in dietary molybdenum (Mo) concentration in *T. colubriformis*-challenged sheep were closely mirrored by changes in intestinal antibody, granulocyte numbers in the blood and jejunal mucosa and *in vitro* worm-specific proliferation of lymphocytes (McClure *et al.*, 1999). Most other studies involving mineral nutrition have not attempted to describe the underlying mechanisms causing increased resistance. It is known that intestinal parasitism can adversely affect mineral metabolism, particularly P, and there are data to indicate that resistance to intestinal *Trichostrongylus vitrinus* infection in sheep offered a low-P diet (1.88 g kg^{-1} DM) can be lower than on a comparable normal P ration (2.75g kg^{-1} DM) (Coop and Field, 1983). Total worm burdens were reduced by about 87% and faecal nematode egg counts lowered in sheep that were offered the higher-P ration and 'trickle'-infected for 14 weeks. Whether this is due to P deficiency *per se* or a reduced intake of MP consequent on P deficiency is, as yet, uncertain. Low P intake would be compounded by the reduction in P absorption which is a consequence of intestinal parasitism (Wilson and Field, 1983). The normal recycling of P to the rumen is reduced and Coop and Field (1983) found rumen P concentrations of only 87 mg l^{-1}, which is below the levels at which microbial protein production is impaired.

There is also evidence for the influence of trace elements on resistance to nematode infection. Suttle *et al.* (1992) showed that the addition of Mo to the diet of sheep infected with *T. vitrinus* reduced the total worm burdens by 23%. There was evidence for some direct effect on the worms, in addition to indirect effects through enhancement of the immune response. As indicated above, resistance to larval establishment and MMC populations were optimized at a dietary Mo concentration of 6–10 mg Mo kg^{-1} DM. There is also evidence for reduction in faecal egg counts in lactating sheep at pasture when treated with a cobalt bullet (T.M. Gruner and A.R. Sykes, unpublished). Untreated sheep had elevated methylmalonic acid concentrations, indicating impairment of the propionate-to-glucose pathway, a consequence of which would be increased use of amino acids for gluconeogenesis. Copper, given as Cu oxide wire particles, one of the currently available methods of Cu supplementation in ruminants (see Lee *et al.*, Chapter 13, this volume), reduced abomasal nematode populations in sheep by 56–96% (Bang *et al.*, 1990a), but there was no significant effect on the establishment of intestinal nematode populations. The effectiveness of the Cu particles, however, probably depends on an abomasal pH that ensures Cu solubilization (Bang *et al.*, 1990b) and the Cu oxide particles may not be as effective in an established abomasal nematode infection with consequent elevation of pH of the contents. The role of other trace elements, such as zinc, selenium and cobalt, in modifying parasitic infections has been investigated in small-animal models, but little consistent information is available for ruminants.

Resilience

A pivotal study was undertaken by Bown *et al.* (1991b) to investigate which dietary components had a major influence on the resilience and resistance of the host to parasitic infection. In sheep 'trickle'-infected with the intestinal nematode *T. colubriformis*, they attempted to replace the protein estimated to be lost by the host in GI secretions, by infusing either casein or isoenergetic amounts of glucose into the abomasum. These authors showed that, primarily, infection induced a protein deficiency and that the resilience of the animals to a defined larval intake could be improved by protein, but not by energy, infusion. Subsequent studies have investigated the effects of supplementation of diets with rumen-undegradable protein (Kyriazakis *et al.*, 1996; van Houtert and Sykes, 1996; Datta *et al.*, 1998) or urea (Wallace *et al.*, 1998; Knox and Steel, 1999) on the productivity of ruminants. The data showed that depressions in growth rate and wool production and the pathophysiological consequences of infection could be alleviated by the provision of additional MP. The response to urea supplementation was partly attributable to stimulation of feed intake, presumably as a result of increased ruminal cellulose digestion, but also via increased microbial protein synthesis in the rumen.

Relevant to these findings is the observation that individually penned sheep infected with *T. colubriformis* and offered a choice between isoenergetic foods with a high (206 g kg^{-1} DM) or a low (86 g kg^{-1} DM) protein concentration, consumed a higher proportion of the high-protein diet than uninfected controls (Kyriazakis *et al.*, 1994, 1996). Presumably this enabled the sheep to 'adjust' their protein intake to partially offset the parasite-induced increase in protein requirements. However, there are examples where increased dietary protein intake has not improved the resilience of sheep to GI nematode infection. Calculations of likely rumen degradation of food protein and likely microbial protein production suggest that, in some experiments, the difference in MP supply to tissues between supplemented and unsupplemented sheep was probably too small to affect resilience. In other studies, there is insufficient nutritional information available to make a valid assessment. The beneficial effects of dietary protein supplementation tested with parasitized housed sheep have been confirmed in controlled grazing trials where liveweight gain of young parasitized sheep was increased by the addition of sunflower meal (van Houtert *et al.*, 1995b) or fish meal and sunflower meals (van Houtert *et al.*, 1996).

There is limited information on the effect of mineral supply on resilience of sheep to parasitic infection. Coop and Field (1983) showed increased liveweight gain of sheep infected with intestinal *T. vitrinus* when the P concentration of the ration was increased from 1.88 g kg^{-1} DM (low P) to 2.75 g kg^{-1} DM (moderate P). Improvements in resilience have been observed following supplementation of sheep infected with *T. vitrinus* with a diet that contained a higher concentration of Mo (0.05 mmol kg^{-1} DM) (Suttle *et al.*, 1992).

Application of Dietary Supplementation

As highlighted in the introduction, dietary supplementation is being considered as one component in a sustainable control strategy aimed at enhancing the natural ability of the host to combat a parasitic challenge and so reduce the need for frequent chemotherapeutic intervention. However, in many livestock enterprises and areas of the world with limited resources, it may not be practical or economical to feed high-quality rumen-undegradable protein to small ruminants. Production systems are frequently based on low-quality roughage to provide digestible carbohydrate and are also often deficient in degradable N. Several alternative nutritional approaches are being investigated. Studies using urea–molasses feed blocks as a low-cost supplement have shown that this additional source of energy and non-protein N can satisfy the requirements of rumen microorganisms and increase the efficiency of fermentation, thus improving the digestion and utilization of the available diet and consequently the resistance and resilience of sheep and goats to GI nematode infections, particularly where the basic diet comprises low-quality forages (Knox and Zahari, 2000). Feed intake can also be enhanced. This technology has application for many smallholder farmers in resource-poor areas where GI parasitism is a major contributor to low productivity of livestock.

Recently, there has been interest in feeding forages that have the ability to increase the postrumen availability of dietary protein, which may indirectly enhance the immune response. Condensed tannins (CT) are phenolic secondary plant metabolites that have a high affinity for macromolecules, such as proteins, and hence can partially protect dietary protein from rumen degradation, thus increasing amino acid availability in the small intestine. There is accumulating evidence that sheep parasitized with GI nematodes can have reduced faecal egg counts or lower worm burdens, or both, and increased resilience when grazing on forages such as sulla or trefoil species (Table 14.2) with a high CT content (Niezen *et al.*, 1995, 1998). However, the effects may depend on the species of nematode present and the impact of the forage on feed intake and digestibility. Studies in housed sheep that were

Table 14.2. Agriculturally useful forage plants, which contain CT and have shown potential for improving resilience/resistance to GI nematode infection in sheep.

Botanical name	Common name
Lotus uliginosus (pedunculatus)	Greater bird's-foot trefoil
Lotus corniculatus	Bird's-foot trefoil
Hedysarum coronarium	Sulla
Onobrychis viciifolia	Sainfoin

experimentally infected with *T. colubriformis* larvae and offered a CT extract incorporated into the feed showed reduced worm burdens and a lower faecal egg count compared with sheep fed a comparable low or moderate level of protein without CT (Athanasiadou *et al.*, 2000a; Butter *et al.*, 2000). In addition to the indirect action of CT, there is recent evidence which indicates that they may exert direct anthelmintic effects on GI parasites (Athanasiadou *et al.*, 2000b). Further research is required to assess the most appropriate means of incorporating tanniferous forages into grazing strategies, as many of the plants which show promise are not tolerant to high grazing pressure and some will not persist in more northern temperate climates. Forages with a low tolerance for grazing could possibly be used for short periods of grazing as deworming paddocks or be ensiled or conserved and fed to ewes as a supplement during the periparturient period.

References

Abbott, E.M., Parkins, J.J. and Holmes, P.H. (1988) Influence of dietary protein on the pathophysiology of haemonchosis in lambs given continuous infections. *Research in Veterinary Science* 45, 41–49.

Athanasiadou, S., Kyriazakis, I., Jackson, F. and Coop, R.L. (2000a) Consequences of long-term feeding with condensed tannins on sheep parasitised with *Trichostrongylus colubriformis*. *International Journal for Parasitology* 30, 1025–1033.

Athanasiadou, S., Kyriazakis, I., Jackson, F. and Coop, R.L. (2000b) Effects of short-term exposure to condensed tannins on adult *Trichostrongylus colubriformis*. *Veterinary Record* 146, 728–732.

Balic, A., Bowles, V.M. and Meeusen, E.N.T. (2000) The immunobiology of gastrointestinal nematode infections in ruminants. *Advances in Parasitology* 45, 181–241.

Bang, K.S., Familton, A.S. and Sykes, A.R. (1990a) Effect of copper oxide wire particle treatment on establishment of major gastrointestinal nematodes in lambs. *Research in Veterinary Science* 49, 132–137.

Bang, K.S., Familton, A.S. and Sykes, A.R. (1990b) Effect of ostertagiasis on copper status in sheep: a study involving use of copper oxide wire particles. *Research in Veterinary Science* 49, 306–314.

Bermingham, E.N., McNabb, W.C., Reynolds, G.W., Waghorn, G.C., Sutherland, I.A., Revell, D.K. and Roy, N.C. (2000) Whole-body irreversible loss rate of cysteine and valine in sheep with or without a *Trichostrongylus colubriformis* infection. *Asian–Australasian Journal of Animal Sciences* 13, 196–199.

Bown, M.D., Poppi, D.P. and Sykes, A.R. (1989) The effects of a concurrent infection of *Trichostrongylus colubriformis* and *Ostertagia circumcincta* on calcium, phosphorus and magnesium transactions along the digestive tract of lambs. *Journal of Comparative Pathology* 101, 11–20.

Bown, M.D., Poppi, D.P. and Sykes, A.R. (1991a) Nitrogen transactions along the digestive tract of lambs concurrently infected with *Trichostrongylus colubriformis* and *Ostertagia circumcincta*. *British Journal of Nutrition* 66, 237–249.

Bown, M.D., Poppi, D.P. and Sykes, A.R. (1991b) The effect of post-ruminal infusion of protein or energy on the pathophysiology of *Trichostrongylus colubriformis* infection and body composition in lambs. *Australian Journal of Agricultural Research* 42, 253–267.

Butter, N.L., Dawson, J.M., Wakelin, D. and Buttery, P.J. (2000) Effect of dietary tannin and protein concentration on nematode infection (*Trichostrongylus colubriformis*) in lambs. *Journal of Agricultural Science, Cambridge* 134, 89–99.

Coop, R.L. and Field, A.C. (1983) Effect of phosphorus intake on growth rate, food intake and quality of the skeleton of growing lambs infected with the intestinal nematode *Trichostrongylus vitrinus*. *Research in Veterinary Science* 35, 175–181.

Coop, R.L. and Holmes, P.H. (1996) Nutrition and parasite interaction. *International Journal for Parasitology* 26, 951–962.

Coop, R.L. and Kyriazakis, I. (1999) Nutrition–parasite interaction. *Veterinary Parasitology* 84, 187–204.

Coop, R.L., Huntley, J.F. and Smith, W.D. (1995) Effect of dietary protein supplementation on the development of immunity to *Ostertagia circumcincta* in growing lambs. *Research in Veterinary Science* 59, 24–29.

Coop, R.L., Kyriazakis, I., Huntley, J.F., Jackson, E. and Jackson, F. (1997) The influence of protein and amino acid on the resilience of sheep to intestinal parasitism. In: *Proceedings 4th International Congress for Sheep Veterinarians, Armidale, Australia*. University of New England, Armidale, pp. 196–198.

Datta, F.U., Nolan, J.V., Rowe, J.B. and Gray, G.D. (1998) Protein supplementation improves the performance of parasitised sheep fed a straw-based diet. *International Journal for Parasitology* 28, 1269–1278.

Datta, F.U., Nolan, J.V., Rowe, J.B., Gray, G.D. and Crook, B.J. (1999) Long-term effects of short-term provision of protein-enriched diets on resistance to nematode infection and liveweight gain and wool growth in sheep. *International Journal for Parasitology* 29, 479–488.

Donaldson, J., van Houtert, M.F.J. and Sykes, A.R. (1998) The effect of nutrition on the periparturient parasite status of mature ewes. *Animal Science* 67, 523–533.

Donaldson, J., van Houtert, M.F.J. and Sykes, A.R. (2001) The effect of dietary fishmeal supplementation on parasite burdens of periparturient sheep. *Animal Science* 72, 149–158.

Dynes, R.A., Ankersmit, A.E.L., Poppi, D.P., Barrell, G.K. and Sykes, A.R. (1990) Studies on the physiological basis of appetite depression in nematode infection in sheep. *Proceedings of the New Zealand Society of Animal Production* 50, 249–253.

Dynes, R.A., Poppi, D.P., Barrell, G.K. and Sykes, A.R. (1998) Elevation of feed intake in parasite-infected lambs by central administration of a cholecystokinin receptor antagonist. *British Journal of Nutrition* 79, 47–54.

Fox, M.T. (1997) Pathophysiology of infection with gastrointestinal nematodes in domestic ruminants: recent developments. *Veterinary Parasitology* 72, 285–308.

Gregory, P.C., Wenham, G., Poppi, D., Coop, R.L., MacRae, J.C. and Miller, S.J. (1985) The influence of a chronic subclinical infection of *Trichostrongylus colubriformis* on gastrointestinal motility and digesta flow in sheep. *Parasitology* 91, 381–396.

Horbury, S.R., Mercer, J.G. and Chappell, L.H. (1995) Anorexia induced by the parasitic nematode *Nippostrongylus brasiliensis*: effects on NPY and CRF gene expression in the rat hypothalamus. *Journal of Neuroendocrinology* 7, 867–873.

Houdijk, J.G.M., Kyriazakis, I., Jackson, F., Huntley, J.F. and Coop, R.L. (2000) Can an increased intake of metabolizable protein affect the periparturient relaxation in immunity against *Teladorsagia circumcincta* in sheep? *Veterinary Parasitology* 91, 43–62.

Houdijk, J.G.M., Kyriazakis, I., Coop, R.L. and Jackson, F. (2001a) The expression of immunity to *Teladorsagia circumcincta* in ewes and its relationship to protein nutrition depend on body protein reserves. *Parasitology* 122, 661–672.

Houdijk, J.G.M., Kyriazakis, I., Jackson, F. and Coop, R.L. (2001b) The relationship between protein nutrition, reproductive effort and breakdown in immunity to *Teladorsagia circumcincta* in periparturient ewes. *Animal Science* 72, 595–606.

Jones, W.O. and Symons, L.E.A. (1982). Protein synthesis in the whole body, liver, skeletal muscle and kidney cortex of lambs infected by the nematode *Trichostrongylus colubriformis*. *International Journal for Parasitology* 12, 295–301.

Kahn, L.P., Knox, M.R. and Gray, G.D. (1999) Enhancing immunity to nematode parasites in pregnant and lactating sheep through nutrition and genetic selection. In: *Recent Advances in Animal Nutrition in Australia*, Vol. 12. University of New England, Armidale, Australia, pp. 15–22.

Kahn, L.P., Walkden-Brown, S.W. and Lea, J.M. (2000) Dietary enhancement of resistance to *Trichostrongylus colubriformis* in merino weaners. *Asian–Australasian Journal of Animal Sciences* 13, 68–71.

Kambara, T., McFarlane, R.G., Abell, T.J., McAnulty, R.W. and Sykes, A.R. (1993) The effect of age and dietary protein on immunity and resistance in lambs vaccinated with *Trichostrongylus colubriformis*. *International Journal for Parasitology* 23, 471–476.

Knox, M.R. and Steel, J.W. (1999) The effects of urea supplementation on production and parasitological responses of sheep infected with *Haemonchus contortus* and *Trichostrongylus colubriformis*. *Veterinary Parasitology* 83, 123–135.

Knox, M. and Zahari, M.W. (2000) Urea–molasses blocks for parasite control. *FAO Animal Production and Health Papers* 141, 23–38.

Kyriazakis, I., Oldham, J.D., Coop, R.L. and Jackson, F. (1994) The effect of subclinical intestinal nematode infection on the diet selection of growing sheep. *British Journal of Nutrition* 72, 665–677.

Kyriazakis, I., Anderson, D.H., Oldham, J.D., Coop, R.L. and Jackson, F. (1996) Long-term subclinical infection with *Trichostrongylus colubriformis*: effects on food intake, diet selection and performance of growing lambs. *Veterinary Parasitology* 61, 297–313.

Kyriazakis, I., Tolkamp, B.J. and Hutchings, M.R. (1998) Towards a functional explanation for the occurrence of anorexia during parasitic infection. *Animal Behaviour* 56, 265–274.

Leyva, V., Henderson, A.E. and Sykes, A.R. (1982) Effect of daily infection with *Ostertagia circumcincta* larvae on food intake, milk production and wool growth in sheep. *Journal of Agricultural Science, Cambridge* 99, 249–259.

MacRae, J.C. (1993) Metabolic consequences of intestinal parasitism. *Proceedings of the Nutrition Society* 52, 121–130.

MacRae, J.C., Smith, J.S., Sharman, G.A.M., Corrigall, W. and Coop, R.L. (1982) Energy metabolism of lambs infected with *Trichostrongylus colubriformis*. In: Ekern, A. and Sundstol, E. (eds) *Energy Metabolism of Farm Animals*. European Association of Animal Production Publication No. 29, Agricultural University of Norway, Ås, Norway, pp. 112–115.

McAnulty, R.W., Familton, A.S., Sedcole, R.D. and Sykes, A.R. (2001) Changes in the resistance of the ewe to infection with *Teladorsagia circumcincta* during late pregnancy and lactation. *Animal Science* 72, 159–168.

McClure, S.J., McClure, T.J. and Emery, D.L. (1999) Effects of molybdenum intake on primary infection and subsequent challenge by the nematode parasite *Trichostrongylus colubriformis* in weaned Merino lambs. *Research in Veterinary Science* 67, 17–22.

Niezen, J.H., Waghorn, T.S., Charleston, W.A.G. and Waghorn, G.C. (1995) Growth and gastrointestinal nematode parasitism in lambs grazing either lucerne (*Medicago sativa*) or sulla (*Hedysarum coronarium*) which contains condensed tannins. *Journal of Agricultural Science, Cambridge* 125, 281–289.

Niezen, J.H., Robertson, H.A., Waghorn, G.C. and Charleston, W.A.G. (1998) Production, faecal egg counts and worm burdens of ewe lambs which grazed six contrasting forages. *Veterinary Parasitology* 80, 15–27.

Poppi, D.P, MacRae, J.C., Brewer, A.C., Dewey, P.J.S. and Walker, A. (1985). Calcium and phosphorus absorption in lambs exposed to *Trichostrongylus colubriformis*. *Journal of Comparative Parasitology* 95, 453–464.

Poppi, D.P., MacRae, J.C., Brewer, A. and Coop, R.L. (1986) Nitrogen transactions in the digestive tract of lambs exposed to the intestinal parasite *Trichostrongylus colubriformis*. *British Journal of Nutrition* 55, 593–602.

Robinson, J.J. (1990) Pastoral industries in the 21st century. *Proceedings of the New Zealand Society of Animal Production* 50, 345–359.

Rowe, J.B., Nolan, J.V., de Chaneet, G., Teleni, E. and Holmes, P.H. (1988) The effect of haemonchosis and blood loss into the abomasum on digestion in sheep. *British Journal of Nutrition* 59, 125–139.

Suttle, N.F., Knox, D.P., Jackson, F., Coop, R.L. and Angus, K.W. (1992) Effects of dietary molybdenum on nematode and host during *Trichostrongylus vitrinus* infection in lambs. *Research in Veterinary Science* 52, 224–229.

Sykes, A.R. (1994) Parasitism and production in farm animals. *Animal Production* 59, 155–172.

Sykes, A.R. and Coop, R.L. (1976) Intake and utilisation of food by growing lambs with parasitic damage to the small intestine caused by daily dosing with *Trichostrongylus colubriformis* larvae. *Journal of Agricultural Science, Cambridge* 86, 507–515.

Sykes, A.R. and Coop, R.L. (1977) Intake and utilisation of food by growing sheep with abomasal damage caused by daily dosing with *Ostertagia circumcincta* larvae. *Journal of Agricultural Science, Cambridge* 88, 671–677.

Sykes, A.R., Coop, R.L and Angus, K.W. (1975) Experimental production of osteoporosis in growing lambs by continuous dosing with *Trichostrongylus colubriformis*. *Journal of Comparative Pathology* 85, 549–559.

Sykes, A.R., Coop, R.L. and Angus, K.W. (1977) The influence of chronic *Ostertagia circumcincta* infection on the skeleton of growing sheep. *Journal of Comparative Pathology* 87, 521–529.

Symons, L.E.A. (1985) Anorexia: occurrence, pathophysiology and possible causes in parasitic infections. *Advances in Parasitology* 24, 103–133.

van Houtert, M.F.J. and Sykes, A.R. (1996) Implications of nutrition for the ability of ruminants to withstand gastrointestinal nematode infections. *International Journal for Parasitology* 26, 1151–1167.

van Houtert, M.F.J., Barger, I.A., Steel, J.W., Windon, R.G. and Emery, D.L. (1995a) Effects of dietary protein intake on responses of young sheep to infection with *Trichostrongylus colubriformis*. *Veterinary Parasitology* 56, 163–180.

van Houtert, M.F.J., Barger, I.A. and Steel, J.W. (1995b) Dietary protein for young grazing sheep: interactions with gastrointestinal parasitism. *Veterinary Parasitology* 60, 283–295.

van Houtert, M.F.J., Barger, I.A. and Steel, J.W. (1996) Supplementary feeding and gastrointestinal parasitism in young grazing sheep. *Proceedings of the New Zealand Society of Animal Production* 56, 94–98.

Wallace, D.S., Bairden, K., Duncan, J.L., Eckersall, P.D., Fishwick, G., Gill, M., Holmes, P.H., McKellar, Q.A., Murray, M., Parkins, J.J. and Stear, M.J. (1998) The influence of dietary supplementation with urea on resilience and resistance to infection with *Haemonchus contortus*. *Parasitology* 116, 67–72.

Waller, P.J. (1997) Anthelmintic resistance. *Veterinary Parasitology* 72, 391–412.

Waller, P.J. (1999) International approaches to the concept of integrated control of nematode parasites of livestock. *International Journal for Parasitology* 29, 155–164.

Wilson, W.D. and Field, A.C. (1983) Absorption and secretion of calcium and phosphorus in the alimentary tract of lambs infected with daily doses of *Trichostrongylus colubriformis* or *Ostertagia circumcincta* larvae. *Journal of Comparative Pathology* 93, 61–71.

Yu, F., Bruce, L.A., Calder, A.G., Milne, E., Coop, R.L., Jackson, F., Horgan, G.W. and MacRae, J.C. (2000) Subclinical infection with the nematode *Trichostrongylus colubriformis* increases gastrointestinal tract leucine metabolism and reduces availability of leucine for other tissues. *Journal of Animal Science* 78, 380–390.

15 Deleterious Substances in Grazed Pastures

G.C. WAGHORN[1], N.R. ADAMS[2] AND D.R. WOODFIELD[1]

[1]*AgResearch Limited, Grasslands Research Centre, Palmerston North, New Zealand;* [2]*CSIRO Livestock Industries, Wembley, Western Australia, Australia*

Deleterious substances can reduce the nutritive value (NV) of a forage or pasture for grazing animals. These substances are often toxins, which increase mortality, decrease productivity or reduce the quality or wholesome nature of animal products and hence toxins can be deleterious to the animal, the consumer or both. The range of toxic substances is extensive, especially in native or unimproved forages or shrubs. Improved pastures, the main focus of this chapter, also have diverse toxins from fungal (mycotoxins), plant (phytotoxins) and bacterial origins. In addition to affecting sheep, many toxins also affect cattle and non-ruminants.

This chapter reviews forage toxins from a grazing perspective, identifies some major causes of ill health and poor productivity in sheep, considers the impact of intensive grazing practices upon their incidence and discusses the role of the rumen and tissues in altering the toxicology of some compounds. The list of substances that are deleterious to sheep is extensive. It is also important to appreciate that, even in improved pastures, ingestion of weed species can occur, especially in times of feed deficit.

Two main categories of toxins will be considered in some detail; fungal alkaloids, associated with temperate grasses, and oestrogenic compounds, often associated with clovers. Consideration will also be given to photosensitizing agents, cyanogens, phenolic compounds (tannins), bloat and nitrite (NO_2^-) poisoning. Most toxins associated with weeds will not be discussed in detail, as this topic has been comprehensively reviewed by Cheeke (1998).

Why are Plants Toxic?

Protection against herbivory is often suggested as the reason forages produce or are associated with toxic substances, but the threat to plants from insect and microbial predation is often greater than consumption by large animals. In some instances, plants may have evolved with fungi to reduce the impact of insect damage. For example, *Neotyphodium lolii* infection of perennial ryegrass (*Lolium perenne*) affords protection against the Argentine stem weevil (*Listronotus bonariensis*) and other insects, but has tremorgenic effects (staggering) on sheep (Easton, 1999). Likewise, the presence of condensed tannins in some legumes (e.g. *Lotus* spp.) protects against consumption, but, given a choice, sheep prefer leaves containing high concentrations of tannin to stems containing more structural fibre but less tannin.

Some innocuous plant components can become toxic following exposure to the rumen microflora, e.g. the production of equol from formononetin present in red clover (*Trifolium pratense*), with consequent reduced fertility. More often rumen microflora deactivate potentially toxic plant compounds.

Selection and Use of Improved Varieties

Past improvements in temperate forages have focused on agronomic factors, such as dry matter (DM) yield, disease resistance, seasonal growth and persistence, with little attention to NV (Woodfield, 1999). The use of *in vitro* digestibility and the advent of near-infrared reflectance spectroscopy (NIRS) have improved selection for nutritional characteristics (Casler, 1999), but until recently toxins in forages have received little attention. Notable exceptions include cyanoglycosides in white clover, oestrogenic compounds in subterranean and red clover and alkaloids in phalaris. Animal disorders associated with fungal endophytes have also been the focus of considerable international research for the past decade.

Intensive temperate agriculture has contributed to pastoral toxicity problems. Attempts to maximize profit by grazing high-producing monocultures or binary mixtures, aided by liberal fertilizer and irrigation, have created ideal conditions for fungal growth. The reduction in dietary choice and intensive grazing may force animals to eat more dead matter accumulated at the canopy base. The dead matter, stems and sheaths of grasses have poor NV and contain the highest concentrations of fungi in swards (Di Menna *et al.*, 1992). In addition, when grazing pressure is high, the reduced choice may lead animals to select pasture weeds containing high levels of toxins, such as ragwort (*Senecio jacobaea*) or Paterson's curse (*Echium plantagineum*).

Veterinary Indications of Toxicosis

Instances of ill health in livestock are often due to either inadequate diet (quantity and quality) or ingestion of excessive quantities of toxic material. Understanding the toxicosis also requires a knowledge of the diet eaten, as distinct from that which is on offer. The effects of some toxicoses are easily recognized (e.g. photosensitivity), but in many instances toxins cause subclinical conditions, indicated only by diminished appetite and poor productivity (e.g. endophyte toxicity). Other toxicoses are apparent only through diminished fertility in apparently healthy animals.

A diverse range of deleterious substances is found in pastures (Table 15.1). Alkaloids and glycosides account for many deleterious effects but even fundamental compounds, such as chlorophyll and protein, can be toxic. Alkaloids are of fungal or plant origin and are classified on the basis of heterocyclic ring structures; many are used in human medicine. Glycosides are derived from plants, and the active (aglycone) portion is released by enzyme action following cell damage; their effects can be exacerbated by trampling, frost or chewing.

Aetiology and Metabolism of Toxic Compounds

Once selected, the plant is chewed with copious saliva and about 60% of cell contents are released and exposed to a diverse array of ruminal bacteria, protozoa and fungi, which may either decrease or increase the toxicity of ingested compounds. In general, ruminants are more tolerant of toxins than non-ruminant animals (Cheeke, 1998), suggesting that deactivation is the more prevalent outcome, but there are notable exceptions. For example, oestrogenic compounds impair fertility following rumen modification of formononetin present in subterranean and red clovers. Similarly, when the tropical legume leucaena (*Leucaena leucocephala*) is consumed, the toxic amino acid mimosine is degraded to goitrogenic dihydroxypyridine compounds, unless bacteria capable of degrading mimosine and its metabolites (e.g. *Synergistes jonesii*) are present in the rumen. Other examples of increased toxicity include conversion of ingested nitrates (NO_3^-) to nitrites (NO_2^-) and hydrolysis of cyanogenic glycosides to release cyanide.

Toxins can also impair microbial or rumen function; for example, dietary condensed tannins can result in significant reductions in fibre digestibility (Barry and Manley, 1984) and voluntary intake. Toxins such as saponins may also cause intestinal damage (irritants or lesions), especially of the microvilli, or inhibition of enzyme activity. Effects of trypsin inhibitors derived from beans are well known, but diarrhoea in sheep affected by pyrrolizidine alkaloids derived from ryegrass endophyte fungi suggests impaired absorption or hypermotility, leading to a rapid digesta passage to the faeces.

Dietary toxins that affect sheep may not affect other ruminants, and vice versa. Goats are more tolerant of dietary tannins than sheep, while sheep are more tolerant of ragwort toxin than cattle. These differences may be attributable to ruminal and/or postabsorptive characteristics of different species.

The liver is the first and most important organ able to intercept and detoxify metabolites absorbed from the gastrointestinal tract. Hepatic detoxification is often brought about by inducible, non-specific mixed-function oxidases (MFO), which are able to oxidize, alter or reduce toxi-

Table 15.1. Common toxins in temperate pastures (grasses, legumes, weeds).

Toxin	Sources	Structure	Principal effects on sheep
Alkaloids	Synthesized by plants and fungi	Usually basic, synthesized from amino acids and classified on heterocyclic ring structure	Often very toxic, causing irreversible liver damage
Pyrrolizidine	Ragwort, fescue endophyte Paterson's curse	Based around two five-sided rings	Irreversible liver damage, hepatic copper accumulation
Indole	Ergots in fescue, phalaris and ryegrass endophyte	Derivatives of tryptophan based around five- and six-sided rings	Vasoconstriction, hyperthermia, poor performance, incoordination
Quinolizidine	Lupins	Two six-sided rings	Respiratory paralysis, damage to central nervous system
Indolizine	Fungi in red clover	Five- and six-sided rings	Profuse salivation
Glycosides	Plant metabolites	Carbohydrate linked to a glycone moiety	Wide-ranging, dependent on properties of aglycone
Cyanogenic	White and sub. clovers, sorghum	Ruminal hydrolysis yields cyanide	Cellular respiratory inhibitor
Goitrogenic	Brassicas	Glucosinolates yielding (iso)thiocyanates, nitriles	Reduces thyroid function, goitre, poor growth
Saponins	Legumes (lucerne)	Steroid or triterpenoid aglycone	Foaming ruminal contents, bloat
Nitropropanol	Vetches (*Astragalus* spp.)	Yields 3-nitro-1-propanol	Methaemoglobinaemia, nerve damage
Isoflavones	Red and subterranean clovers	Flavanoid based on three six-sided rings	Oestrogenic activity, infertility
Cytoplasmic protein	Plant cytoplasm	Soluble, non-toxic unless in excess	Can cause bloat, high ammonia production, exacerbates effects of liver damage
Phylloerythrin	Metabolite of chlorophyll	Cyclic structure comprising five-sided rings	Photosensitization after liver damage
S-methylcysteine sulphoxide	Brassicas	Amino acid derivative	Haemolytic anaemia
Oxalates	Weed species (e.g. *Rumex*)	Oxalic acid	Impaired mineral (esp. calcium) absorption
Condensed tannin	Some legumes (e.g. lotus)	Polymerized flavonoid units	High concentrations impair rumen microbial activity and amino acid absorption
Hypericin	St John's wort	Multiple six-sided rings	Photosensitization

cants to less harmful compounds. A principal component of MFO is the cytochrome P450 system, which hydroxylates many toxic substances. This system alters reactive functional groups on toxins (e.g. OH, SH, NH_2) to facilitate conjugation and urinary excretion. Some toxins can impair liver function – for example, pyrrolizidine alkaloids from sources such as ragwort or the mycotoxin sporodesmin. Damage reduces liver capacity for utilizing absorbed nutrients or detoxifying ammonia from high-protein diets and increases susceptibility to other toxins. Some toxins are unaffected by the liver enzymes and pass into the systemic circulation to affect a wide range of organs.

Phytotoxicoses in Improved Temperate Forages

Plant varieties with potentially toxic metabolites have occasionally been released. Very successful programmes have been undertaken to reduce the phyto-oestrogen content of subterranean clover and red clover, as well as cyanoglycosides in white clover (Stern *et al.*, 1983; Caradus and Woodfield, 1997; Rumball *et al.*, 1997), but the most basic component of plants, chlorophyll, can still cause photosensitization in some instances. The use of animal trials in field and laboratory conditions will minimize the likelihood of further errors.

Photosensitization

Photosensitization can be broadly categorized into primary and secondary types. Primary photosensitization is due to the ingestion and absorption of photodynamic agents that reach the skin through the systemic circulation. Examples of plants in this category include St John's wort (*Hypericum perforatum*), found in many roadside pastures and waste areas, and buckwheat (*Fagopyrum esculentum*), grown as either a grain or a forage crop. Other examples include celery (*Apium* spp.) and spring parsley (*Petroselinum crispum*), grazed in rangelands (Cheeke, 1998).

Photosensitivity symptoms are most severe in light (non-pigmented) skin, typical of sheep. Absorption of light photons excites photodynamic agents in the skin (e.g. phylloerythrin (also known as phytoporphyrin)) to yield free radicals, which react with dermal proteins and cell membranes. This results in extreme sensitivity of the affected skin, which is alleviated by avoidance of sunlight, but secondary effects include reddening, serous oozing and thickening, sloughing and necrosis of the skin. Animals may refuse to feed and ewes may prevent lambs from sucking sensitive teats.

Ruminants are most commonly affected by secondary photosensitization. This is associated with liver damage, so that photodynamic compounds are not detoxified in sufficient quantity by the liver and pass into the systemic circulation. The most common situation is probably due to phylloerythrin, which is a ruminal degradation product of chlorophyll, usually removed by the liver and excreted in the bile. When liver function or biliary flow is compromised, the phylloerythrin initiates photodynamic reactions in the skin. The effects may be immediate, if the forage contains sufficient chlorophyll, or delayed until animals are grazing lush green pasture. Toxins capable of causing liver damage include sporodesmin from the fungus *Pithomyces chartarum*, which can be very common in New Zealand improved pastures in warm humid weather, or the *Phomopsis leptustromiformis* parasite common to *Lupinus* species.

Other forms of photosensitization, not necessarily associated with liver disease but of an unknown aetiology, include photosensitization in lambs fed lucerne (*Medicago sativa*), either fresh or as hay, burr medic (*Medicago polymorpha*), bird's-foot trefoil (*Lotus corniculatus*), clovers (*Trifolium* spp.) and cicer milkvetch (*Astragalus cicer*) (Parton *et al.*, 2001). Photosensitization without liver damage is well known with lambs grazing rape, with oedema of the ears and neck and sometimes necrosis of the ears.

Clinical or subclinical photosensitization represents an important cost to the sheep industry. Liver damage will reduce potential productivity of the flock, even after regeneration, and render these animals more susceptible to mild challenges in the future. It is essential to provide shade and remove the flock from the source of photosensitization. Prevention through avoidance of photosensitizing agents or hepatotoxins is paramount but may be difficult when the feed and toxin are inseparable.

Phyto-oestrogens

Many legumes contain compounds that bind weakly to the mammalian oestrogen receptor. These compounds impair the fertility of ewes and, to a lesser extent, cattle, but have little effect on male animals. Very high concentrations of phyto-oestrogens in subterranean clover can cause classical 'clover disease' in ewes, with dramatic signs, including prolapse of the uterus, dystocia, mammary development in ewes and wethers, enlarged bulbourethral glands of wethers (Plate 15.1) and very low lambing rates. Such obvious clinical problems are now rare, but low-level infertility appears to be widespread.

Two types of infertility have been described in sheep. Ewes grazing oestrogenic pasture have suppressed ovarian function, so that twinning rate and even ovulation itself are suppressed. The ability to conceive may be reduced through impaired sperm transport through the cervix and sometimes increased embryonic mortality is reported. However, the most significant effect is reduced twinning rate. Smith *et al.* (1979) reported that feeding ewes material containing 25 mg kg^{-1} coumestans reduced their ovulation rate by 25%. Indeed, the only effect of phyto-oestrogens may be a reduced number of twins born 5 months after grazing the oestrogenic pasture. Since twinning rate also depends on nutritional status, such losses would not be observed unless the phyto-oestrogenic content was being monitored. This form of infertility is temporary, resolving within 4–6 weeks after the ewes are removed from the oestrogenic pasture.

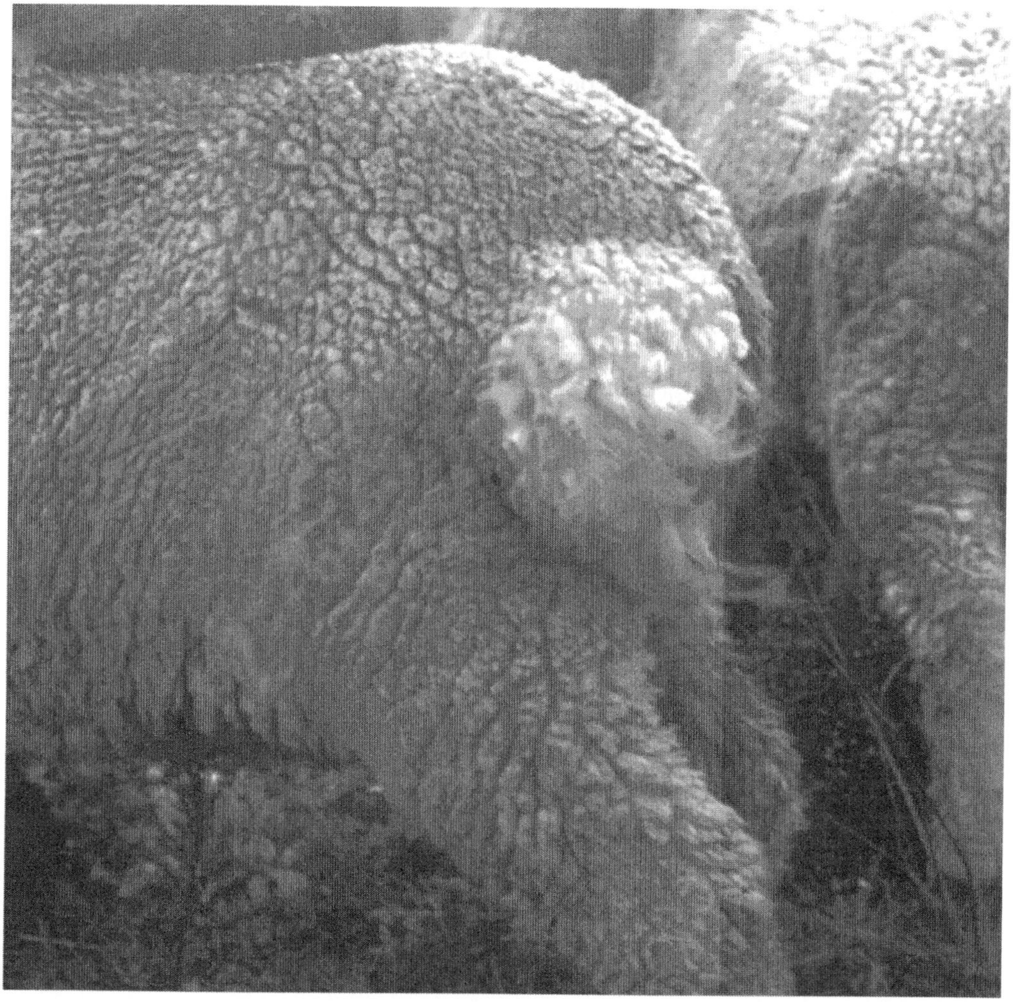

Plate 15.1. Enlarged bulbo-urethral gland in a wether sheep as a result of grazing pasture containing a highly oestrogenic variety of subterranean clover (*Trifolium subterraneum*). The enlargement was sufficient to cause some pressure necrosis on the skin overlying the gland.

The second form of infertility in ewes occurs after grazing oestrogenic pastures for periods of at least 4 months. This infertility is both permanent and cumulative, becoming worse with each year of exposure. The major clinical sign is failure to conceive; ovulation and twinning rates are normal but damage to the cervix prevents normal sperm transport in permanently infertile ewes. A low level of this infertility is widespread in Western Australia (Adams *et al.*, 1988), but has not been described elsewhere. The highly seasonal rainfall in Western Australia has resulted in strong dependence on subterranean clover as the pasture legume, and many of the original subterranean clover varieties had high formononetin concentrations.

Diagnosis of infertility due to phyto-oestrogens is not difficult; however, most cases of reproductive loss due to phyto-oestrogens are not diagnosed. Relationships between oestrogenicity and reproductive loss are reasonably well established, so it is possible to estimate the degree of reproductive loss due to phyto-oestrogens by measuring the oestrogenic activity in the feed (Adams, 1995). The most reliable means of estimating oestrogenicity is through bioassay, because phyto-oestrogens may undergo extensive metabolism. The metabolic pathways vary between ruminants and non-ruminants, so it is better to assess oestrogenicity in the species of interest. For sheep, measuring the increase in teat length of wethers over a 7–10-day period provides a quick, cheap and sensitive bioassay, although it is not very precise. However, the chemical identity and metabolism of the common phyto-oestrogens have now been described, so chemical assay is a useful guide to diagnosis. These diagnostic methods are suitable for temporary infertility, but permanent infertility may occur even years after the sheep have been exposed to oestrogenic pasture, so measurement of pasture oestrogenicity is only useful as supporting evidence. Accurate diagnosis of permanent oestrogenic infertility in ewes depends on identification of histopathological changes in the cervix (Adams, 1990).

Oestrogenic compounds appear to increase the resistance of the plant against disease. The significant oestrogenic compounds involved in infertility are isoflavones and coumestans. Concentrations of the oestrogenic isoflavones are under genetic control, as indicated in Table 15.2, so that their concentration depends primarily on the clover variety. Environmental conditions, such as temperature and nutrient supply, have a lesser effect on isoflavone concentrations. Varieties of subterranean clover and red clover have been developed that contain sufficient genistein or biochanin A to maintain competitiveness in the sward, but are low in formononetin so as to minimize reproductive problems (Rumball *et al.*, 1997).

Table 15.2. Summary of major oestrogens in pasture.

Class of phyto-oestrogen	Chemical compound	Control in the plant	Plant species affected
Isoflavone	Genistein Daidzein Biochanin A Formononetin	Genetic control	Subterranean clover Red clover Soybean Berseem clover
Coumestans	Coumestrol 4′-Methoxycoumestrol Repensol Trifoliol Sativol	Response to disease	Lucerne Medics White clover Soybean
Fungal oestrogens	Zearalenone Zearalenol	*Fusarium* fungi	Dead plant material

In contrast to the isoflavones, the concentration of coumestans depends primarily on the response by plants to environmental conditions, particularly attack by insects or fungi. Genotype is important only to the extent that it determines the overall sensitivity of the plant to infestation. The environmental impact is illustrated by the findings of Hall (1984) that samples of lucerne grown in inland Australia had low coumestrol concentrations, whereas most lucerne samples grown in more humid coastal regions of Australia contained sufficient coumestrol to cause reproductive problems in sheep. In annual medics, coumestans usually accumulate during the senescence and death of the plant, so concentrations are higher in dry pastures.

Isoflavone phyto-oestrogens are extensively metabolized in the rumen (Cox and Braden, 1974). After an adaptation period of 7–10 days, the rumen flora are able to break down genistein, biochanin A and daidzein to non-oestrogenic metabolites. As a result, these compounds have only a short-term effect on fertility of sheep. However, formononetin is transformed to the oestrogenic isoflavan equol, which is absorbed by the animal from the rumen, so that in ruminants formononetin is the major isoflavone of concern. Coumestans undergo little metabolism in the rumen, so the animal is less able to adapt to their presence.

Fusarium fungi growing on moist dead plant material may produce the oestrogenic compound zearalonone. This causes prolonged oestrus, lowered ovulation rates and temporary infertility in a high proportion of ewes. Although zearalonone is also used as a growth promotant, the presence of this compound in animal products can adversely affect trade with some countries.

Cyanogens

Cyanogens are ubiquitous in plants, but are only considered to be cyanogenic if the concentration exceeds 10 mg kg^{-1} fresh weight (Davis, 1991). Common cyanogenic forages include sorghum (*Sorghum vulgare*), Sudan grass (*Sorghum sudanense*), their hybrid 'Sudax', cynodon grasses (e.g. Bermuda grass) and white clover (*Trifolium repens*). Some weed species also contain very high cyanogenic glycoside concentrations (Parton *et al.*, 2001).

Cyanide is released from the glycosides by hydrolysis subsequent to rupture of cellular vacuoles (containing the glycosides) in the presence of cytosolar hydrolytic enzymes. Hence foliar damage caused by wilting, trampling, chewing or freezing will enhance the release of cyanide. The near-neutral pH of the rumen is optimal for enzyme activity, so ruminants are more sensitive to cyanide than non-ruminants. However, cyanide is readily detoxified, so toxicity occurs only when intake is rapid and excessive.

Hydrogen cyanide (HCN) is readily transported into animal cells, where it inactivates the respiratory cytochrome oxidase system. This effectively halts oxygen utilization, resulting in anoxia in all tissues, with brain and heart failure the primary causes of death. Signs of cyanide poisoning are dyspnoea (laboured breathing), excitement, staggering, convulsions and coma. These symptoms occur only when the cyanide absorption is very high and exceeds the tissue capacity for detoxification through conversion to thiocyanate, which is excreted in the urine. The lethal level is about 2 mg HCN kg^{-1} body weight (BW) in ruminants.

Methods for minimizing the risk of cyanide poisoning vary with the type of forage on offer. Avoidance of cyanogenic weeds (such as *Poa aquatica*) is obvious, while the toxicity of Sudan grass and sorghum is lower after flowering. White clovers with reduced cyanide levels are available. Cyanide concentrations in grasses tend to be highest in new foliage and are increased by nitrogenous fertilizers and some herbicides. Frosting and wilting increase the cyanide content and the rate of ingestion has a major impact on the likelihood of toxicosis. Hungry animals should not be given free access to these forages, and treatment – usually removal from toxic pastures – must be initiated very rapidly to prevent deaths of affected animals (Parton *et al.*, 2001).

Condensed tannins

Detrimental effects of condensed tannins in temperate improved swards are rare, except under poor growing conditions, which result in high tannin concentrations in the DM and reduced choice for the grazing animal. Condensed tannins occur mainly in dicotyledonous plants, especially *Lotus* spp., sulla (*Hedysarum coronarium*), sainfoin (*Onobrychis viciifolia*), dock (*Rumex obtusifolius*), lespedeza (*Serecia lespedeza*) and leucaena (*L. leucocephala*). They comprise up to 100 g kg^{-1} of DM in temperate forages but may reach 300 g kg^{-1} of DM in tropical forages and shrubs (Jackson *et al.*, 1996). They are often present in succulent portions of plants (leaves), which are sought after by grazing ruminants, especially when grasses are of poor quality.

When dietary concentrations exceed about 40–80 g kg^{-1} of DM, animal growth can be impaired due to low intake, but deaths occur only after prolonged grazing of forage having concentrations in excess of 100 g kg^{-1} of DM. The hydroxyl moieties in condensed tannins bind with plant, microbial and animal proteins, reducing the efficiency of microbial digestion in the rumen and also reducing absorption of amino acids from the intestine. Effects are more serious in non-ruminants than in ruminants (Waghorn *et al.*, 1999).

Distinct from condensed tannins are the hydrolysable tannins. These are readily hydrolysed to yield potentially toxic compounds (e.g. gallic acid), but they are not present in pastures, only in tree leaves and browse.

Recent studies have demonstrated the beneficial attributes of low concentrations of dietary condensed tannins for sheep (Waghorn *et al.*, 1999). Tannins are able to reduce excess losses of protein to microbial degradation in the rumen by reducing proteolysis, so a higher proportion of plant protein reaches the intestine and increases net amino acid absorption relative to equivalent diets without tannin. Low levels of condensed tannins will also reduce the incidence of bloat by preventing the production of a stable foam in the rumen following the rapid ingestion of high-quality forage, particularly legumes.

Oxalates

Oxalates in species such as sheep sorrel (*Rumex acetosella*), buffel grass (*Cenchrus ciliaris*), setaria (*Setaria sphacelata*) and sour sob (*Oxalis pes-caprae*) have caused poisoning and deaths in sheep (Seawright, 1982). Oxalates occur as oxalic acid or as salts in these plants and are largely degraded to carbonate and formate in the rumen, or precipitated as the calcium salt. However, when ingested in sufficient quantity, oxalates may be absorbed and reduce plasma calcium concentration. Absorbed oxalates also damage capillaries, leading to pulmonary oedema and oxalate-crystal precipitation in the kidneys. Symptoms of toxicity resemble hypocalcaemia, with staggering and recumbence.

Tissue damage and death occur after prolonged feeding on forages containing oxalate, or feeding diets containing an excess of 20 g kg^{-1} oxalate in the DM (McKenzie *et al.*, 1988). Death usually results from kidney damage.

Nitrate–nitrite

Nitrate–nitrite toxicity is a common and often lethal consequence of forage having high concentrations of nitrate (NO_3^-) in the DM (5–10 g kg^{-1}). This is usually associated with highly fertilized soils, especially when moisture causes rapid plant growth following a dry period. Nitrates accumulate in stems of rapidly growing plants, especially in overcast conditions (which favour nitrogen uptake but not photosynthesis). Nitrite poisoning has been associated with ryegrass species, brassicas (rape, turnip, choumoellier), as well as lucerne, barley, wheat and maize. Water containing over 200 mg kg^{-1} NO_3^- is also potentially hazardous. Toxicosis is brought about by intraruminal conversion of NO_3^- to NO_2^-, which is usually further reduced to ammonia, unless concentrations are very high, in which case absorbed NO_2^- associates with haemoglobin to form methaemoglobin, resulting in death through tissue anoxia. Horses and other non-ruminants are less susceptible to NO_3^- poisoning, because they do not convert NO_3^- to NO_2^- in the digestive tract. Nitrate poisoning can be very rapid or take several hours, depending on the source of NO_3^-. Pregnant animals may abort. Treatment is to limit access to high-NO_3^- feeds.

Species-specific toxicoses

Phalaris

Phalaris toxicoses are a significant problem in Australia, where sheep graze phalaris (*Phalaris aquatica*, formerly *Phalaris tuberosa*)-dominant pastures, and on *Phalaris arundinacea* (reed canary grass) pastures in the USA. The three unrelated toxicoses associated with *P. aquatica* include staggers, cardiac sudden death and polioencephalomalacic sudden death (PE) (Bourke, 1998a). Potentially toxic concentrations of NO_3^- and cyanide have also been reported in *P. aquatica* pastures associated with sudden death in sheep (Bourke, 1992), so a range of situations, often affected by climate, may cause significant health problems for sheep. In contrast, toxicosis associated with *P. arundinacea* is not usually lethal, but high concentrations of hordenine have been associated with poor palatability and indole alkaloid concentrations exceeding 2 g kg^{-1} of the DM with diarrhoea and ill thrift (Cheeke, 1998).

Phalaris staggers is a nervous disorder that affects sheep and cattle, and is caused by methylated tryptamines and β-carboline alkaloids, which occur in all commercial phalaris varieties. While these alkaloids are present in phalaris plants throughout the year, the incidence and severity of phalaris staggers, the time of onset and the reversibility of symptoms are extremely variable. The most common control of phalaris staggers is through cobalt prophylaxis by slow-release cobalt ruminal pellets or pasture sprays (Bourke, 1998b), which facilitate rumen microbial capacity for detoxification. Selection for reduced toxin concentrations remains an option for long-term control. Low dimethyltryptamine alkaloid selections, such as var. Sirolan (Oram and Edlington, 1996), still caused phalaris staggers, due to elevated concentrations of *N*-methyltyramine alkaloids and β-carboline, which inhibit the hepatic monoamine oxidase system and reduce the animal's capacity to detoxify absorbed alkaloids (McKenna and Towers, 1984). Sheep affected by phalaris staggers can display tremors, twitching, head nodding, leg weakness, lack of coordination, collapse and struggling to rise. The nervous symptoms of phalaris staggers can persist from several days to several months, and death or permanent disability can occur (Bourke, 1998b).

Cardiac sudden death affects sheep and horses (Bourke, 1998a) and is caused primarily by *N*-methyltyramine (Anderton *et al.*, 1994). It is characterized by difficulty in breathing, sudden collapse and frequently death of a few sheep when mobs are gathered, moved or disturbed. Incidence is highest in autumn, coinciding with new-season regrowth of phalaris, particularly after drought. Long-term control may be provided by phalaris varieties with low *N*-methyltyramine content (Oram and Edlington, 1996). In the absence of such varieties, the best management is to minimize disturbances of affected mobs, since most animals will survive without ill effects.

Polioencephalomalacic sudden death affects sheep, resulting in the sudden death overnight of a high proportion of animals between 12 and 48 h of starting to graze toxic phalaris-dominant pastures (Bourke, 1998a). The toxin responsible for PE is not known; however, Bourke (1998a) suggests that it is probably a direct antagonist of either thiamine or pyridoxine, since it rapidly compromises the integrity of blood vessels supplying the central portion of the brain. Failure of these blood vessels to supply oxygen and nutrients results in rapid degeneration of the brain and ultimately death. The PE is often worst when very hungry mobs of sheep are moved on to phalaris-dominant pastures with short new-season regrowth after periods of drought or frost.

Annual ryegrass

Annual ryegrass (*Lolium rigidum*) toxicity is a significant problem in South Australia and Western Australia and in South Africa. This neurological disease of sheep can be responsible for hundreds of deaths when grazing toxic pasture. The symptoms are superficially similar to ryegrass staggers (see below), with neurological disturbances, high-stepping gait and convulsions, but annual-ryegrass toxicity is lethal, involving damage to the brain (especially the cerebellum) from 2 days to 12 weeks after grazing toxic pasture (Chapman, 1989). Lesions are brought about by highly toxic glycolipids (corynetoxins), which inhibit the activity of enzymes responsible for *N*-glycosylation of glycoproteins (Jago and Culvenor, 1987).

Annual-ryegrass toxicity requires interaction between a plant nematode (*Anguina agrostis* or *Anguina funesta*) and a pathogenic bacterium (*Clavibacter toxicus*), possibly in association with a bacteriophage. When annual-ryegrass seedlings become infected with *A. agrostis*, the larvae are carried on the growing tip and burrow into the developing flower to form a gall, in which the adult nematode lays eggs. The eggs hatch into larvae, which can remain dormant for several years. The nematode is non-toxic and the galls are brown or black, unless the nematodes are infected with *Clavibacter* (possibly in association with a bacteriophage (Ophel *et al.*, 1993)), which produces corynetoxins. The presence of these bacteria is indicated by a yellow slime on the seed heads, which gives a yellowness to ryegrass fields and indicates a potentially toxic situation. Corynetoxins are not detoxified by rumen fermentation and there is no treatment for sheep suffering from annual-ryegrass toxicity.

No practical methods exist for controlling *Clavibacter*, and the best way to prevent annual-ryegrass toxicity is by breaking the nematode life cycle, either by eradicating annual ryegrass by cropping or by preventing flowering. The risk of toxicity in a sward is reduced when galls are shed late in the season and, provided stocking rates are low, it is possible to graze previously toxic pastures late in the season (Chapman, 1989).

Kikuyu

Kikuyu (*Pennisetum clandestinum*) is a widely grown tropical forage, which may contain a variety of deleterious substances, including oxalates, saponins and nitrates (Pienaar *et al.*, 1993). Outbreaks of kikuyu poisoning in sheep (and other animals) have been reported in New Zealand, Australia and South Africa. The aetiology is not understood and, although some evidence suggests mycotoxins may be responsible, other evidence suggests this is unlikely (Cheeke, 1998). Invasions of army worm have also been implicated in kikuyu poisoning in some cases (Smith and Martinovich, 1973), but not others. Symptoms include salivation, sham drinking, cessation of ruminal and intestinal motility and severe dehydration. There is no effective treatment and mortality may be high.

Brassicas

Although not strictly pastures, brassica species, such as turnips, kale and rape, are sown with grass or used in grazing systems. All of these contain two sulphur-containing compounds (the amino acid *S*-methylcysteine sulphoxide (SMCO) and glucosinolates). The presence of these compounds, and especially their degradation products, can lower growth rates and lead to haemolytic anaemia (SMCO) and goitre or goitrogenic effects (glucosinolates).

The SMCO can account for as much as 40–60 g kg^{-1} of the DM and is metabolized in the rumen to release dimethyldisulphide, which is absorbed and reduced to an inactive form by glutathione peroxidase. When excess dimethyldisulphide is absorbed, haemolytic anaemia develops, with reduced haemoglobin concentrations and the appearance of precipitated, oxidized haemoglobin granules in the erythrocytes (Heinz bodies). Symptoms of haemolytic anaemia may not develop until animals have grazed brassicas for 3–4 weeks, and include poor performance, loss of appetite, diarrhoea and jaundice. Extended exposure to high concentrations of SMCO will result in death and in liver and kidney damage in surviving sheep. Surviving animals will make a complete recovery 3–4 weeks after removal from brassica pasture.

The SMCO content of brassicas increases during winter and is exacerbated by nitrogenous fertilizers. Growth on low-sulphur soils has been reported to lower the SMCO content of brassicas (McDonald *et al.*, 1981); both a gradual introduction and supplementation with pasture are likely to minimize the toxic effects.

The glucosinolates are hydrolysed by plant or microbial enzymes in the rumen to yield glucose, as well as isothiocyanate, nitrile or thiocyanate, depending upon the structure of the aglycone portion of the molecule. These compounds may interfere with thyroid function through a range of reactions, and are exacerbated by low dietary iodine concentration, leading to goitre. Interference with thyroid function is manifest by reducing iodine uptake by the thyroid gland or interference with iodination of tyrosine and reducing thyroxine secretion.

Symptoms of glucosinolate toxicity are primarily those of iodine insufficiency; clinical signs include enlargement of the thyroid gland, and up to 60% of newborn lambs have died when their dams have been grazing kale (Sinclair and Andrews, 1958). Prolonged exposure to glucosinolates will reduce productivity, but exposures of several weeks may not be apparent in ewes, although newborn lambs may suffer from goitre (Grace, 1994).

Mycotoxicoses in Forages

Mycotoxins are secondary metabolites produced by fungi associated with vegetative herbage and dead litter. Active research into mycotoxins in forages grew from frequent widespread outbreaks of photosensitization due to facial eczema in sheep in New Zealand and led to the realization of the benefits to pastures as well as detrimental effects on animal production. For example, the ryegrass endophyte *N. lolii* provides protection for the plant from insect attack, improves drought tolerance and may also contribute to improved persistence by deterring excessive grazing. The endophyte is also responsible for ryegrass staggers, requiring researchers to select fungal strains that are able to protect the host plant without impairing animal performance. The extensive and ongoing research effort given to modifying and understanding the perennial-ryegrass endophyte (Woodfield and Matthew, 1999) indicates the complex associations between fungi and forage; simple elimination of fungi may be more detrimental to farming than the risks of toxicoses on animal performance.

Mycotoxins include a wide range of compounds but are usually aromatic, non-immunogenic hydrocarbons of relatively low molecular weight. The principal genera responsible for toxicoses in sheep grazing pasture (Table 15.3) are *Aspergillus*, *Penicillium* and *Fusarium* but also include *Claviceps*, *Stachybotrys*, *Alternaria*, *Myrothecium* and *Pithomyces*. Toxins must survive rumen degradation to be absorbed and affect a range of organs, including the liver, kidneys and nervous system, but also cardiac function, gastrointestinal function and reproduction. Some are carcinogenic or immunosuppressive.

Facial eczema

Facial eczema (pithomycotoxicosis) is the most important mycotoxicosis in New Zealand, where outbreaks affect both sheep and cattle (Smith, 1989). Facial eczema has also been reported from both coasts of the USA, Australia, southern areas of South Africa and parts of South America, France and the UK. The disease occurs in warm moist situations, which favour the growth of *Pithomyces chartarum* in pasture litter. Ingestion of these fungal spores results in rapid absorption of sporodesmin, often leading to severe photosensitization.

Sporodesmin is concentrated in the liver and bile. A series of glutathione-linked oxidation and reduction reactions of sporodesmin generate superoxide and other free radicals, leading to liver damage and secondary photosensitization. This damage prevents excretion of phylloerythin (from chlorophyll), leading to photosensitivity, and endogenous porphyrins accumulate, leading to jaundice. Even severe liver damage rarely leads to deaths and partial regeneration is common, but appetite is greatly reduced and animals become extremely sensitive to sunlight, seeking shade wherever possible. Symptoms of photosensitization include swelling and burning of the ears and head, skin sloughing and inappetence.

Table 15.3. Common mycotoxicoses affecting sheep grazing improved temperate pastures.

Disorder	Fungus	Principal toxin	Forage type/component	Mode of action	Outcome
Facial eczema	*Pithomyces chartarum*	Sporodesmin	Pasture litter	Hepatotoxin, secondary photosensitization	Inappetence, very poor performance, rarely fatal
Ryegrass staggers	*Neotyphodium lolii*	Lolitrem B, ergovaline	*Lolium perenne*, esp. sheath, stem, seed	Neurotoxin, tremorgen	Very poor growth, heat stress, diarrhoea
Tall-fescue toxicosis	*Neotyphodium coenophialum*	Ergovaline, ergopeptides, clavine alkaloids	*Festuca* spp.	Vasoconstrictor	Heat stress, very poor growth, dry gangrene
Fusarium infertility	*Fusarium* spp.	Zearalenone	Pasture litter	Hyperoestrogenism, testicular atrophy	Temporary infertility
Paspalum	*Claviceps paspali* *Claviceps purpurea*	Paspalinines, ergotomine, ergometrine, ergotoxine	Paspalum seed heads	Tremorgen, gangrene, internal bleeding	Staggers, loss of extremities
Kikuyu poisoning	?	?	Kikuyu grass		Depression, drooling, convulsions
Lupinosis	*Phomopsis leptostromiformis*		Lupin stubble	Hepatotoxin	Inappetence, secondary infections, deaths

The severity of the problem in New Zealand has led to a good understanding of conditions likely to trigger an outbreak of facial eczema, as well as procedures for reducing the impact of the toxin. Spores are produced most freely when relative humidity approaches 100%, day temperatures are between 20 and 24°C and night temperatures are over 14°C. These conditions favour rapid development of spores within a 48 h period, so that pasture spore counts are used to indicate danger periods. Counts in excess of 100,000 spores per g of fresh grass are considered dangerous. The severity is affected by a range of factors, including stocking rate, closeness of grazing, previous exposure and sheep breed.

The effects of facial eczema can be controlled by reducing the intake of spores or by treating animals with zinc to reduce liver injury. Administration of zinc must be 20–30 times the nutritional requirements and be given before the sporodesmin challenge. Treatment in New Zealand is now by slow-release intraruminal bullet, although drenching with a zinc oxide slurry is also effective. A daily dose of 25 mg Zn kg^{-1} BW (usually as ZnO) for sheep provides protection without inducing toxicity or residue problems in the animal product or pasture. Spraying pastures with benzimidazole fungicides will render them safe for grazing for 6 weeks, provided rainfall does not occur within 3 days of spraying. Lax grazing, to reduce intake of spores from dead material, may also alleviate the impact of toxicity, but administration of zinc salts has been the most effective means for providing protection for animals.

There are genetic differences between breeds and between individuals in their susceptibility to facial eczema. Merinos appear more resistant to sporodesmin than British sheep breeds (Smith *et al.*, 1980) and heritability of resistance to facial eczema has been calculated as 0.42, so that selection for improved resistance to facial eczema is a possible means for reducing the costs of this problem (Smith, 1989).

Ryegrass staggers

Ryegrass staggers affects animals grazing perennial-ryegrass (*L. perenne*)-dominant pastures and should not be confused with grass staggers (hypomagnesaemia) or annual-ryegrass toxicity. It is a significant problem in New Zealand and parts of Australia where perennial ryegrass is a dominant pasture species. Outbreaks of ryegrass staggers occur mainly in summer and autumn and the neurological impact on coordination, resulting in staggering, head shaking and collapse when sheep become excited, can result in significant mortality from misadventure. Wild-type *N. lolii* produces a range of alkaloids, including lolitrem B and ergovaline, which are responsible for tremorgenic reactions in sheep. Further, it is increasingly apparent that the tremorgens responsible for staggering are also associated with poor animal performance, health and well-being, previously described as ill thrift.

A higher proportion of perennial-ryegrass pastures in New Zealand are infected with *N. lolii* than is apparent in Europe (Easton, 1999). The fungal endophyte improves ryegrass persistence, partly through the effects of peramine, which inhibits feeding (and consequently egg laying and larval development) of the Argentine stem weevil (*L. bonariensis*). An extensive research effort has been undertaken by New Zealand scientists to identify beneficial and detrimental compounds produced by *N. lolii* and to select strains that protect the plant without compromising sheep health. These strains produce very low concentrations of lolitrem B but maintain a high production of peramine.

Endophyte is concentrated in the leaf sheath, reproductive stem and inflorescence with relatively low concentrations in the leaf blade. As new leaves form, the endophyte grows into the blade to only a small degree. The symbiotic association between ryegrass and endophyte is supported by the intracellular location of hyphae, so there are no external indications of the endophyte in the seed or other parts of the plant. Endophyte within the seed embryo maintains the infection in the new seedling, but the viability of the endophyte is reduced if seed is stored for long periods and is compromised by warm conditions prior to germination, so seed falling to the ground and remaining dormant for several months is likely to lose viable endophyte.

Health problems in sheep grazing perennial ryegrass with wild-type endophyte include reduced growth rates (or even weight loss), ryegrass staggers, increased diarrhoea, dags and fly strike, heat stress and reduced plasma prolactin concentrations (Table 15.4). Although ryegrass endophyte does not appear to compromise reproductive performance in ewes, any reduction in ewe feed intake will compromise lamb growth rate (Watson *et al.*, 1999).

Table 15.4. Impact of ryegrass staggers on sheep performance in New Zealand (from Fletcher *et al.*, 1999).

	Number of		Endophyte			
	Trials	Sheep	Wild	Nil	Difference	Significance
Spring grazing						
LW gain (g day^{-1})	3	280	126	168	42	*
Dags (0–5 scale)	2	160	1.5	0.5	–	*
Respiration rate (min^{-1})	3	280	88	79	9	n.s.
Body temperature (°C)	3	360	40.2	40.0	0.2	n.s.
Plasma prolactin (ng ml^{-1})	2	160	103	243	140	**
Summer/autumn grazing						
LW gain (g day^{-1})	5	330	41	112	71	**
Staggers (0–5)	4	300	3.1	0	–	**
Dags (0–5)	3	240	1.5	0.4	–	*
Fly strike (%)	2	180	23	2	21	**
Respiration rate (min^{-1})	3	192	99	73	26	*
Body temperature (°C)	4	300	40.6	40.2	0.4	*
Plasma prolactin (ng ml^{-1})	3	240	63	136	73	**

LW, live weight; *, significant at 5% probability; **, significant at 1% probability; n.s., not significant.

Control of ryegrass staggers is made difficult by the benefits that the endophyte provides for the ryegrass plant. Much of New Zealand farming is carried out in hilly environments best suited to ryegrass/clover pastures, so the strategy adopted in that country has been to select endophytes that produce peramine to benefit the host plant, but which do not produce significant quantities of lolitrem B or ergovaline. Selection of these strains has produced marked improvements in sheep performance (Table 15.4) at equivalent DM yields (Woodfield and Matthew, 1999). Introduction of non-toxic endophytes offers good opportunities for success, because the symbiosis between endophyte and ryegrass is very specific, only allowing a single strain per plant. The main potential problem remains contamination of pastures containing novel endophytes through germination of seed containing wild-type endophyte. This can occur through transfer in hay or after passage of seed through the animal (Hume, 1999).

Tall-fescue toxicoses

Tall fescue (*Festuca arundinacea*) also has an association with an endophyte fungus, *Neotyphodium coenophialum*, leading to a wide range of deleterious effects in grazing animals. These include dry gangrene of lower extremities, reduced feed intakes, low weight gains and milk production and very low plasma prolactin concentrations in sheep and cattle.

There are over 15 million ha of endophyte-infected pastures in North America, and fescue toxicity is also important in Australasia and Argentina. The endophyte benefits the plant through pest and drought resistance and better tolerance of adverse soil and environmental conditions and results in a greener, more vigorous plant than endophyte-free fescue. The endophyte is located primarily in the sheath and inflorescence, rather than the leaf. It has no reproductive phase and, like *N. lolii*, is transmitted via infected seeds.

Although ergovaline and clavine alkaloids are important toxins, the fungus produces a range of modified ergopeptides, as well as loline alkaloids (pyrrolizidine alkaloids). This diversity may account for the greater toxicity of fescue endophyte compared with ryegrass endophyte (Lane *et al.*, 1999) and effects on thermoregulation, reproduction and lipid metabolism (Cheeke, 1998). The vasoconstriction leads to tissue anoxia (dry gangrene) and hyperthermia, due to insufficient capacity for heat loss. Sheep appear less affected by fescue toxicosis than cattle, perhaps because their principal route for heat loss is respiratory rather than through the skin. Nevertheless, hyperthermia is common, with reduced intakes, lameness and loss of extremities under severe conditions.

Fescue toxicity can be prevented by either reducing intake of toxic fescue or feeding non-toxic fescue. Avoidance of seed heads (containing the highest concentrations of alkaloid) can reduce toxicity, as will dilution of fescue with non-toxic forages. Hay made before seed development and treatment of hay by ammoniation have been shown to reduce toxicity. Ensiling tall-fescue forage does not affect its ergovaline content.

Endophyte-free fescue can be grown under good climatic conditions, but in many regions of the USA the presence of endophyte is essential for persistence and forage growth. Selection of endophyte strains containing peramine to deter insects, but with low ergovaline concentrations, represents a promising means for achieving both persistence and animal performance.

Paspalum staggers

Paspalum staggers has been reported in Australia, New Zealand, South Africa, the USA and parts of Europe where *Paspalum dilatatum* (dallis grass) is grown. Paspalum seed heads are frequently infected by *Claviceps paspali*, which produces tremorgens, leading to incoordination, head tremors and collapse when disturbed (Botha *et al.*, 1996). These symptoms are similar to those of ryegrass staggers. Paspalum may also be infected with *Claviceps purpurea*, which grows on several grains and grasses and also forms sclerotinia (ergot bodies) in the seed heads. When sheep consume *C. purpurea*, they develop breathing difficulties, excessive salivation, diarrhoea and bleeding within the digestive tract (Cheeke, 1998), but the avoidance of seed heads, more typical of sheep than cattle, reduces the incidence of ergot poisoning, provided adequate leafy foliage is available.

Symptoms due to the tremorgenic paspalinine are more common than the gangrenous condition in sheep, and removal of sheep from infected pastures will enable complete recovery. This condition also resembles ryegrass staggers, in that rapid movement will induce collapse, but the condition is not lethal.

The gangrenous syndrome arises from derivatives of lysergic and isolysergic acids, including ergotamine (a central nervous system stimulant and depressor), ergometrine and ergotoxine, all of which are powerful arteriolar smooth-muscle constrictors. Arteriolar and capillary constriction results in bleeding and gangrene of the affected part, with clinical signs similar to those of fescue toxicity.

Forage lupins

Lupins can cause toxicity in sheep through either alkaloid poisoning or mycotoxicosis associated with grazing mature lupin stems or stubble. The quinolizidine alkaloid poisoning affects sheep to a greater extent than goats or cattle and can be a major cause of mortality in sheep in western USA. Toxicity increases after flowering, with seeds being especially toxic. Symptoms of toxicity include laboured breathing, with death by respiratory paralysis.

Lupin mycotoxicosis is caused by ingestion of toxins from *P. leptostromiformis*. The fungi reside mainly in lupin stems and become toxic after seed harvest, so sheep grazing lupin stubble are at the greatest risk of toxicity. The fungus has been reported in both wild, high-alkaloid lupin (*Lupinus cosentinii*) and commercially available sweet lupin (*Lupinus angustifolius*). Fungal growth is facilitated by warm, overcast, moist conditions. Stubble may remain toxic for several months, with peak toxicity at the end of summer. Lupinosis has been reported in sheep in Europe, South Africa, the USA, Australia and New Zealand and is an important toxicosis in Australia, where lupins are used extensively as a fodder crop.

Symptoms of lupinosis include lack of appetite, loss of condition and lethargy. Deaths may occur within 2–4 days of sheep being introduced to toxic stubble. Chronic or subacute lupinosis, resulting from liver damage and consumption of lesser amounts of toxin over a long period, can result in a high proportion of a flock having poor performance, with increased susceptibility to disease and other toxins (e.g. photosensitivity). With acute toxicity, the liver is enlarged, fatty and yellow or orange in colour, in contrast to the small, hardened copper- or tan-coloured livers in sheep exposed to chronic toxicity. Liver copper concentrations are elevated, while zinc concentrations are depressed.

Lupinosis can be minimized by grazing stubble soon after seed harvest, before extensive fungal growth occurs. Grazing intensity should be low so that sheep are not forced to eat excessive stem, and animals should be removed from stubble in the event of rain, which increases fungal growth. Treatment should focus on improving appetite, while zinc administration will lower liver copper concentrations and help overcome inappetence.

Conclusion

Although this review has identified wide-ranging toxicoses that affect sheep grazing temperate forages, the advantages provided by yield, quality, palatability and persistence of these forages under a range of growing conditions far outweigh the occasional (and sometimes severe) health problems. These problems are nevertheless important and can affect reproduction and productivity and influence product quality for human usage. Future solutions need to focus on causes and prevention rather than treatment of toxicoses.

Improved communication and cooperation between animal and plant researchers, together with chemists, mycologists and molecular biologists, are essential for the development of improved forage varieties for animal production. Recent research involving teams with such expertise has identified causes of ill thrift, and breeders are producing varieties well suited to high-performance ruminants. However, producers may have to move away from pastures based on only one or two forage species if animal health and productivity are to be sustained with minimal veterinary intervention.

High stocking rates and minimum choice force sheep to eat lower pasture strata and increase the likelihood of toxicoses in flocks grazing intensive pastures. This emphasizes the difficulties faced by farmers attempting to maximize profitability in the face of the vagaries of climate and commodity prices. However, there is an increasing need to achieve this goal in a sustainable manner with good animal welfare, with the implication that toxicoses must be minimized in a consumer-driven market.

References

Adams, N.R. (1990) Permanent infertility in ewes exposed to plant estrogens. *Australian Veterinary Journal* 67, 197–201.

Adams, N.R. (1995) Detection of the effects of phytoestrogens on sheep and cattle. *Journal of Animal Science* 73, 1509–1515.

Adams, N.R., Sanders, M.R. and Ritar, A.J. (1988) Estrogenic damage and reduced fertility in ewe flocks in south Western Australia. *Australian Journal of Agricultural Research* 39, 71–77.

Anderton, N., Cockrum, P.A., Walker, D.W. and Edgar, J.A. (1994) Identification of a toxin suspected of causing sudden death in livestock grazing phalaris pastures. In: Colegate, S.M and Dorling, P.R. (eds) *Plant-associated Toxins, Agricultural, Phytochemical and Ecological Aspects*. CAB International, Wallingford, UK, pp. 269–274.

Barry, T.N. and Manley, T.R. (1984) The role of condensed tannins in the nutritional value of *Lotus pedunculatus* for sheep. 2. Quantitative digestion of carbohydrates and proteins. *British Journal of Nutrition* 51, 493–504.

Botha, C.J., Kellerman, T.S. and Fourie, N. (1996) A tremorgenic mycotoxicosis in cattle caused by *Paspalum distichum* (L.) infected by *Claviceps paspali*. *Journal of the South African Veterinary Association* 67, 36–37.

Bourke, C.A. (1992) Toxins in pasture plants – phalaris toxicity. *Animal Production in Australia* 19, 399–401.

Bourke, C.A. (1998a) Factors affecting the incidence of the PE 'sudden death' form of *Phalaris aquatica* poisoning in sheep. *Proceedings of Australian Agronomy Conference* 9, 326–329.

Bourke, C.A. (1998b) The association of soil cobalt with the incidence of the 'staggers' form of *Phalaris aquatica* poisoning in livestock. *Proceedings of Australian Agronomy Conference* 9, 330–332.

Caradus, J.R. and Woodfield, D.R. (1997) World checklist of white clover varieties II. *New Zealand Journal of Agricultural Research* 40, 115–206.

Casler, M.D. (1999) Breeding for improved quality: potentials and problems. In: *Proceedings of the XVIII International Grassland Congress*. Association Management Centre, Calgary, pp. 323–330.

Chapman, H.M. (1989) Annual ryegrass toxicity. In: *Second International Congress for Sheep Veterinarians*. Sheep and Beef Cattle Society of New Zealand, Massey University, Palmerston North, pp. 268–276.

Cheeke, P.R. (1998) *Natural Toxicants in Feeds, Forages and Poisonous Plants*. Interstate Publishers, Danville, Illinois, 479 pp.

Cox, R.I. and Braden, A.W.H. (1974) The metabolism and physiological effects of phyto-oestrogens in livestock. *Proceedings of the Australian Society of Animal Production* 10, 122–129.

Davis, R.H. (1991) Cyanogens. In: DeMello, J.P., DeMello, F., Duffus, C.M. and Duffus, J.M. (eds) *Toxic Substances in Crop Plants*. Royal Society of Chemistry, Cambridge, pp. 202–225.

Di Menna, M.E., Mortimer, P.H., Prestidge, R.A., Hawkes, A.D. and Sprosen, J.M. (1992) Lolitrem B concentrations, counts of *Acremonium lolii* hyphae and the incidence of ryegrass staggers in lambs on plots of *A. lolii*-infected ryegrass. *New Zealand Journal of Agricultural Research* 35, 211–217.

Easton, H.S. (1999) Endophyte in New Zealand pastures, an overview. In: Woodfield, D.R. and Matthew, C. (eds) *Ryegrass Endophyte: an Essential New Zealand Symbiosis*. Grasslands Research and Practice Series No. 7, New Zealand Grassland Association, Palmerston North, pp. 1–10.

Fletcher, L.R., Sutherland, B.L. and Fletcher, G.C. (1999) The impact of endophyte on the health and productivity of sheep grazing ryegrass-based pastures. In: Woodfield, D.R. and Matthew, C. (eds) *Ryegrass Endophyte: an Essential New Zealand Symbiosis*. Grasslands Research and Practice Series No. 7, New Zealand Grassland Association, Palmerston North, pp. 11–19.

Grace, N.D. (1994) *Managing Trace Element Deficiencies*. New Zealand Pastoral Agriculture Research Institute, Palmerston North, 70 pp.

Hall, D.G. (1984) Coumestrol content of lucerne in New South Wales. *Animal Production in Australia* 15, 689.

Hume, D.E. (1999) Establishing and maintaining a toxin-free pasture: a review. In: Woodfield, D.R. and Matthew, C. (eds) *Ryegrass Endophyte: an Essential New Zealand Symbiosis*. Grasslands Research and Practice Series No. 7, New Zealand Grassland Association, Palmerston North, pp. 123–132.

Jackson, F.S., Barry, T.N., Lascano, C. and Palmer, B. (1996) The extractable and bound condensed tannin content of leaves from tropical tree, shrub and forage legumes. *Journal of the Science of Food and Agriculture* 71, 103–110.

Jago, M.V. and Culvenor, C.C.J. (1987) Tunicamycin and corymetoxin poisoning in sheep. *Australian Veterinary Journal* 64, 232–235.

Lane, G.A., Tapper, B.A. and Davies, E. (1999) Ergot alkaloids additional to ergovaline in endophyte-infected perennial ryegrass and tall fescue in New Zealand. In: Woodfield, D.R. and Matthew, C. (eds) *Ryegrass Endophyte: an Essential New Zealand Symbiosis*. Grasslands Research and Practice Series No. 7, New Zealand Grassland Association, Palmerston North, pp. 95–100.

McDonald, R.C., Manley, T.R., Barry, T.N., Forss, D.A. and Sinclair, A.G. (1981) Nutritional evaluation of kale (*Brassica oleracea*) diets. 3. Changes in plant composition induced by soil fertility practices, with special reference to SMCO and glucosinolate concentrations. *Journal of Agricultural Science, Cambridge* 97, 13–23.

McKenna, D.J. and Towers, G.H.N. (1984) Biochemistry and pharmacology of tryptamines and β-carbolines: a mini review. *Journal of Psychoactive Drugs* 16, 347–358.

McKenzie, R.A., Bell, A.M., Storie, G.J., Keenan, F.J., Cornack, K.M. and Grant, S.G. (1988) Acute oxalate poisoning of sheep by buffel grass (*Cenchrus ciliaris*). *Australian Veterinary Journal* 65, 26.

Ophel, K.M., Bird, A.F. and Kerr, A. (1993) Association of bacteriophages particles with toxin production by *Clavibacter toxicus*, the causal agent of annual ryegrass toxicity. *Phytopathology* 83, 676–681.

Oram, R.N. and Edlington, J.P. (1996) Breeding non-toxic phalaris (*Phalaris aquatica* L.). *Proceedings of Australian Agronomy Conference* 8, 450–453.

Parton, K. and Chambers, J.P. (2001) *Veterinary Clinical Toxicology*. Publication No. 208, Veterinary Continuing Education, Massey University, Palmerston North, 393 pp.

Pienaar, J.P., Tainton, N.M. and van Ryssen, J.B.J. (1993) Factors affecting the voluntary feed intake of sheep grazing *Pennisetum clandestinum* (kikuyu) pastures: observations from forage analysis. *African Journal of Range and Forage Science* 10, 140–144.

Rumball, W., Keogh, R.G., Miller, J.E. and Claydon, R.B. (1997) 'Grasslands G27' red clover (*Trifolium pratense* L.). *New Zealand Journal of Agricultural Research* 40, 369–372.

Seawright, A.A. (1982) *Animal Health in Australia*, Vol. 2. *Chemical and Plant Poisons*. Australian Bureau of Animal Health, Australian Government Publishing Service, Canberra, 290 pp.

Sinclair, D.P. and Andrews, E.D. (1958) Prevention of goitre in new-born lambs from kale fed ewes. *New Zealand Veterinary Journal* 6, 87–98.

Smith, B.L. (1989) Mycotoxicoses associated with grassland farming of sheep. In: *Second International Congress for Sheep Veterinarians*. Sheep and Beef Cattle Society of New Zealand, Massey University, Palmerston North, pp. 255–267.

Smith, B.L. and Martinovich, D. (1973) Kikuyu poisoning of cattle. 2. Epizootiological Aspects. *New Zealand Veterinary Journal* 21, 85–89.

Smith, B.L., Stanbridge, T.A. and Embling, P.P. (1980) Sheep breed differences in pento-barbitone sleeping time and response to experimental sporodesmin intoxication. *New Zealand Veterinary Journal* 28, 35–36.

Smith, J.F., Jagusch, K.T., Brunswick, L.F.C. and Kelly, R.W. (1979) Coumestans in lucerne and ovulation in ewes. *New Zealand Journal of Agricultural Research* 22, 411–416.

Stern, W.R., Gladstones, J.S., Francis, C.M., Collins, W.J., Chatel, D.L., Nicolas, D.A., Gillespie, D.J., Wolfe, E.C., Southwood, O.R., Beale, P.E. and Curnow, B.C. (1983) Subterraneum clover improvement: an Australian programme. In: *Proceedings XIV International Grassland Congress, Lexington, Kentucky*. Westview Press, Boulder, Colorado, pp. 116–119.

Waghorn, G.C., Reed, J. and Ndlovu, L.R. (1999) Condensed tannins and herbivore nutrition. *Proceedings of the XVIII International Grassland Congress*, Vol. III. Association Management Centre, Calgary, pp. 153–166.

Watson, R.H., Keogh, R.G. and McDonald, M.F. (1999) Ewe reproductive performance and growth rate of suckling lambs on endophyte-infected perennial ryegrass pasture. In: Woodfield, D.R. and Matthew, C. (eds) *Ryegrass Endophyte: an Essential New Zealand Symbiosis*. Grasslands Research and Practice Series No. 7, New Zealand Grassland Association, Palmerston North, pp. 19–26.

Woodfield, D.R. (1999) Genetic improvements in New Zealand forage cultivars. *Proceedings of the New Zealand Grassland Association* 61, 3–7.

Woodfield, D.R. and Matthew, C. (eds) (1999) *Ryegrass Endophyte: an Essential New Zealand Symbiosis*. Grasslands Research and Practice Series No. 7, New Zealand Grassland Association, Palmerston North, 168 pp.

16 The Nutritional Management of Grazing Sheep

M. FREER

CSIRO Plant Industry, GPO Box 1600, Canberra, Australian Capital Territory, Australia

Introduction

When sheep managers or their advisers attempt to apply the wealth of nutritional information reviewed in the earlier chapters of this book, they face a number of difficulties. These spring largely from the highly variable feeding environment of grazing animals and the relatively low level of control on nutrient intake that can be exercised by the manager. This chapter will discuss the problems in applying the results of research on grazing sheep to nutritional management and describe some of the tools that are being developed to overcome these problems.

For example, although nutritional management must start with knowledge of the intake of nutrients, both the quantity and quality of the herbage diet selected are virtually impossible to measure directly and slow and expensive to estimate indirectly. Coleman and Henry (Chapter 1), Weston (Chapter 2) and Forbes and Mayes (Chapter 3, this volume) have analysed the numerous pasture and animal interactions that affect nutrient intake, but the manager has to attempt to apply this information to a continually changing scene of pasture attributes and animal requirements.

Within this scene, the manager seeks the stocking rate that will strike the best balance between optimum nutrient intake per animal and the efficient and sustainable use of the pasture resource. At this stocking rate, the supply of pasture nutrients will usually be inadequate for sheep requirements for some part of the year and the manager must decide whether to provide supplements or to tolerate a weight loss that may be regained later. When supplements are offered, there is a degree of substitution for pasture (see Dove, Chapter 6, this volume), which is difficult to predict but important in its effects on nutrient intake and the economics of supplementary feeding. Decisions on the composition of the supplement, particularly in respect of protein, will depend not only on the selected pasture diet but also on the amount of microbial protein synthesized (see Mackie *et al.*, Chapter 4, and Annison *et al.*, Chapter 5, this volume). They may also depend on the need for specific amino acids for wool or meat production (see Hynd and Masters, Chapter 8, and Oddy and Sainz, Chapter 11, this volume). For pregnant or lactating ewes with a variable nutrient intake (see Robinson *et al.*, Chapter 9, and Treacher and Caja, Chapter 10, this volume), the manager's feeding policy will be affected by the partition of nutrients between maternal weight loss or gain and the growth of the fetus or the production of milk.

Therefore, however sound the scientific basis for the systems of nutrient requirements for sheep that have been accepted in different countries, e.g. those of the National Research Council (NRC, 1985), the Standing Committee on Agriculture (SCA, 1990) and the Agricultural and Food Research Council (AFRC, 1993), it is difficult to apply them directly to grazing animals. In response, computer programs have recently been developed that attempt to integrate the same nutritional information in a way that enables the performance of specified grazing animals to be predicted from a defined feed base. Such models then become the basis of decision-support tools, for use by farmers or their advisers.

Grazing Models

A decision-support tool based on a model of the grazing animal can be designed to help either with tactical problems in the day-to-day feeding management of grazing sheep or with strategic problems that concern the efficient long-term meshing of animal requirements and feed supply at a specific location, through adjustments to stocking rate, mating date, fodder conservation, etc. Both types of tool have at their core a model of the grazing sheep responding to its feed supply; this chapter will discuss the simulation procedures that have been developed to predict these responses. Although this discussion will not be directly concerned with research models, whose proper place is within the earlier chapters in this volume (see, for example, Oddy and Sainz, Chapter 11), research models will always have an important role as the source of increased complexity in management models, but only where this is found to be essential. The major constraint is that increased complexity within the model will usually be matched by a requirement for greater detail in the inputs, so the process cannot usefully advance beyond the ability of the user to quantify these inputs.

This constraint is less severe in a strategic tool built round a dynamic model in which many of the variables related to herbage composition and sward structure are generated day by day by a pasture growth module, rather than being estimated by the user. In the same way, it follows that, in the dynamic model, many of the current values for animal variables, e.g. milk production and wool growth, flow from the simulation of the animal's earlier nutritional history. But, for tactical tools, where the same inputs rely on the user's estimates of the current state of the grazing system, progress in model development must depend to a large degree on finding ways of improving these estimates.

In contrast to the large number of decision-support tools developed for ruminants in stalls or feedlots, few are commercially available for the nutritional management of grazing sheep. Two examples, NUTBAL (Stuth *et al.*, 1999; Grazingland Animal Nutrition Laboratory, Texas A&M University, USA) and GrazFeed (Freer *et al.*, 1997; Horizon Agriculture Pty Ltd, www.hzn.com.au/grazfeed.htm), will be used here to illustrate the conceptual problems involved. Both have been designed as tactical packages to predict the productivity of animals grazing a specified pasture and to assess the need for supplements to reach a target level of productivity. The animal model within GrazFeed is also used in the strategic packages GrassGro (Moore *et al.*, 1997) and FarmWi$e (Moore, 2001), where it is combined with soil-moisture and pasture-growth modules, driven by daily weather records, to simulate pasture production at specified sites. GrassGro is typically used for long-term predictions of productivity and risk in response to changes in animal or pasture management. In FarmWi$e, the biological model is directed by a flexible whole-farm management structure and is used for the optimization of management. SheepO (McPhee, 1996) has some features in common with GrassGro, but with a simpler pasture growth model, and is typically used for predictions over 1 year at a time. Some examples of validation exercises with these tools are presented in McPhee (1996) and Stuth *et al.* (1999).

The sheep model in NUTBAL is based on the US system of nutrient requirements (NRC, 1985), whereas the GrazFeed model is an implementation of the Australian recommendations for ruminants (SCA, 1990). However, application of the feeding standards provides only part of the answer to the simulation of the productivity of grazing sheep. There remain many problem areas, some to do with the inadequacy of current knowledge and others to do with the difficulty of relating current knowledge to features of the animal's grazing environment that can be readily measured. The main problems are grouped below under the general headings of predicting nutrient intake by grazing sheep, predicting the partition of absorbed and recycled nutrients and predicting the effect of nutrition on the quality or commercial value of the product. The ways in which the animal models in current management tools deal with these difficulties are discussed, with some indication of the extent to which research models offer prospects for improvement.

Predicting Nutrient Intake

The GrazFeed model

The inputs to the grazing model must describe the sheep and the grazed pasture in a way that allows the constraints to feed intake and the influence of diet selection, discussed by Weston (Chapter 2), and Forbes and Mayes (Chapter 3, this volume), to be adequately simulated. In GrazFeed, intake is predicted as the product of the potential intake of food, when limited by neither quantity nor quality (i.e. dry matter (DM) digestibility (DMD) of a grass diet at least 0.8), and the relative intake (or proportion of the potential intake) that the particular feed source offers the animal. The predicted intake of nutrients is then partitioned between the estimated requirements for maintenance and productive purposes. Only a few of the predictive equations are displayed in this chapter, but a spreadsheet program (SheepExplorer) is freely available from the following website to enable the interested reader to explore the effect of a range of inputs on all the major functions: www.pi.csiro.au/grazplan.

Potential intake

To enable the model to be used generally for all genotypes, all stages of maturity and all body conditions, the prediction of potential intake, as with several other predicted attributes, is scaled to: (i) the mature weight (SRW) of the sheep when in average body condition; (ii) its relative size (RS) (i.e. stage of development); and (iii) its relative condition (RC). Relative size, which has a maximum value of 1.0 at maturity, is defined as the ratio of 'normal' weight (NW) to SRW, where NW is the lesser of the following two variables: (i) the weight for age of a 'well-grown' animal of SRW (Brody, 1945); and (ii) the highest weight reached by the sheep so far. Relative condition is defined as the ratio of current weight (CW) to NW and it follows that CW is the product of SRW, RC and RS.

For a sheep with a specified SRW, a quadratic function relates potential intake to RS, with a peak at 85% maturity. For mature sheep in better than average condition, potential intake continues to decline with falling energy demand, as a function of RC rather than RS. Immature sheep that lose weight fall in RC but not RS and hence potential intake does not decline. As their maintenance requirement depends on CW, compensatory growth will occur when feeding conditions improve. During lactation, potential intake by the ewe increases according to a function that follows the lactation curve but lags behind it by some 14 days. For single- or twin-rearing ewes, respectively, potential intake may reach peak values of 1.65 or 1.9 times the level appropriate for the same ewe when not lactating. The specification of potential intake as a function of the sheep's current nutrient demand is comparable to the concept of Weston (Chapter 2, this volume) for a constraint set by the animal's capacity to use energy.

In hot weather that persists day and night, potential intake is reduced, but it is increased when ambient temperature is below the sheep's lower critical temperature. If, on low-quality pasture, later computations indicate that the intake of rumen-degradable protein is less than the estimated requirements for microbial growth, potential intake is reduced by the ratio of the two and feed intake is recalculated. It is assumed that recycling of urea to the rumen will satisfy microbial needs at the lower intake level, but quantitative information on the recycling process under grazing conditions is still sketchy. Providing a supplement containing sufficient urea or degradable protein will restore potential intake to its original level.

Relative intake

Where herbage is abundant, intake will be limited mainly by quality factors that determine its rate of disappearance from the reticulorumen (see Weston, Chapter 2, this volume) and are negatively related to structural carbohydrate levels and shear strength. Selective grazing of the youngest plant material will tend to maximize the quality of the diet and hence the amount eaten. As the weight or height of herbage falls, however, both the harvesting ability of the animal and its scope for selection decline, leading to a decline in feed intake. Prediction of relative intake must, therefore, account for the effects of the accessibility of the herbage (relative availability), its quality (relative ingestibility) and those interactions between the two that determine diet selection.

In the GrazFeed model, relative availability, on a scale of 0–1, is the product of the predicted relative rate of grazing (g h^{-1}) and the predicted relative time spent grazing (min day^{-1}), each related exponentially to herbage weight (t DM ha^{-1}). Both components of the computation are modified by mean herbage height if this differs from the standard of 3 cm for each t DM ha^{-1}. Relative ingestibility is linearly related to DMD; at DMD = 0.8 it has a value of 1.0 for temperate grasses and 1.17 for legumes, since, at the same DMD, sheep consume about 17% more legume (Freer and Jones, 1984). The mean value for relative ingestibility will thus depend on the specified proportions of grass and legume in the available herbage.

The problem, in designing a tactical tool, is to find the best compromise between research-based knowledge of the constraints to relative intake and the trained user's ability to relate them to the visual appearance or the rapidly assessable status of the sward. For example, the GrazFeed program asks the user for a relatively simple description of the pasture: the weight, height and digestibility of the green and dead fractions of the herbage, and the proportion of legume. The model then attempts to convert these inputs into a profile of the pasture that matches the way that the herbage may be perceived by the selectively grazing animal. Using arbitrary polynomial functions, the specified green and dead herbage is distributed between six pools, each with a characteristic DMD from 0.8 down to 0.3 (for examples, see Table 16.1), the herbage in each digestibility pool ranging from 0.05 above to 0.05 below the mean. In a strategic tool such as GrassGro, this distribution is generated through the pasture-growth and maturation module, rather than depending on the user's assessment of the pasture.

Conceptually, the sheep first attempts to satisfy its potential intake from the most digestible pool available. The extent to which it is able do this, i.e. the relative intake (*R*), offered by this pool is determined by the relative availability (*F*) of the pool multiplied by the relative ingestibility (*Q*) of the herbage in it. The relative intake offered by the second pool again depends on the availability and ingestibility of this material but applies

Table 16.1. Estimation of daily feed intake by a Merino castrate weaner of 36 kg (with a potential intake of 1.6 kg DM) and the digestibility of its selected diet from a pasture with estimated weights of 500 kg DM ha^{-1} of green herbage and 200 kg DM ha^{-1} dead herbage, of mean digestibilities 0.72 and 0.45, respectively, with 10% legume.

	Herbage pool					
	1	2	3	4	5	6
Mean dry matter digestibility	0.8	0.7	0.6	0.5	0.4	0.3
Relative ingestibility	1.02[a]	0.85	0.68	0.51	0.34	0.17
Weight of herbage (kg DM ha^{-1})	197	219	105	75	73	31
Relative availability[b]	0.34	0.25	0.08	0.05	0.04	0.01
Relative intake	0.34	0.21	0.05	0.02	0.01	0.00
Cumulative relative intake	0.64					
Intake of herbage (kg DM)	1.02					
Digestibility of diet[c]	0.73					

[a]Greater than 1.0 because herbage included 10% legume.
[b]After adjusting for the proportion of appetite already satisfied by more-digestible pools.
[c]Weighted average of the herbage eaten from all pools.

only to the proportion of the potential intake that was not satisfied by the first pool. This process continues until all pools have contributed to the cumulative value of the relative intake or until the potential intake, modified by the mean ingestibility of the selected diet, has been reached. The general computation of relative intake, R_d, from digestibility pool d uses the following function.

$$R_d = F_d Q_d \tag{1}$$

where:

$$F_d = \left(1 - \sum_{k=1}^{d-1} F_k\right) T_d G_d$$

$T_d = 1 + 0.6\exp(-(1 + 0.35\o_d)(0.0012 H_d B_d)^2)$
$G_d = 1 - \exp(-(1 + 0.35\o_d)0.0012 H_d B_d)$
$B_d, \o_d$ = weight of herbage (kg DM ha^{-1}) and proportion, in pool d
H_d = mean height of herbage/standard height for weight, in pool d
$Q_d = 1 - 1.7\min(1,(0.8 - (1 - P)S) - DMD_d) + 0.17P$
P = proportion of legume in the herbage
S = 0.0 and 0.16 for C3 and C4 grasses, respectively

Figure 16.1 shows the predicted values of T, G and F for the first digestibility pool, in relation to the weight of herbage in the pool. The effect of an increase in the relative height (H) of the herbage would be to move the asymptotic values for each variable to the left and thereby increase relative availability; conversely, a reduction in relative height would reduce relative availability.

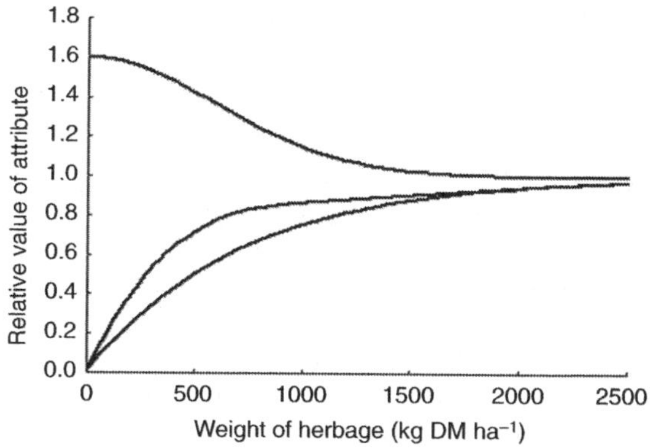

Fig. 16.1. Relative availability and its component attributes (calculated for the first digestibility pool, where the unsatisfied capacity of the sheep has a relative value of 1.0) in relation to the weight of herbage dry matter. The upper line is the relative time spent grazing (T), the lowest line is the relative rate of eating (G) and the middle line is the relative availability (F).

The diet selected as a result of this process has a mean digestibility and crude protein concentration that are almost invariably higher than those of the available herbage (see Table 16.1) and the degree of selection increases with the weight of herbage. It is virtually impossible to test experimentally the algorithms used for distributing herbage between the digestibility pools, because of the technical difficulty of sorting herbage on this basis. However, these functions generate degrees of diet selection on temperate pastures that are similar to those in published results (Hamilton *et al.*, 1973; Wales *et al.*, 1998).

A more flexible system may be needed for tropical (C4) grasses, which appear to vary more widely in the scope they offer for selective grazing. In *Paspalum dilatatum*, for example, Stockdale (1999) found little difference between green plant parts in their content of metabolizable energy (ME). On the other hand, in *Cenchrus ciliaris* (buffel grass), S.R. McLennan (Moorooka, Queensland, 1997, personal communication) found differences in digestibility between green leaf and green stem (at least 30 percentage units) that were much wider than would be expected in a C3 grass. Structural differences between temperate swards and some tropical pastures (Stobbs, 1973) may also need to be recognized through adjustment to the specified height of the herbage. In some cases, relatively small amounts of green leaf may be readily available through their attachment to tall stems.

Although, as mentioned above, relative ingestibility is directly related to the proportion of legume in the pasture, it is assumed that the proportion of legume in the selected diet will be the same as that in the available herbage (Newman *et al.*, 1992). More quantitative information on the question of whether or not grazing sheep actively select for legume may come from the alkane-based techniques described by Forbes and Mayes (Chapter 3, this volume).

The procedure for predicting relative intake depends on the ability of the user to make a quantitative assessment of a particular pasture, a skill that has been widely extended through southern Australia by PROGRAZE training courses (Bell and Allan, 2000). This ability must be reinforced by regular calibration of weight and digestibility estimates, a constraint that applies equally to estimates of weight made visually or by electronic probe (Vickery *et al.*, 1980). Moreover, the calibration of herbage weight must use the standard cutting technique for which the model's functions are scaled – namely, a shearing hand-piece run as close to the soil surface as possible.

At present, digestibility remains the primary indicator of relative ingestibility, mainly because of its current acceptance by users, but allowance must be made, where possible, for differences between herbage species. Intake functions established for temperate grasses that use the C3 photosynthetic pathway are not applicable to tropical (C4) grasses (Minson, 1982). The computation listed above in Equation (1) recognizes that, although the digestibility of a C4 grass may be about 15 percentage units lower than that of a C3 grass at the same stage of development, its relative ingestibility may be the same. Calculations based on measurements by D.B. Coates (Townsville, Queensland, 1998, personal communication) on a number of C4 grasses showed a linear relationship ($r^2 = 0.81$) between relative ingestibility and DMD. This regression had a similar slope to the common line for C3 grasses, but an increase of 0.26 in the value of the intercept. It is likely that further attempts to characterize individual pasture species will depend on the development of herbage-quality indicators that are more closely related than digestibility to relative ingestibility. Well-calibrated measurements by near-infrared spectroscopy (NIRS) and estimates of shear strength (see Coleman and Henry, Chapter 1, this volume) may become feasible alternatives for the rapid assessment of herbage quality.

If the sheep are grazing in an intensive rotational system, the weight of available herbage may change significantly in a 24 h period; intake predicted from the initial amount would then be an overestimate. Relative intake in this case is calculated five times during the day, after deducting from the available herbage the weight of herbage eaten and the weight that is assumed to be wasted by trampling and fouling, up to that point. A comparison of predicted intakes by intensively grazed dairy cows, with intakes estimated by Wales *et al.* (1998), indicated that the amount 'wasted' was as great as the amount eaten; corresponding estimates of 'wastage' have not been made for intensively grazed sheep. It is not clear whether this 'wastage' results solely from trampling and fouling or partly as a behavioural response in animals accustomed to frequent moves to fresh pasture.

Substitution of supplement for pasture

Although there are relatively few reliable measurements of concurrent intakes of supplement and pasture, it is clear that substitution rate (i.e. the depression in pasture DM intake per unit increase in supplement DM intake) is not constant for a particular supplement, but varies with the quantity and quality of the pasture (see Dove, Chapter 6, this volume). The procedure adopted in GrazFeed for predicting the effect of a supplement on the relative intake of pasture is based on the assumption that the animals will select the supplement before herbage of the same or poorer quality, i.e. relative ingestibility (Q). In other words, the supplement is inserted as an additional pool at the appropriate point in the hierarchy of digestibility pools before relative intake is computed. For example, a supplement with $Q = 0.9$ (calculated in a similar way to herbage, with a maximum value of 1.0), will be selected after 0.09 of the herbage in the second pool (which, in the absence of legume, has Q of mean 0.83, covering a range from 0.745 to 0.915), but before the remaining 0.91 of that pool.

In the calculation of relative intake set out in Equation (1), the contribution of the herbage in each digestibility pool depends on the proportion, UC_d, of the potential intake that has not been satisfied by higher-quality pools, where $UC_d = 1.0 - \sum_{k=1}^{d-1} F_k$. The way in which the contribution of the supplement (F_s) to the total relative intake is computed is crucial to the prediction of the substitution rate, because it affects UC_d and hence the intake from the next lower pool of herbage. This contribution is under four constraints: (i) the value of UC_d remaining; (ii) the ingestibility (Q_s) of the supplement; (iii) the amount offered (O_s) as a proportion of the animal's potential intake (I_{max}); and (iv) the ME concentration of the supplement. The contribution (and hence the substitution rate) is reduced for milking ewes, depending on the day of lactation (A), and for an increase in the ratio of protein concentration (CP_s) to organic-matter digestibility (OMD_s) in the supplement.

$$UC_d = \max\left(0, 1 - \sum_{k=1}^{d-1} F_k - \frac{F_s}{M.P}\right) \qquad (2)$$

$$\text{where } F_s = \min\left(\frac{O_s}{I_{max} Q_s}, UC_d, \frac{10.5}{M/D_s}\right)$$

$M = 1 + 1.5\exp(-(A/21)^2)$ for lactating ewes, otherwise $= 1.0$
$P = \max(1, 1.7 - 0.1(OMD_s/CP_s))$

Table 16.2 shows how the feeding of a supplement to sheep on the pasture described in Table 16.1 would affect the calculation of relative intake. Over a wide range of herbage weights and supplement quality, predicted substitution rates (Fig. 16.2) resulting from similar calculations show general agreement with experimental results reported by Allden (1981), Milne *et al.* (1981) and Stockdale *et al.* (1997). However, the general procedure needs more experimental data, resulting from a wider application of the techniques described by Dove (Chapter 6, this volume). In particular, the procedure needs to cope with situations where the animal's preference for a supplement is determined by other attributes than relative ingestibility. At present, the user of the program merely has the option of overriding the standard procedure, thus ensuring that the supplement is consumed before all pools of herbage, if experience or the method of feeding suggests that this is more appropriate.

Table 16.2. Estimation of daily feed intake by a Merino castrate weaner of 36 kg (with a potential intake of 1.6 kg DM) with the same pasture conditions as in Table 16.1, but with the inclusion of a supplement of 300 g day^{-1} of a mixture (80 : 20) of wheat and lupins.

	Feed pool							
	1	Suppl.	1	2	3	4	5	6
Mean dry matter digestibility	0.8	0.91	0.8	0.7	0.6	0.5	0.4	0.3
Relative ingestibility	1.02[a]	1.0	1.02	0.85	0.68	0.51	0.34	0.17
Weight of herbage (kg DM ha^{-1})	118		79	219	105	75	73	31
Relative availability[b]	0.21	0.17	0.09	0.21	0.05	0.01	0.00	0.00
Relative intake (RI)	0.22	0.17	0.09	0.18	0.03	0.00	0.00	0.00
Cumulative RI of herbage	0.52							
Intake of herbage (kg DM)	0.83							
Digestibility of herbage diet[c]	0.75							
Substitution rate[d]	0.44							

[a]Herbage in this pool (with 10% legume) has a mean relative ingestibility of 1.02 (see Equation (1)), with a range from 0.932 to 1.017.
[b]After adjusting for the proportion of appetite already satisfied by more-digestible pools.
[c]Weighted average of the herbage eaten from all pools.
[d]Depression in herbage intake (0.12 kg DM)/intake of supplement (0.27 kg DM).

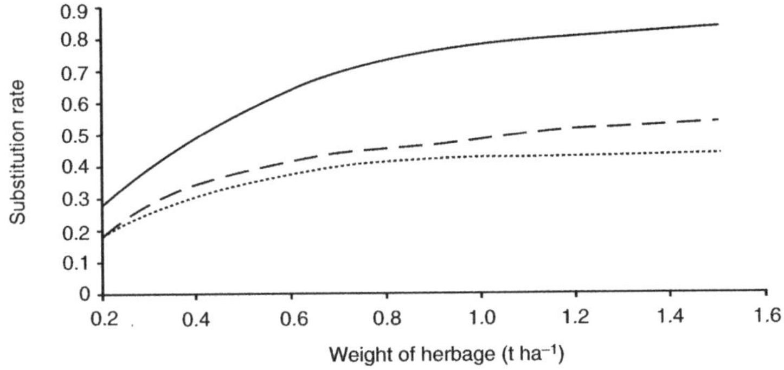

Fig. 16.2. Predicted substitution rate when a supplement of 300 g wheat is offered to a non-lactating ewe (solid line) or a ewe in early lactation (dotted line) grazing a pasture with a mean dry matter digestibility (DMD) of 0.72, compared with a non-lactating ewe (dashed line) grazing a pasture of mean DMD 0.52.

Sheep grazing semiarid rangelands

The predictive functions in the GrazFeed model are intended to apply generally to pastures of grasses and forbs, but are not suitable for semiarid rangelands, where animals graze browse plants in a highly selective way (see O'Reagain and McMeniman, Chapter 12, this volume). Under these conditions, the NUTBAL model may be more useful.

The NUTBAL model

Quite a different approach is taken in the NUTBAL model (Stuth *et al.*, 1999) to the prediction of pasture intake – one that relies much less on the need to assess the available pasture directly. The procedure is based on the assumption that, when intake is not limited by the quantity of herbage, the daily output of faecal DM is a constant proportion of the fat-corrected body weight of a specified animal in a stable physiological state (Forbes, 1980; Ellis *et al.*, 1988). To compute feed intake, the estimate of faecal output is divided by the indigestibility of the diet, estimated by NIRS on faecal samples.

The baseline limiting value for faecal output as a proportion of the fat-corrected body weight in a non-breeding mature ewe is taken as 0.011 (Ellis *et al.*, 1988). Adjustments are made for growing, pregnant and lactating animals and for deficiencies in rumen-degradable protein. For sheep that are not in average body condition, the body weight used in the calculation is corrected to a standard condition.

Further adjustments to the upper limit of faecal output are made for extremes of temperature beyond the thermal neutral zone of the animal and if it seems likely that mud will restrict grazing activity. Also, the limit is adjusted downwards if the weight of standing forage (t DM ha^{-1}) is judged to be low enough to restrict intake.

Users of the program are advised to submit recent faecal samples from the flock of sheep for NIRS at intervals of 5–30 days, depending on the rate of change of grazing conditions. Digestibility of the selected diet is then predicted from equations derived by Lyons and Stuth (1992) from a comparison of conventional laboratory estimates of digestibility with NIRS values on faeces for a broad spectrum of forage types.

NUTBAL would have particular advantages for extensive grazing of highly variable pastures, on which direct assessment is difficult, or of semi-arid rangelands, where the effects of selective browsing on intake and diet selection have not yet been quantified. In these situations, also, the time-lag in analysing faecal samples would generally be less important than in more intensive grazing systems, where management adjustments often need to be effected rapidly.

Partition of Absorbed and Recycled Nutrients

The loss and recovery of body weight in response to fluctuations in feed supply is a regular seasonal feature of the nutrition of grazing sheep. The proportion of a deficit in nutrient intake that will be met by the nutrients released through tissue catabolism, rather than by reduced fetal development, milk production or wool growth, varies directly with the condition of the animal and with the priority of the tissue being synthesized. For example, milk production in early lactation is more likely to be maintained close to its potential, despite the inability of the ewe to consume adequate nutrients, than it is in late lactation, when there is a greater tendency to restore body condition.

Predicting the effects of the partition of nutrients during periods of dietary stress and recovery also depends on information on the energy and protein content of catabolized and restored body tissue. In the growing sheep, the energy and protein contents of empty bodyweight gain are predicted in the GrazFeed model (Freer *et al.*, 1997) as functions of relative size. The energy content increases in sigmoid fashion from about 9 to a maximum of about 27 MJ kg^{-1} gain, and protein decreases from about 200 to about 70 g kg^{-1} gain. There is good evidence (Searle *et al.*, 1972) that the composition of weight loss is similar to that of gain. However, in mature sheep (Sanson *et al.*, 1993) and cattle (Wright and Russel, 1984), the ratio of fat to protein in these gains and losses is directly related to the condition of the animal. The data of Wright and Russel (1984) were used to develop the following general equations for predicting the energy value of empty bodyweight change, EVC (MJ kg^{-1}), and its protein content, PCC (g kg^{-1}), from the animal's relative condition, RC.

$$EVC = 13.2 + 13.8RC \quad (3)$$

$$PCC = 0.187 - 0.115RC \quad (4)$$

The condition of the mature sheep therefore affects the amount of protein mobilized during a period of negative energy balance. For sustaining milk production or wool growth, this protein is indistinguishable from the metabolizable protein (MP) absorbed from the gut, its efficiency of use depending on the suitability of its amino acid composition for the particular end-product. Revell *et al.* (1999), for example, showed that the efficiency of use of recycled protein for wool synthesis is closely related to the N : S ratio in the mobilized tissue and hence its content of sulphur-containing amino acids.

For a mature ewe in average condition, with a predicted energy value for empty bodyweight loss of 27 MJ kg^{-1}, the estimated value for liveweight loss is 24.8 MJ kg^{-1} (assuming that gut contents account for 0.09 of liveweight change). These predictions appear to break down in early lactation when the expected loss of body tissue may be accompanied by an increased retention of water, both in the empty body and in the gut contents. As discussed by Treacher and Caja (Chapter 10, this volume), highly variable estimates, up to 100 MJ kg^{-1} liveweight loss, have been recorded in early lactation. As values of this order must indicate that water is replacing body tissue, it is clear that liveweight change is a poor guide to energy change. There is inadequate information at present to predict the extent and duration of this anomaly and it is not known whether it is a feature of lactating animals only or of any animals losing tissue rapidly.

Partition during lactation

Geenty and Sykes (1986) observed in experiments with grazing ewes that all the sheep, irrespective of differences in nutrition during pregnancy or in milk production, were in negative energy balance during the first 6 weeks of lactation, even when offered ample herbage. As it is an unavoidable feature of many extensive grazing systems that ewes lamb on to pastures offering only a restricted intake of energy, this problem is likely to have a severe effect on the ewe's milk production unless the ewe is in good body condition (Robinson *et al.*, 1999). The simulation of milk production in the GrazFeed model attempts to account for the changing pattern of energy partition as lactation progresses, in relation to the ewe's potential production, energy intake and body condition.

The potential production of milk on a particular day of lactation, expressed as the ME value of the milk for the young, MY_{max}, is predicted from Equation (5), which is based on that of Wood (1969). Wood's equation has been rewritten to relate MY_{max} to stage of lactation, A (days), expressed as a proportion of the time to peak lactation. The predicted MY_{max} is scaled for the mother's mature weight (SRW) and relative size (RS) and the number of young and is related to her body condition at parturition (RC_b), in accord with results from Grainger *et al.* (1982).

$$MY_{max} = 0.486\ SRW^{0.75}\ RS\ RC_b\ LB\ M \exp(1 - M) \qquad (5)$$

where:

$$M = (A + 2)/22$$

For ewes with twins, 0.486 is replaced by 0.778. These parameters are appropriate for a ewe of a prime-lamb breed; for Merino ewes, they are replaced by 0.389 and 0.622, respectively.

After the time of peak lactation, MY_{max} is reduced if current milk production consistently fails to reach the potential. In the dynamic version of the model in the GrassGro package, this adjustment, LB, is recalculated daily as a function of the 10-day running mean of the ratio of actual to potential milk production. The same factor is used to make a corresponding adjustment to the potential intake of feed. It is one of the limitations of a 1-day tactical model that GrazFeed holds no direct information on earlier milk production, so the adjustment is computed from the estimated loss of energy reserves since parturition.

Milk production may fall below the potential either because it exceeds the lamb's ability to consume it, as predicted from Dove (1988), or because the ewe's intake of ME is insufficient to achieve the potential. From the intake of ME that is in excess of the ewe's maintenance requirement (ME_{xs}), expressed as a proportion (MR) of the ME needed to achieve MY_{max}, Equation (6) computes the milk production (MY) that can be sustained at any stage of lactation, A (days). This logistic function reproduces a diminishing response to energy inputs at high levels of production (Hulme *et al.*, 1986) when body reserves are being restored. On the other hand, it recognizes that a relatively high level of milk production may be maintained even in severely underfed animals in early lactation, through the mobilization of body reserves. The degree to which this is achieved is determined by the animal's current RC (Robinson *et al.*, 1999). Figure 16.3 shows how the predicted value of MY, as a proportion of potential milk yield, is directly related to the condition of the ewe and inversely related to

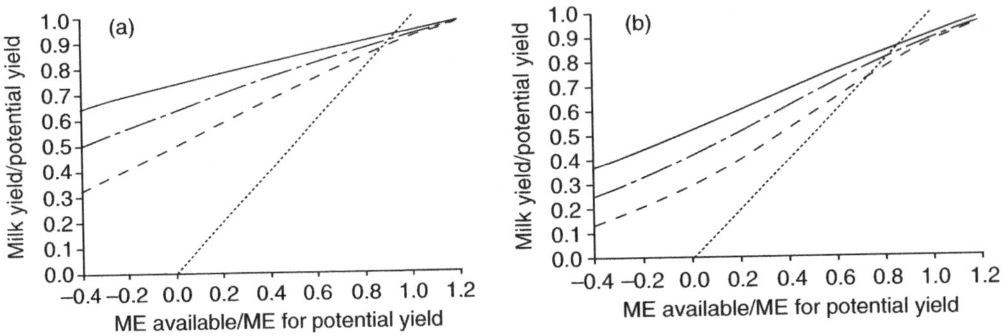

Fig. 16.3. Predicted milk yield as a proportion of potential yield, in relation to the available ME (after deducting the maintenance requirement) as a proportion of the ME required for the potential yield (a) on day 15 of lactation and (b) on day 90 of lactation, for ewes with relative body condition of 1.1 (solid line), 1.0 (dot–dash line) or 0.9 (dashed line), compared with the 1 : 1 relationship (dotted line).

the time since parturition. The value of *MY* represents the actual yield of milk (as ME for the young), unless a lower ceiling is set by the lamb's voluntary intake or by a deficiency of MP, derived either from the diet or from the possible mobilization of body tissue.

$$MY = \frac{1.17\,MY_{max}}{1.0 + \exp(-(-1.6 + 4.0MR + 0.008AD(MR - 0.012AD) - 3.0RC(MR - 0.6RC)))} \quad (6)$$

where:

$AD = \max(A, MR/44)$

Compensatory gain in growing sheep

Feed restriction and loss of weight, followed by rapid regain (compensation) when conditions improve, are part of the normal seasonal pattern in the growth of weaned sheep in most extensive grazing systems. Decisions on whether it is worth supplementing the animals to avoid the loss of weight depend on the efficiency with which the sheep are able to return to their normal growth path. In the GrazFeed model, the potential intake of food by these lambs when they start to regain weight remains a function of their relative size before feed was restricted. As a result, the intake of nutrients in excess of their maintenance requirement, which is a function of their current weight, is greater than it would be in a lamb that had not undergone restriction, and therefore they gain at a faster rate.

However, this is only part of the picture. As discussed by Oddy and Sainz (Chapter 11, this volume), protein accretion and hence water retention proceed at a faster than normal pace during the early stages of recovery from underfeeding. As a result, the regained tissue has a lower than normal energy value, although the efficiency of energy retention is not depressed. Similarly, the authors of Chapter 11 have reviewed work suggesting that the composition of weight gain in animals close to maintenance may contain an unusually high proportion of protein to fat if the postruminal supply of amino acids is increased. At present, the scale and duration of these changes in composition are not well enough defined for incorporation in the grazing model.

Future Development

The current grazing model performs a reasonably satisfactory simulation of sheep performance in a conventionally managed grazing system on temperate pastures, in terms of the gross outputs of weight gains by adults and young and their growth of wool (see, e.g. Stuth *et al.*, 1999). Improvements will come, in particular, from better data for the prediction of intake from different pasture species, substitution rates for supplements and the partition of nutrients in sheep with low levels of intake relative to their nutrient requirements.

New technologies are directing attention to possibilities for increasing productivity or the quality (i.e. value) of the product through manipulation of the diet, either through genetic manipulation of the feed base or through the provision of specifically targeted nutrients as supplements. These changes are aimed, in particular, at remedying the low levels of MP absorbed, relative to the CP concentration in high-quality herbage. This protein is highly degraded in the rumen and at too rapid a rate in relation to the availability of energy sources to be efficiently incorporated into microbial protein, most being lost to the sheep as urinary urea. Moreover, the digestible fraction of the microbial CP (MCP) has an amino acid profile not best suited to the synthesis of wool, meat or milk.

The superiority of legumes over grasses and of spring over autumn herbage in the energy : protein synchrony achieved in the rumen, resulting in more efficient use of ME for weight gain, is already recognized in the functions for predicting k_g and the synthesis of MCP. Evidence for a similar effect on k_l is still rather sketchy. Pasture breeding aimed at increasing the concentration of water-soluble carbohydrates may lead to cultivar-specific values for k_g. Work on increasing the content of specific amino acids in undegraded dietary protein shows most potential for wool growth (see below) but could possibly be extended to meat and milk production. However, Oddy and Sainz (Chapter 11, this volume) indicate that responses in weight gain in ruminant lambs have, so far, been variable. They suggest that improvements to the efficiency of conversion of nutrients to commercial meat, particularly meat of a more acceptable composition, depend on a better understanding of the mechanisms of animal growth.

Most of these possibilities are still at the stage of experimental exploration and, even when perfected, will probably have relatively little impact on the many flocks that graze extensively on native pastures, with minimal supplementary feeding. However, in more intensive systems, competitive advantage will increasingly lie with meeting specifications for product quality and can be expected to involve achieving higher yields of finer wool with greater staple strength, lean lamb meat and ewe milk of specified composition. To the extent that these targets can be met through nutritional changes rather than improvements to the animal genotype, the nature of the changes may suggest a need for increased complexity in the animal model, so as to follow the path of individual nutrients, rather than just ME and MP. Simulation at this level, aimed at predicting the effects of feed composition and treatment on the absorption and metabolism of individual amino acids and short-chain fatty acids, is an active field of research (Nagorcka *et al.*, 2000). While the practical implementation of such a model would be relatively straightforward for housed sheep on feed of known composition, there is no way, at present, of specifying in sufficient detail the composition of that part of the diet of grazing sheep that is selected from the pasture. Given this major constraint, we need to ask how well current grazing models could simulate effects of nutritional management on product quality and what improvements are feasible. At present, most of the possible approaches discussed in earlier chapters are still the subject of experimental study, but wool quality provides some examples of changes that can be made.

The three main nutritional options for improving the growth and quality of wool are: increasing the absorption of sulphur-containing amino acids, increasing the ratio of length to diameter in the growing fibre and increasing staple strength (see Hynd and Masters, Chapter 8, this volume). In grazing sheep, most of the absorbed protein is of microbial origin and the GrazFeed model predicts the gross efficiency of conversion to wool as 1.16 times the ratio of the average weight of the shorn fleece to the mature weight of the sheep (typically *c.* 0.1 for a Merino), up to a ceiling set by the ME intake, as shown in Fig. 8.3 (see Chapter 8, this volume). If the intake of slowly degradable high-sulphur amino acids is increased, either by genetic modification of pasture plants (McNabb *et al.*, 1993) or supplementary feeds (White *et al.*, 2000a) or by treatment of the supplements, then the estimate of efficiency can be adjusted by increasing the specified fleece weight. This will increase the slope and the plateau levels of the lines in Fig. 8.3. There are few data at present to guide the extent of the adjustment, but White *et al.* (2000b) found that the daily addition of 2 g of protected methionine to a variety of diets increased gross efficiency of wool growth by 0.02–0.04.

Fibre diameter is predicted when the animal model is used in the dynamic GrassGro tool, as a function of the user-specified mean diameter for the genotype, assuming a constant relationship between fibre length and diameter (see Hynd and Masters, Chapter 8, this volume). If a supplement or other nutritional treatment can be shown to increase the ratio of fibre length to diameter in a predictable way for the whole diet, then this adjustment could be included. The same authors indicate that staple strength depends mainly on the variability in fibre diameter along the staple but, although this characteristic is readily predictable from the seasonal variation in nutrient inputs, quantifying the relationship is still at the experimental stage.

References

AFRC (1993) *Energy and Protein Requirements of Ruminants*. CAB International, Wallingford, UK, 143 pp.

Allden, W.G. (1981) Energy and protein supplements for grazing livestock. In: Morley, F.H.W. (ed.) *Grazing Animals*. World Animal Science B1, Elsevier, Amsterdam, pp. 289–308.

Bell, A.K. and Allan, C.J. (2000) PROGRAZE – an extension package in grazing and pasture management. *Australian Journal of Experimental Agriculture* 40, 325–330.

Brody, S. (1945) *Bioenergetics and Growth*. Rheinhold, NewYork, 1203 pp.

Dove, H. (1988) Estimation of the milk intake of lambs from the turnover of deuterium- or tritium-labelled water. *British Journal of Nutrition* 60, 375–387.

Ellis, W.C., Wylie, M.J. and Matis, J.H. (1988) Dietary–digestive interactions determining the feeding value of forages and roughages. In: Ørskov, E.R. (ed.) *Feed Science*. Elsevier, Amsterdam, pp. 177–229.

Forbes, M.J. (1980) A model of the short-term control of feeding in the ruminant: effects of changing the animal or feed characteristics. *Appetite* 1, 21–41.

Freer, M. and Jones, D.B. (1984) Feeding value of subterranean clover, lucerne, phalaris and Wimmera ryegrass for lambs. *Australian Journal of Experimental Agriculture and Animal Husbandry* 24, 156–164.

Freer, M., Moore, A.D. and Donnelly, J.R. (1997) GRAZPLAN: decision support systems for Australian grazing enterprises. II. The animal biology model for feed intake, production and reproduction and the GrazFeed DSS. *Agricultural Systems* 54, 77–126.

Geenty, K.G. and Sykes, A.R. (1986) Effect of herbage allowance during pregnancy and lactation on feed intake, milk production, body composition and energy utilization at pasture. *Journal of Agricultural Science, Cambridge* 106, 351–357.

Grainger, C., Wilhelms, G.D. and Mcgowan, A.A. (1982) Effect of body condition at calving and level of feeding in early lactation on milk production of dairy cows. *Australian Journal of Experimental Agriculture and Animal Husbandry* 22, 9–17.

Hamilton, B.A., Hutchinson, K.J., Annis, P.C. and Donnelly, J.B. (1973) Relationships between the diet selected by grazing sheep and the herbage on offer. *Australian Journal of Agricultural Research* 24, 271–277.

Hulme, D.J., Kellaway, R.C., Booth, P.J. and Bennett, L. (1986) The CAMDAIRY model for formulating and analysing dairy cow rations. *Agricultural Systems* 22, 81–108.

Lyons, R.K. and Stuth, J.W. (1992) Fecal NIRS equations predict diet quality of free ranging cattle. *Journal of Range Management* 48, 380–382.

McNabb, W.C., Higgins, C.M., Tabe, L.M. and Higgins, T.J.V. (1993) The transfer of genes encoding proteins with high nutritional value into pasture legumes. In: *Proceedings of the XVII International Grassland Congress*. New Zealand Grassland Association, Tropical Grasslands Society of Australia, NZ Society of Animal Production, Australian Society of Animal Production (Queensland Branch) and NZ Institute of Agricultural Science, Palmerston North, p. 1085.

McPhee, M.J. (1996) SheepO version 4.0: a sheep management package. *Environmental Software* 11, 105–112.

Milne, J.A., Maxwell, T.J. and Souter, W. (1981) Effect of supplementary feeding and herbage mass on the intake and performance of grazing ewes in early lactation. *Animal Production* 32, 185–195.

Minson, D.J. (1982) Effects of chemical and physical composition of herbage eaten upon intake. In: Hacker, J.B. (ed.) *Nutritional Limits to Animal Production from Pasture*. Commonwealth Agricultural Bureaux, Farnham Royal, UK, pp. 167–182.

Moore, A.D. (2001) FarmWi$e: a flexible decision support tool for grazing systems management. In: *Proceedings 19th International Grassland Congress, Brazil, 11–21 February 2001*. Brazilian Society of Animal Husbandry, São Pedro, pp. 1045–1046.

Moore, A.D., Donnelly, J.R. and Freer, M. (1997) GRAZPLAN: decision support systems for Australian grazing enterprises. III. Pasture growth and soil moisture submodels and the GrassGro DSS. *Agricultural Systems* 55, 535–582.

Nagorcka, B.N., Gordon, G.L.R. and Dynes, R.A. (2000) Towards a more accurate representation of fermentation in mathematical models of the rumen. In: McNamara, J.P., France, J. and Beever, D.E. (eds) *Modelling Nutrient Utilization in Farm Animals*. CAB International, Wallingford, UK, pp. 37–48.

Newman, J.A., Parsons, A.J. and Harvey, A. (1992) Not all sheep prefer clover: diet selection revisited. *Journal of Agricultural Science, Cambridge* 119, 275–283.

NRC (1985) *Nutrient Requirements of Sheep*, 6th revised edn. National Academy Press, Washington, DC, 99 pp.

Revell, D.K., Baker, S.K. and Purser, D.B. (1999) Nitrogen and sulfur mobilised from body tissue can be used for wool growth. *Australian Journal of Agricultural Research* 50, 101–108.

Robinson, J.J., Sinclair, K.D., Randel, R.D. and Sykes, A.R. (1999) Nutritional management of the female ruminant: mechanistic approaches and predictive models. In: Jung, H.-J.G. and Fahey, G.C. (eds) *Nutritional Ecology of Herbivores*. American Society of Animal Science, Savoy, Illinois, pp. 550–608.

Sanson, D.W., West, T.R., Tatman, W.R., Riley, M.L., Judkins, M.B. and Moss, G.E. (1993) Relationship of body composition of mature ewes with condition score and body weight. *Journal of Animal Science* 71, 1112–1116.

SCA (1990) *Feeding Standards for Australian Livestock. Ruminants*. Standing Committee for Agriculture and CSIRO, Melbourne, 266 pp.

Searle, T.W., Graham, N.McC. and O'Callaghan, M. (1972) Growth in sheep. I. The chemical composition of the body. *Journal of Agricultural Science, Cambridge* 79, 371–382.

Stobbs, T.H. (1973) The effect of plant structure on the intake of tropical pastures. 1. Variation in the bite size of grazing cattle. *Australian Journal of Agricultural Research* 24, 809–819.

Stockdale, C.R. (1999) Effects of season and time since defoliation on the nutritive characteristics of three irrigated perennial pasture species in northern Victoria 1. Energy, protein and fibre. *Australian Journal of Experimental Agriculture* 39, 555–565.

Stockdale, C.R., Dellow, D.W., Grainger, C., Dalley, D. and Moate, P.J. (1997) *Supplements for Dairy Production in Victoria*. Dairy Research and Development Corporation, Glen Iris, Victoria, 95 pp.

Stuth, J.W., Freer, M., Dove, H. and Lyons, R.K. (1999) Nutritional management for free-ranging livestock. In: Jung, H.-J.G. and Fahey, G.C. (eds) *Nutritional Ecology of Herbivores*. American Society of Animal Science, Savoy, Illinois, pp. 696–751.

Vickery, P.J., Bennett, I.L. and Nicol, G.R. (1980) An improved capacitance meter for estimating herbage mass. *Grass and Forage Science* 35, 247–252.

Wales, W.J., Doyle, P.T. and Dellow, D.W. (1998) Dry matter intake and nutrient selection by lactating cows grazing irrigated pastures at different pasture allowances in summer and autumn. *Australian Journal of Experimental Agriculture* 38, 451–460.

White, C.L., Tabe, L.M., Dove, H., Hamblin, J., Young, P., Phillips, N., Taylor, R., Gulati, S., Ashes, J. and Higgins, T.J.V. (2000a) Increased efficiency of wool growth and live weight gain in Merino sheep fed transgenic lupin seed containing sunflower albumin. *Journal of the Science of Food and Agriculture* 81, 147–154.

White, C.L., Young, P., Phillips, N. and Rodehutscord, M. (2000b) The effect of dietary protein source and protected methionine (Lactet) on wool growth and microbial protein synthesis in Merino wethers. *Australian Journal of Agricultural Research* 51, 173–183.

Wood, P.D.P. (1969) Factors affecting the shape of the lactation curve in cattle. *Animal Production* 11, 307–316.

Wright, I.A. and Russel, A.J.F. (1984) The composition and energy content of empty body weight change in mature cattle. *Animal Production* 39, 365–369.

Index

Printed and bound by CPI Group (UK) Ltd, Croydon, CR0 4YY
16/09/2026
14963436-0003